Color Atlas

of

Common Oral Diseases

Third Edition

Color Atlas

of

Common Oral Diseases

Third Edition

Robert P. Langlais, DDS, MS, FACD, FICD
Professor
Department of Dental Diagnostic Science
University of Texas Health Science Center at San Antonio
School of Dentistry
San Antonio, Texas

Craig S. Miller, DMD, MS, FACD
Professor of Oral Medicine,
Department of Oral Health Practice and Department of Microbiology, Immunology and Molecular Genetics
College of Dentistry, College of Medicine
University of Kentucky
Lexington, Kentucky

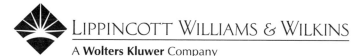
LIPPINCOTT WILLIAMS & WILKINS
A **Wolters Kluwer** Company
Philadelphia · Baltimore · New York · London
Buenos Aires · Hong Kong · Sydney · Tokyo

Editor: John Goucher
Managing Editor: Jacquelyn Merrell
Marketing Manager: Chris Kushner
Project Editor: Paula C. Williams
Designer: Armen Kojoyian
Compositor: Maryland Composition, Inc.
Printer: Quebecor World - Kingsport

The publisher is not responsible (as a matter of product liability, negligence, or otherwise) for any injury resulting from any material contained herein. This publication contains information relating to general principles of medical care which should not be construed as specific instructions for individual patients. Manufacturers' product information and package inserts should be reviewed for current information, including contraindications, dosages, and precautions.

Printed in the United States of America

Library of Congress Cataloging-in-Publication Data

Langlais, Robert P.
   Color atlas of common oral diseases / Robert P. Langlais, Craig S. Miller.—3rd ed.
     p. ; cm.
   Includes index.
   ISBN 0-7817-3385-5 (alk. paper)
    1. Mouth—Diseases—Atlases. 2. Oral medicine—Atlases. I. Miller, Craig S. II. Title.
   [DNLM: 1. Mouth Diseases—pathology—Atlases. 2. Tooth
Diseases—pathology—Atlases. WU 17 L282c 2002]
   RC815 .L35 2002
   617.5′22′00222—dc21

                             2002016206

The publishers have made every effort to trace the copyright holders for borrowed material. If they have inadvertently overlooked any, they will be pleased to make the necessary arrangements at the first opportunity.

To purchase additional copies of this book call our customer service department at **(800) 638-3030** or fax orders to **(301) 824-7390**. International customers should call **(301) 714-2324**.

Visit Lippincott Williams & Wilkins on the Internet: http://www.lww.com. Lippincott Williams & Wilkins customer service representatives are available from 8:30 am to 6:00 pm, EST, Monday through Friday, for telephone access.

                                                   04
2 3 4 5 6 7 8 9 10

To our wives,
Denyse and Sherry

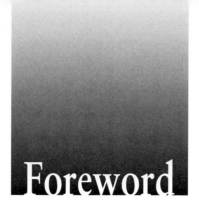

Foreword

Practicing oral medicine—that is, diagnosing and treating oral manifestations of local or systemic diseases—is often a difficult challenge for the practitioner. This complexity stems from the many conditions that directly or indirectly affect the mouth and adjacent structures and the entailing spectrum of signs and symptoms that often make a differential diagnosis quite difficult.

The organized approach that helps to simplify this aspect of oral health care delivery demands careful history taking, methodical oral examinations, recognition of normal structures and deviations from normal, and the ability to form a differential diagnosis—a priority list of conditions or diseases that the findings suggest. The differential diagnosis forms the basis for performing tests that should lead to a definitive diagnosis and the appropriate treatment plan. These steps are important for standards of care, optimal patient health and function, protecting the clinician from censure, and nurturing meaningful referrals.

An important step of the diagnostic sequence, not to be overlooked, is the dental hygienist, who often sees the patient first. Because many signs and symptoms may represent malignant disease, precancerous lesions, or infectious conditions, it is incumbent upon the dental hygienist to recognize deviations from normal, identify patients who may have these disorders, and inform the dentist of the clinical findings.

The third edition of *Color Atlas of Common Oral Diseases* by Drs. Langlais and Miller greatly assists in the diagnostic process by providing an updated and organized approach to conditions that afflict the mouth. Chapters on normal anatomy, specific tissues, different sites, and clinical features of color and form are presented with many high-quality color illustrations and radiographs that have been carefully selected to represent features of conditions or diseases.

The accompanying text is abbreviated to present concise overviews with emphasis on the clinical description of oral lesions, which allows a useful understanding of the entity in question. The book also includes a brief glossary of useful terms that describe clinical findings, tables summarizing the characteristics of each group of disorders, and a separate listing of prescriptions useful in the management of these problems.

Because it is so difficult to master the complex variations of signs and symptoms associated with the multitude of oral manifestations of disease, a visual approach is one of the most helpful aids. Thus, the third edition of the *Atlas* will be of significant help to clinicians at all levels of experience in creating a differential diagnosis, establishing a diagnosis, and forming a basis for a rational approach to managing and resolving patient problems.

Sol Silverman, Jr, MA, DDS

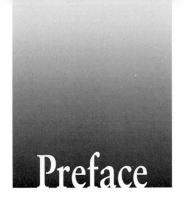

Preface

The 3rd edition of *Color Atlas of Common Oral Diseases* is a thorough revision of the second edition and includes many significant improvements. New diagrams, drawings, illustrations, and clinical cases, including many radiographs, have been added. The entire book now contains 600 color and radiographic images. Illustrations are arranged according to clinical appearance to facilitate the construction of a differential diagnosis and to learn by pattern recognition. Each color page has eight illustrations so that disorders closely related by appearance or cause can be easily compared. In this edition, the sequence of entities has been slightly rearranged so that the reader begins with normal anatomy and progresses to disease. Specific sections on normal radiographic anatomy, dental anomalies, disorders of the gingiva and periodontium, caries and caries progression, and jaw cysts and tumors have been added. Throughout the text there is new information concerning the etiology of diseases including specific gene defects and pathophysiologic abnormalities as well as new treatment approaches. Select illustrations also have been replaced with better examples to more accurately represent the common presentation of disease, which in turn should enhance the reader's understanding.

The goal of this atlas continues to be to provide an affordable text that has high-quality color illustrations and the salient clinical features of common oral diseases for those who are studying or attempting to identify oral disorders. The *Atlas* fulfills our philosophy of having a practical book that makes learning easy and fun by categorizing conditions on the basis of appearance, using excellent examples of diseases and including appendices of glossaries, prescriptions, and self-assessment tests. These appendices are the result of our daily teaching experiences in which we have found that students benefit from a reference that not only explains the condition but also has prescriptions for proper management. We encourage students to explore all aspects of this textbook, including the appendices. All students should benefit from the glossary of terms, tables of common oral conditions, prescriptions arranged by management of disorders, and the self-assessment test. As before, the appendix of prescriptions was written to simulate actual prescriptions. Also, the most current American Heart Association guidelines for antibiotic prevention of infective endocarditis are found in Appendix II.

For this edition our publisher has kindly allowed us to substitute new or better cases on existing pages and has agreed to increase the size of the color pictures without increasing the page size. To do this we compressed the legends, but in turn added more comments about the illustrations in the corresponding text. Images from the same patient are now indicated with symbols (*) by each figure legend. Also, for the first time we have cross-referenced illustrations on other pages to further increase the scope of our illustrative material.

One of the significant new additions is the section on radiographic dental anomalies. This section covers many common entities seen in daily dental practice. The inclusion of this section has allowed us to increase the number of anomalies primarily seen in radiographs. We have also added several new pages on the description and radiographic appearance of cysts and tumors of the jaws. The clinical and radiographic sections on dental caries and periodontal disease have also been expanded.

The expansion of this edition was made with specific curricular content issues in mind so that for the first time this text may be considered as the recommended oral pathology text in oral/dental hygiene training programs as well as for dental students in the areas of oral pathology and in radiographic interpretation. We hope that this edition will continue to be useful to students of dental assisting, dental hygiene, and dentistry, as well as postgraduate dentists, hygienists, dental practitioners, and dental specialists whose goal it is to become more knowledgeable about oral diseases.

We would like to remind faculty members and any other interested parties that we plan to continue to give away the color slides and radiographs of all of the conditions illustrated in this edition, as well as a CD of all of our PowerPoint title slides to those who attend our annual summer workshop. Each year at the workshop the authors present continuing educational seminars that progressively cover the information in the *Atlas*. Complete coverage takes 3 years. **Strong interest in this course has come from faculty in dental hygiene programs.** We continue to encourage their attendance as well as all other interested parties who teach oral assessment, oral diagnosis, oral medicine, or oral pathology. Details are printed on the inside cover of this text. We believe that the educational information and material provided at the summer workshop is a tremendous value to educators whose goal it is to help students, hygienists, and dentists master this most important subject.

Finally, we wish to express our thanks to all health care professionals who have referred patients to our clinics and provided illustrations found in this text.

Robert P. Langlais
Craig S. Miller

For persons involved in education, the authors have the complete set of illustrations available for purchase as color slides. Details on the purchase of these slides are available by contacting

Craig S. Miller, DMD, MS
MN 118, Oral Medicine
University of Kentucky College of Dentistry
800 Rose
Lexington, KY 40536-0297
cmiller@pop.uky.edu
FAX 859-323-9136

Information regarding the annual summer conference that provides continuing education of material found in this text can also be obtained by contacting Dr. Miller at the address listed on this page.

Acknowledgments

We are extremely grateful to our many colleagues who have graciously provided material for publication in this atlas. Without their contributions, this fine quality text would not have been possible. We are also grateful to all practicing dentists and physicians who have referred patients throughout the years to the Department of Dental Diagnostic Science Referral Clinic.

To Professor Sol Silverman, who completely reviewed this text and wrote the foreword, we extend our thanks for his valuable comments and contributions. In addition, we are grateful for the many illustrations Dr. Silverman has provided, which can be seen throughout this text.

April Cox and Al Julian of the Photographic Services Section of Education Resources of The University of Texas Health Science Center receive a special thank you for their masterful job of cropping and recreating the proper color balance on our illustrations. We are especially grateful for the incredible efforts made by April Cox, who personally reviewed each color slide for possible color modifications and/or correction. We are also grateful to Albert Preciado and the entire Photography Unit, whose photography skills are evident throughout this work.

Finally, we would like to thank our wives, Denyse and Sherry, for their continuing support throughout this project. Authorship of a high-quality text requires numerous off-duty hours; without the understanding of these two most important people in our lives, this work might never have been completed.

We also wish to express our appreciation to the following persons for contribution of their clinical photographs and radiographs used in this text:

Dr. Kenneth Abramovitch
Dr. A.M. Abrams
Dr. Marden Alder
Dr. Robert Arm
Dr. Ralph Arnold
Dr. Tom Aufdemorte
Dr. Bill Baker
Dr. Douglas Barnett
Dr. Pete Benson
Dr. Howard Birkholz
Dr. Steve Bricker
Dr. Dale Buller
Dr. Israel Chilvarquer
Dr. Jerry Cioffi
Dr. Laurie Cohen
Dr. John Coke

Dr. Herman Corrales
Dr. James Cottone
Dr. Robert Craig, Jr
Dr. Stephen Dachi
Dr. Maria de Zeuss
Dr. Anna Dongari
Dr. S. Brent Dove
Dr. David Freed
Dr. Franklin Garcia-Godoy
Dr. Birgit Glass
Dr. Tom Glass
Dr. Michael Glick
Dr. Kirsten Gosney
Dr. Ed Heslop
Dr. Michael Huber
Dr. Sheryl Hunter
Dr. J.L. Jensen
Dr. Ron Jorgenson
Dr. Jerald Katz
Dr. George Kaugers
Dr. Eric Kraus
Dr. Olaf Langland
Dr. Al Lugo
Dr. Curt Lundeen
Dr. Carson Mader
Dr. Nancy Mantich
Dr. Tom McDavid
Dr. John McDowell
Dr. Monique Michaud
Dr. Dale Miles
Dr. David Molina
Dr. Charles Morris
Dr. Rick Myers
Dr. Christoffel Nortjé
Dr. Pirkka Nummikoski
Dr. Linda Otis
Dr. Garnet Pakota
Dr. Roger Rao
Dr. Tom Razmus
Dr. Spencer Redding
Dr. Terry Rees
Dr. Michele Saunders
Dr. Stanley Saxe
Dr. Tom Schiff
Dr. Jack Sherman
Dr. Sol Silverman
Dr. Larry Skoczylas
Dr. D.B. Smith
Dr. John Tall
Dr. Geza Terezhalmy
Dr. Mark Thomas
Dr. Martin Tyler
Dr. Margo Van Dis
Dr. Michael Vitt
Dr. Elaine Winegard
Dr. Donna Wood

Figures Courtesy Page

Fig. 1.5	Dr. Kirsten Gosney	Fig. 32.4	Dr. James Cottone and Dr. Steve Bricker	Fig. 45.7	Dr. Stephen Dachi
Fig. 2.2	Dr. James Cottone	Fig. 32.5	Dr. James Cottone	Fig. 46.7	Dr. Geza Terezhalmy
Fig. 2.8	Dr. Linda Otis	Fig. 32.6	Dr. Pete Benson		
				Fig. 49.2	Dr. Bill Baker
Fig. 3.3	Dr. Kirsten Gosney	Fig. 33.7	Dr. Jack Sherman	Fig. 49.4	Dr. Dale Miles
Fig. 3.4	Dr. Kirsten Gosney	Fig. 33.8	Dr. Tom Aufdemorte	Fig. 49.8	Dr. Ken Abramovitch
Fig. 3.7	Dr. Ralph Arnold				
		Fig. 34.1	Dr. Kenneth Abramovitch	Fig. 51.7	Dr. Spencer Redding
Fig. 11.1	Dr. Sheryl Hunter	Fig. 34.3	Dr. James Cottone	Fig. 51.8	Dr. James Cottone
Fig. 11.2	Dr. Christoffel Nortjé	Fig. 34.7	Dr. Anna Dongari		
Fig. 11.4	Dr. Ron Jorgenson			Fig. 52.5	Dr. Linda Otis
Fig. 11.5	Dr. Franklin Garcia-Godoy	Fig. 35.3	Dr. Maria de Zeuss	Fig. 52.6	Dr. Ed Heslop
Fig. 11.6	Dr. Ron Jorgenson	Fig. 35.4	Dr. Stanley Saxe	Fig. 52.7	Dr. Tom Razmus
Fig. 11.7	Dr. Ron Jorgenson	Fig. 35.5	Dr. Ralph Arnold	Fig. 53.3	Dr. Margot van Dis
Fig. 11.8	Dr. Al Lugo	Fig. 35.6	Dr. Ralph Arnold	Fig. 53.4	Dr. Margot van Dis
				Fig. 53.5	Dr. Larry Skoczylas
Fig. 12.6	Dr. Kenneth Abramovitch	Fig. 36.1	Dr. Monique Michaud	Fig. 53.6	Dr. Larry Skoczylas
		Fig. 36.2	Dr. Monique Michaud		
		Fig. 36.5	Dr. Roger Rao	Fig. 54.3	Dr. Robert Craig, Jr
Fig. 13.3	Dr. Rick Myers	Fig. 36.6	Dr. Roger Rao	Fig. 54.7	Dr. Robert Craig, Jr
Fig. 13.6	Dr. Ralph Arnold	Fig. 36.7	Dr. Larry Skoczylas		
Fig. 13.8	Dr. Israel Chilvarquer			Fig. 55.2	Dr. Birgit Glass
		Fig. 37.4	Dr. Kenneth Abramovitch	Fig. 55.5	Dr. Tom Razmus
Fig. 16.7	Dr. Geza Terezhalmy	Fig. 37.7	Dr. Sol Silverman		
		Fig. 37.8	Dr. Michael Huber	Fig. 56.2	Dr. James Cottone
Fig. 17.3	Dr. Jerry Katz			Fig. 56.4	Dr. James Cottone
Fig. 17.7	Dr. Pirkka Nummikoski	Fig. 38.2	Dr. Bill Baker		
Fig. 17.8	Dr. Pirkka Nummikoski	Fig. 38.8	Dr. Pete Benson	Fig. 57.2	Dr. Geza Terezhalmy
				Fig. 57.6	Dr. James Cottone
Fig. 18.2	Dr. Charles Morris	Fig. 39.5	Dr. Jerry Cioffi	Fig. 57.8	Dr. Ken Abramovitch
		Fig. 39.6	Dr. Jerry Cioffi		
Fig. 19.6	Dr. Ralph Arnold	Fig. 39.7	Dr. Tom Aufdemorte	Fig. 58.2	Dr. David Freed
Fig. 19.8	Dr. David Molina			Fig. 58.3	Dr. Linda Otis
		Fig. 40.3	Dr. Curt Lundeen	Fig. 58.4	Dr. Linda Otis
Fig. 20.3	Dr. Birgit Glass				
		Fig. 41.1	Dr. Nancy Mantich	Fig. 59.3	Dr. Nancy Mantich
Fig. 22.7	Dr. Birgit Glass	Fig. 41.6	Dr. Christoffel Nortjé	Fig. 59.4	Dr. Tom McDavid
		Fig. 41.8	Dr. John McDowell	Fig. 59.5	Dr. Dale Miles
Fig. 23.3	Dr. Ralph Arnold			Fig. 59.6	Dr. Curt Lundeen
		Fig. 42.1	Dr. Linda Otis	Fig. 59.7	Dr. Geza Terezhalmy
Fig. 25.1	Dr. Kenneth Abramovitch	Fig. 42.8	Dr. Geza Terezhalmy	Fig. 59.8	Dr. Michael Vitt
Fig. 25.6	Dr. Garnet Pakota			Fig. 60.6	Dr. Tom McDavid
		Fig. 44.2	Dr. Dale Miles	Fig. 60.7	Dr. Charles Morris
Fig. 26.3	Dr. Robert Arm	Fig. 44.3	Dr. Geza Terezhalmy	Fig. 60.8	Dr. Charles Morris
Fig. 26.8	Dr. Christoffel Nortjé	Fig. 44.4	Dr. Olaf Langland		
		Fig. 44.7	Dr. Dale Miles	Fig. 61.6	Dr. Tom McDavid
Fig. 29.3	Dr. Charles Morris				
Fig. 29.4	Dr. Tom McDavid	Fig. 45.1	Dr. Tom McDavid	Fig. 62.4	Dr. Birgit Glass
Fig. 29.5	Dr. Ralph Arnold	Fig. 45.2	Dr. Dale Buller	Fig. 62.5	Dr. Jerry Cioffi
Fig. 29.8	Dr. Mark Thomas	Fig. 45.3	Dr. J.L. Jensen		
		Fig. 45.4	Dr. S. Brent Dove	Fig. 63.1	Dr. Curt Lundeen
Fig. 32.3	Dr. Ed Heslop	Fig. 45.5	Dr. James Cottone	Fig. 63.2	Dr. Tom McDavid

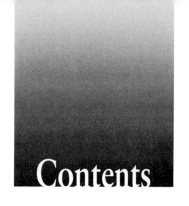

Contents

Section I

Anatomic Landmarks

Landmarks of the Oral Cavity

Lips (Fig. 1.1) The lips externally border the oral cavity. They are covered by parakeratotic mucosa, beneath which is fibrovascular tissue that lacks adnexal structures. Deeper are muscles that control lip movement (orbicularis oris, levator, and depressor oris). The color of lips depends on the pigmentation of the patient. The junction of the lips with the labial mucosa is the **wet line**, the point of contact of the upper and lower lips. The **vermilion** is the portion external to the wet line. The **vermilion border** is the junction of the lip with the skin. The lips should be everted and palpated during oral examination. The surface should be smooth, nonscaly, uniform in color, and free of fissures, ulcerations, nodules, and masses; the border smooth and well delineated.

Labial and Buccal Mucosa (Figs. 1.2 and 1.3) The labial mucosa is the internal lining of the lip; the buccal mucosa is the inner lining of the cheeks. Each is covered by thin, pink parakeratotic epithelium. The mucosa may be brownish-pink or pink with small red capillaries nourishing the region. **Minor salivary gland ducts** empty onto its surface. When the lip is everted, the surface is covered by punctate orifices that exude mucinous saliva. The buccal mucosa extends bilaterally from the labial mucosa to the retromolar pad and pterygomandibular raphe. The presence of fat within the buccal connective tissue can make it appear yellow or tan. Accessory salivary glands are present in this region. The **caliculus angularis** is a normal pinkish papule located buccally at the commissure.

Parotid Papilla (Fig. 1.4) The parotid papilla is the terminal end of **Stenson's duct**, the excretory duct of the parotid gland. It is a triangular, raised, pink papule on the buccal mucosa adjacent to the maxillary first molars bilaterally. To assess its function, the gland is milked by drying the papilla with gauze, pressing the fingers below the mandible, and extending pressure upward and over the gland. In health, clear saliva should flow from the duct.

Floor of the Mouth (Fig. 1.5) The floor of the mouth is the region below the anterior half of the tongue. It consists of thin, pink parakeratinized epithelium, connective tissue, salivary glands, and associated nerves and vessels. The U-shaped boundaries of the floor are the alveolar mucosa anterolaterally and the ventral tongue surface posteriorly. The anterior half is smooth and uniform, the posterior half is bisected by the **lingual frenum**. Between the two halves is an elevated area under which **Wharton's duct** of the submandibular gland lies. This duct terminates anteriorly in an elevated papule called the **sublingual caruncle** through which saliva flows. Along the posterior length of this elevation are multiple small openings of the **ducts of Ravini** that carry saliva from the sublingual salivary gland. Beneath these structures lies the **mylohyoid muscle**.

Hard Palate (Fig. 1.6) The hard palate is the superior aspect of the oral cavity. It is composed of squamous epithelium, connective tissue, minor salivary glands and ducts (in the posterior two thirds only), periosteum, and the palatine processes of the maxilla. Anatomically, it consists of several structures. The **incisive papilla** is behind the maxillary incisors. It is a raised, pink ovoid structure that overlies the nasopalatine foramen. The **rugae** are located slightly posterior to the incisive papilla, in the anterior third of the palate. These fibrous ridges run laterally from the midline to within several millimeters of the attached gingiva of anterior teeth. The alveolar bone that supports the palatal aspect of the posterior teeth is called the lateral vault. In the center of the hard palate is the **median palatal raphe**, the yellow-white junction of the right and left palatine processes.

Soft Palate (Fig. 1.7) The soft palate has more minor salivary glands and lymphoid and fatty tissue than the hard palate. It also lacks bony support. The soft palate functions during mastication and swallowing. It is elevated by the levator palati and tensor palati muscles; motor innervated by cranial nerves IX and X. The **median palatal raphe** is more prominent and thicker in the soft palate. Just lateral to the raphe are the **fovea palatinae**. The fovea are 2-mm excretory ducts of minor salivary glands. They are landmarks of the junction between the hard and soft palates. At the midline and distal aspect of the soft palate is the **uvula**.

Oropharynx and Tonsils (Fig. 1.8) The oropharynx is composed of two tonsillar pillars and the posterior pharyngeal wall. The **uvula** borders its anterior aspect; the anterolateral aspect is bordered by the **tonsillar pillars (fauces)**. The **anterior tonsillar pillar** is formed by the palatoglossus muscle that runs downward, outward, and forward to the base of the tongue. The **posterior pillar** is larger and runs downward, outward, and posteriorly. It is formed by the palatopharyngeus muscle. The **tonsils** are lymphoid tissue within the pillars. They are dome-shaped structures with cryptic invaginations for capturing microbes. In health, they are generally held within the pillars. They enlarge during adolescence (a lymphoid growth period) and during infectious, inflammatory, and neoplastic processes. Islands of tonsillar tissue are seen on the surface of the posterior pharyngeal wall. **Waldeyer's ring** is the ring of adenoid tissue formed by the lingual, pharyngeal, and faucial tonsils.

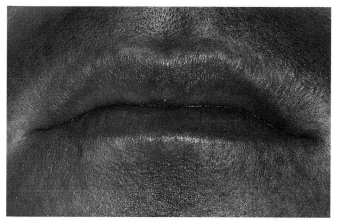

Fig. 1.1. **Lips:** normal, healthy appearance.

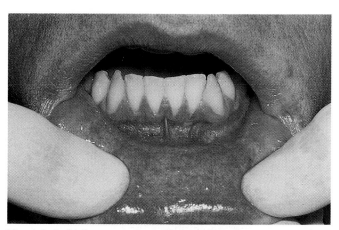

Fig. 1.2. **Labial mucosa:** inner lining of the lips.

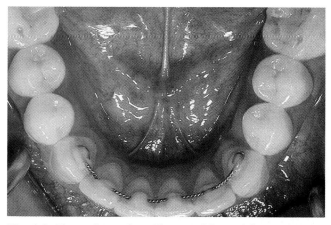

Fig. 1.3. **Buccal mucosa:** and caliculus angularis.

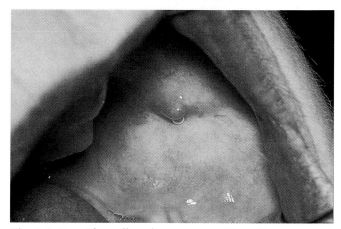

Fig. 1.4. **Parotid papilla:** adjacent to maxillary first molar.

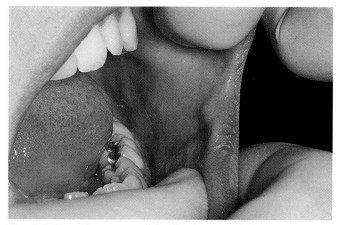

Fig. 1.5. **Floor of mouth:** with central lingual frenum.

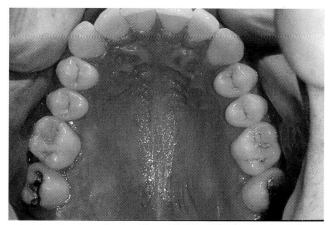

Fig. 1.6. **Hard palate:** incisive papilla and rugae in anterior third.

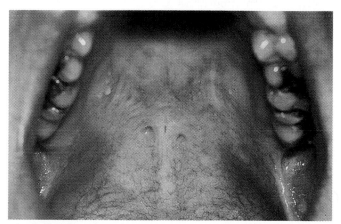

Fig. 1.7. **Soft palate:** fovea palatinae and median palatal raphe.

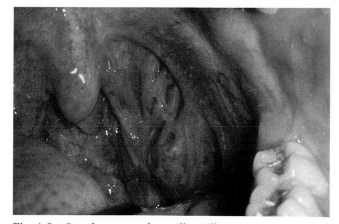

Fig. 1.8. Oropharynx and tonsillar pillars.

Landmarks of the Tongue and Variants of Normal

Normal Tongue Anatomy (Figs. 2.1–2.5) The tongue is a compact muscular organ covered by a protective layer of stratified squamous epithelium. It functions primarily in deglutition, taste, and speech. The dorsum of the tongue has numerous mucosal projections that form papillae. There are four types of projections: filiform, fungiform, circumvallate, and foliate papillae. **Filiform papillae** are the smallest but the most numerous. They are slender, hairlike, cornified stalks that may appear red, pink, or white, depending on the degree of daily irritation experienced. In a patient with good oral hygiene, the papillae appear pink. The dorsum of the tongue contains fewer **fungiform papillae** than filiform papillae. The fungiform papillae are brighter red, and broader than the latter. Fungiform papillae are noncornified, round, or mushroom-shaped; they are slightly elevated and contain taste buds. These papillae are most numerous on the lateral border and anterior tip of the tongue. Fungiform papillae sometimes contain brown pigmentation, especially in melanoderms.

The largest papillae are the **circumvallate papillae**. They appear as 2- to 4-mm pink papules arranged in a V-shaped row along the sulcus terminalis at the posterior aspect of the dorsum of the tongue. They are surrounded by a narrow trench and also contain taste buds. The dorsum contains 8 to 12 circumvallate papillae, which anatomically divide the tongue into two unequal sections: the anterior two thirds and the posterior third.

If the lateral border of the posterior region of the tongue is examined carefully, the **foliate papilla** can be identified. These papillae are leaflike projections oriented as vertical folds. Foliate papilla are more prominent in children and young adults than in older adults. Corrugated hypertrophic lymphoid tissue (lingual tonsil) extending into this area from the posterior dorsal root of the tongue may sometimes be mistakenly called foliate papillae. The **plica fimbriata** are linear projections on the ventral surface of the tongue. The plica fimbriata occasionally have a brown pigmentation.

Fissured Tongue (Plicated Tongue, Scrotal Tongue) (Fig. 2.6) Fissured tongue is a variation of normal tongue anatomy that consists of a single midline fissure, double fissures, or multiple fissures of the dorsal surface of the anterior two thirds of the tongue. Various fissural patterns, lengths, and depths have been observed. The cause is unknown, but fissured tongue is probably developmental, increases with age, and may be associated with xerostomia.

Fissured tongue affects about 1 to 5% of the population. The frequency of the condition is equal in men and women. Fissured tongue occurs commonly in patients with Down's syndrome and in combination with geographic tongue. It is a component of the Melkerson-Rosenthal syndrome (fissured tongue, cheilitis granulomatosa, and unilateral facial nerve paralysis). The fissures may become secondarily inflamed and cause halitosis as a result of food impaction; thus, brushing the tongue to keep the fissures clean is recommended. The condition is benign.

Ankyloglossia (Fig. 2.7) The lingual frenum is normally attached to the ventral tongue and genial tubercles of the mandible. If the frenum fails to attach properly to the tongue and genial tubercles but instead fuses to the floor of the mouth or lingual gingiva and the ventral tip of the tongue, the condition is called ankyloglossia, or "tongue-tie." This congenital condition is characterized by an abnormally short and malpositioned lingual frenum and a tongue that cannot be extended or retracted. The fusion may be partial or complete. Partial fusion is more common. If the condition is severe, speech may be disturbed. Surgical correction and speech therapy are necessary if speech is defective or if a mandibular denture or removable partial denture is planned. The estimated frequency of ankyloglossia is one case per 1,000 births.

Lingual Varicosity (Phlebectasia) (Fig. 2.8) Lingual varicosities, or venous dilatations, are a common finding in elderly adults. The condition has no direct association with peripheral varicosities or with compromised venous return to the heart. The cause of these vascular dilatations is either a blockage of the vein by an internal foreign body, such as a plaque, or the loss of elasticity of the vascular wall as a result of aging. Intraoral varicosities most commonly appear superficially on the ventral surface of the anterior two thirds of the tongue and may extend onto the lateral border and floor of the mouth. Men and women are affected equally.

Varicosities appear as red-blue to purple, fluctuant nodular growths. Individual varices may be prominent and tortuous or small and punctate. Palpation elicits no pain but can disperse the blood from the vessel, thereby flattening the surface appearance. Diascopy causes varices to blanch. When many lingual veins are prominent, the condition is called "phlebectasia linguae" or "caviar tongue." The lip and labial commissure are other frequent sites of phlebectasia. Treatment of this condition is not required.

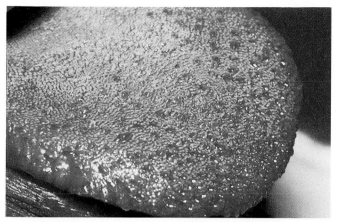

Fig. 2.1. Filiform and fungiform papillae of tongue.

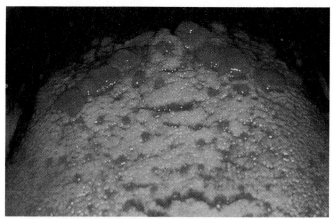

Fig. 2.2. Circumvallate papillae forming a V-shaped row.

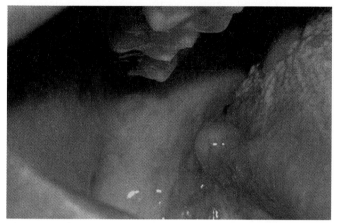

Fig. 2.3. Foliate papilla: posterolateral aspect of tongue.

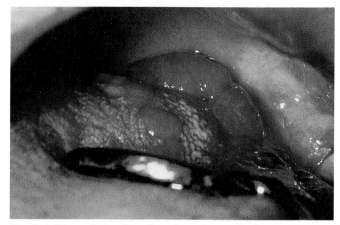

Fig. 2.4. Lingual tonsil at dorsolateral aspect of tongue.

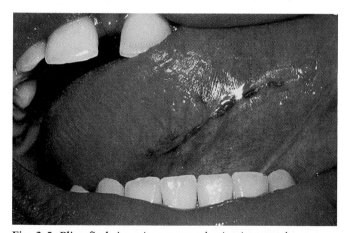

Fig. 2.5. Plica fimbriata, in person who is pigmented.

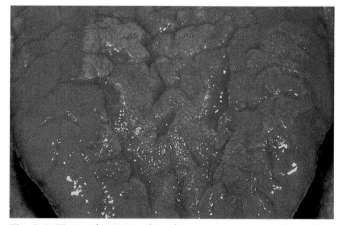

Fig. 2.6. Fissured tongue: dorsal aspect.

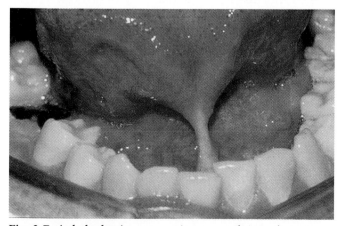

Fig. 2.7. Ankyloglossia; not causing a speech impediment.

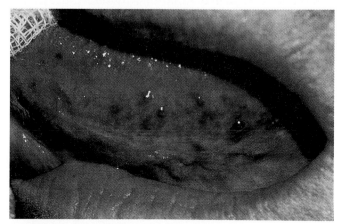

Fig. 2.8. Lingual varicosities; on ventral tongue.

Landmarks of the Periodontium

Periodontium (Figs. 3.1 and 3.2) The periodontium is the tissue that immediately surrounds and supports the teeth in the distal, mesial, buccal, lingual, and apical directions. It consists of alveolar bone, periosteum, periodontal ligament, gingival sulcus, and gingiva; each of these components contributes to stabilizing the tooth within the jaws. The **alveolar bone** is composed of cancellous bone, or spongy bone. It is located between the cortical plates and is permeated by blood vessels and marrow spaces. The **periosteum** is dense connective tissue attached to the outer surface of the alveolar bone. Teeth are anchored to alveolar bone by the connection of the **periodontal ligament** with the **cementum** covering the root and the ligament's attachment to the periosteum. The periodontal ligament covers the tooth root and extends superiorly to the base of the gingival sulcus. The **gingival sulcus** is lined internally by a thin layer of epithelial cells called junctional epithelium. This epithelium provides the barrier to the ingress of bacteria. In health, the gingival sulcus is a crevice less than 3 mm deep. Colonization of bacteria within the sulcus promotes inflammation that breaks down the **epithelial attachment**. A **periodontal pocket** is a gingival sulcus that has experienced apical extension of the epithelial attachment beyond 3 mm because of repeated inflammatory insults and poor oral hygiene. Although accumulation of bacterial plaque is the most important factor influencing the health of the periodontium, position of the tooth within the arch, occlusal loading, parafunctional habits, appliances, drugs, and frenal attachments also affect periodontal health and the development of periodontal pockets.

Alveolar Mucosa and Frenal Attachments (Figs. 3.3 and 3.4) Mucosa is epithelium covering mucus-secreting glands. The **alveolar mucosa** is movable mucosa that overlies alveolar bone and borders the apical extent of the periodontium. It is movable because it is not bound down to the underlying periosteum and bone. The alveolar mucosa is thin and highly vascular. Accordingly, it appears pinkish-red, red, or bright red. On close inspection, small arteries and capillaries can be seen within the alveolar mucosa. These vessels provide nutrients, oxygen, and blood cells to the region. As the mucosa rises from the vestibule away from the periodontium, it is generally identified as either buccal mucosa (if it is located posteriorly) or labial mucosa (if it is located anteriorly).

Frena are muscle attachments at specific locations within the alveolar mucosa. With the lip distended, they appear as arclike rims of flexible tissue. They sometimes produce several fiberlike attachments. Six oral frena have been identified. The **maxillary labial frenum** is located at the midline between the maxillary central incisors, about 4 to 7 mm apical to the interdental region. The **mandibular labial frenum** appears similarly below and between mandibular central incisors within the alveolar mucosa. The **maxillary and mandibular buccal frena** are located within the alveolar mucosa near the first premolar on the right and left sides. Although frena that attach within 3 mm of the cementoenamel junction of a tooth do not directly contribute to periodontal support, they can pull on periodontal tissues and contribute to the development of gingival recession.

Mucogingival Junction (Fig. 3.5) The mucogingival junction is an anatomic landmark representing the border between the unattached alveolar mucosa and the attached gingiva. It is curvilinear and extends around the buccal and lingual aspects of the arches. The prominence of the junction depends on the difference in vascularity and thus the color of the two tissues. It is easily distinguished when the alveolar mucosa is red and the attached gingiva is pink.

Attached Gingiva and Free Marginal Gingiva (Figs. 3.6–3.8) The attached gingiva and free marginal gingiva are close to the tooth. They cover the external aspect of the gingival sulcus. The **attached gingiva** extends coronally from the alveolar mucosa to the free marginal gingiva. It is covered by keratinized epithelium, is bound down to periosteum, and cannot be moved. In health, the attached gingiva is pink and 2 to 7 mm wide. Its surface is slightly convex and stippled, like the surface of an orange. **Interdental grooves** can be seen in the attached gingiva as vertical grooves or narrow depressions located between the roots of the teeth.

The **marginal gingiva** provides the gingival collar around the cervix of the tooth. It is pink and keratinized like the attached gingiva, with a smooth rounded edge. Unlike the attached gingiva, the marginal gingiva is not attached to periosteum nor is it stippled. Its freely movable nature allows a periodontal probe to be passed under it during assessment of pocket depth. Accordingly, it is also termed the **free marginal gingiva**. The junction of the marginal gingiva and the attached gingiva is called the **free gingival groove**.

The **interdental papilla** is the triangular projection of marginal gingiva that extends upward between the teeth. The base of the triangle is nearest the attached gingiva, the apex closest to the interproximal contact of the teeth. The papilla has a buccal and lingual surface. In health, papillae are pink and knife-edge and can barely be moved by the periodontal probe. The presence of inflammation and disease (i.e., gingivitis) alter the color, contour, and consistency of the free marginal gingiva and interdental papillae, causing the marginal gingiva to appear purple, soft, swollen, and tender. Between the buccal and lingual interdental papillae is the **col**, a concave depression of the free marginal gingiva between the teeth.

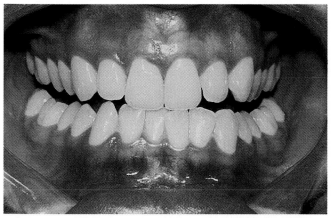

Fig. 3.1. Healthy periodontium: anterior view.

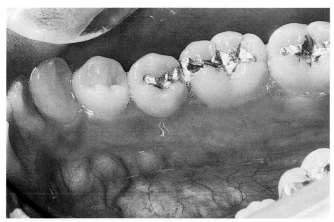

Fig. 3.2. Healthy periodontium: lingual aspect.

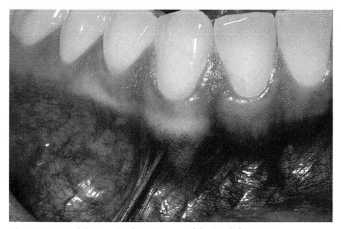

Fig. 3.3. Healthy periodontium and buccal frenum.

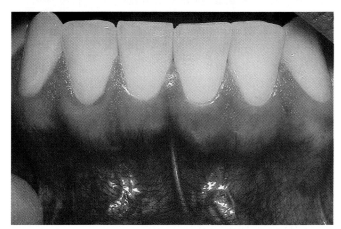

Fig. 3.4. Red alveolar mucosa and labial frenum.

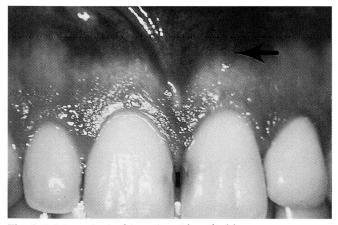

Fig. 3.5. Mucogingival junction: identified by arrow.

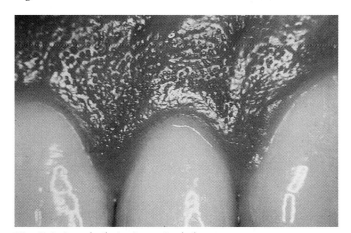

Fig. 3.6. Attached gingiva: stippled texture.

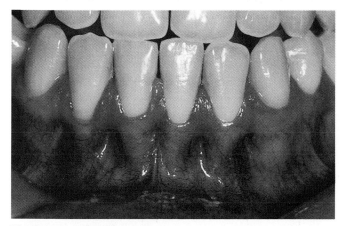

Fig. 3.7. Interdental grooves.

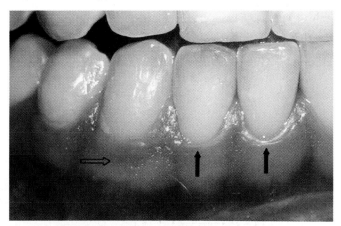

Fig. 3.8. Marginal gingiva and gingival groove, open arrow.

Radiographic Landmarks: Maxilla

Anterior Midline Region (Figs. 4.1 and 4.2) The anterior maxillary film contains several important anatomic structures. The **incisive foramen** is an ovoid depression in the anterior midline of the **hard palate** that overlies the **median palatal suture**. Radiographically, it appears as an ovoid radiolucency that lacks a radiopaque margin. It is located between the roots of the central incisors. It may obscure (but does not resorb) the lamina dura of the central incisor roots. The **median palatal suture** appears as a midline radiolucent line bordered by a radiopaque margin. It runs vertically and apically between the roots of the central incisors to the V-shaped **anterior nasal spine**. The **soft tissue outline of the nose** extends to the apices of the incisors, and the **soft tissue outline of the upper lip** is often seen bisecting the crowns of the central incisors. Alveolar bone appears as fine, interspersed radiopaque **trabeculae** that surround radiolucent **marrow spaces**. The **cementoenamel junction (CEJ)**, or cervical line, of the incisors is seen as a smooth, convex horizontal line delineating the crown and root portions of the tooth. Apically the CEJ is a more subtle convex line delineating the **crest of the alveolar bone**. Between these two entities is a radiolucent band of root structure that is not covered by alveolar bone owing to destruction by periodontal disease.

Anterior Lateral Region (Fig. 4.3) The **superior foramen of the incisive canal** is seen as a round radiolucent landmark within the **nasal fossa** and above the radiopaque line representing the **floor of the nasal fossa**. The radiolucent **incisive canal** runs vertically below the incisive foramen. The **soft tissue outline of the nose** is seen bisecting the roots of the central and lateral incisors. The radiolucent **periodontal ligament space** and radiopaque **lamina dura** surround the roots. The crowns demonstrate a radiopaque **enamel** outer layer, a less dense inner layer of **dentin,** and a centrally located radiolucent **pulp chamber**. Each tooth root has an outer layer of **cementum** that is not normally visible on radiographs, unless excessive amounts, called hypercementosis, are present. Beneath the cementum is the **dentin** of the root that appears immediately adjacent to the radiolucent periodontal membrane space. Centrally within the root is the **root canal space(s)**. In the central and lateral incisors note the **cervical line** crossing the junction between the crown and roots of the teeth. Because of the excess vertical angulation of the beam in this example, the buccal cervical line is projected downward and the lingual cervical line is projected upward much like the buccal and palatal roots of the maxillary first molar. Distal to the lateral incisor is a slightly more radiolucent area called the **lateral fossa**, which is a depression on the labial bone between the lateral and canine roots.

Canine Region (Fig. 4.4) The inverted Y is prominently seen in the canine film. The more-anterior arm of the Y with its superior extension consists of the floor of the nasal cavity (fossa), whereas the more-posterior curved arm is the anterolateral wall of the maxillary sinus. The **soft tissue outline of the nasal mucosa** is delineated superiorly by a thin radiolucent line representing an airspace between the nasal turbinate and nasal mucosa. In this example, the **gingiva** is seen at the **crest of the alveolar ridge** in the edentulous area.

Premolar Region (Fig. 4.5) The **floor of the maxillary sinus** is located above the premolar roots and in this example bisects the molar roots. The normal maxillary sinus floor appears as an irregular, slightly wavy line resembling the slightly broken and irregular line drawn by an artist on textured craft paper. Above the floor and within the lateral sinus wall is the curved radiolucent line representing the **canal of the posterior superior alveolar nerve, artery, and vein**. Notice that this canal has a thin radiopaque margin. Above the second molar root is the radiopaque **zygomatic process of the maxilla** sometimes referred to as the **malar process**. It is the anterior root of the **zygomatic arch**. Sometimes the nasolabial fold can be seen bisecting the root of the first premolar in this film. Note the elongated palatal root of the first molar and the shortened buccal roots owing to incorrect positioning (excessive vertical angulation) of the beam-indicating device (BID or cone) of the x-ray machine during film exposure.

Molar Region (Fig. 4.6) A prominent landmark in the maxillary molar film is the radiopaque U-shaped **zygomatic process of the maxilla**. It delineates the most anterior extent of the **zygomatic arch** (cheek bone) that extends posteriorly beyond the posterior limit of the **maxillary sinus**. The zygomatic arch is buccal and lateral to the maxilla. Distal to the second molar is the **maxillary tuberosity**—a bony structure covered by connective tissue and mucosa.

Tuberosity Region (Figs. 4.7 and 4.8) The anterior or maxillary half of the **zygomatic arch** is delineated from the posterior or temporal portion by the **zygomaticotemporal suture** seen here. Distal to the second molar is the **maxillary tuberosity**, the **lateral pterygoid plate,** and small **hamular process** of the medial pterygoid plate that extends below the lateral pterygoid plate. The **coronoid process** of the mandible is also seen overlying this area (superimposed on the second molar). In the radiograph the **zygomatic arch** extends horizontally across the upper portion of the **maxillary sinus**. Some of these structures may not always be seen with the normal paralleling technique; however, they are seen in special views used to visualize the third molars or regional pathosis.

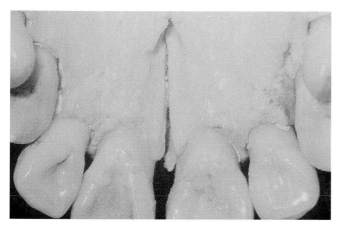

Fig. 4.1. Maxilla: lingual aspect of central incisor region.

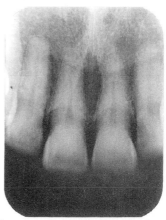

Fig. 4.2. Maxilla: central incisor region radiograph.

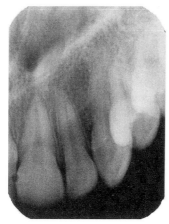

Fig. 4.3. Maxilla: lateral incisor radiograph.

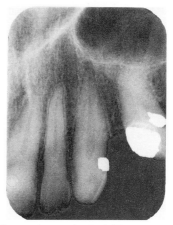

Fig. 4.4. Maxilla: canine periapical film.

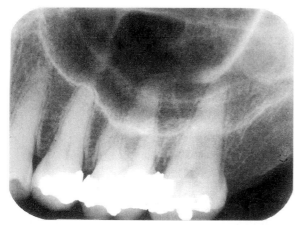

Fig. 4.5. Maxilla: premolar periapical film.

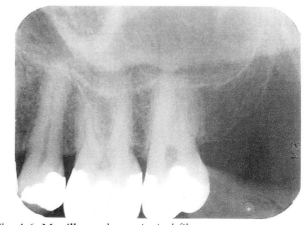

Fig. 4.6. Maxilla: molar periapical film.

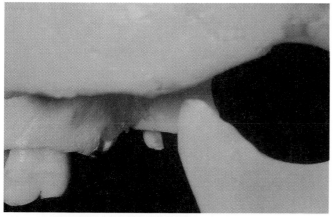

Fig. 4.7. Maxilla: tuberosity region on skull.

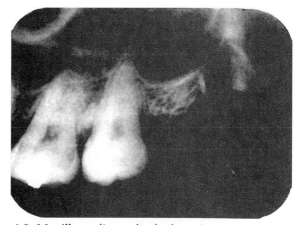

Fig. 4.8. Maxilla: radiograph of tuberosity region.

Radiographic Landmarks: Mandible

Incisor–Canine Region (Figs. 5.1 and 5.2) On the lingual aspect of the mandible, the incisor film reveals the **lingual foramen** below the root apices. This radiolucent landmark is surrounded by the four **genial tubercles**. The superior tubercles serve as the attachment site of the genioglossus muscle, and the inferior pair anchors the geniohyoid muscle. The **inferior border** of the mandible is below this area and is delineated by a thick cortex (outer covering). Radiographically, the **genial tubercles** appear as round doughnut-shaped radiopacities. In this case, the **lingual canal** extends inferiorly from this region. Below this is the **inferior cortex**. The inverted V-shaped thick radiopaque line at the root apices is the **mental ridge** that is located on the buccal aspect of the mandible.

Premolar and Molar Regions (Figs. 5.3 and 5.4) In the photographs of the skull, the **mental foramen** is located at the apex of the second premolar root, and the **external oblique ridge** is highlighted and distal to the second molar. Both are landmarks of the buccal aspect of the mandible. The **internal oblique or mylohyoid ridge** is anterior, more horizontal, and longer than the external oblique ridge. In contrast, it is located on the lingual side of the mandible. Beneath the mylohyoid ridge is a fossa or depression within which lies the submandibular salivary gland.

Premolar Region (Fig. 5.5) Radiographically, the **mental foramen** is a round or ovoid radiolucency about 2 to 3 mm in diameter that lacks a radiopaque corticated margin. It varies in location from the distal aspect of the canine to the distal aspect of the second premolar in the apical region. In this radiograph, a mixed **trabecular pattern** is seen with a denser (more radiopaque) pattern toward the alveolar crest and a looser (more radiolucent) pattern in the apical area. Loose and dense trabecular patterns depend on the number of bone trabeculae present in the region. In this radiograph, the radiopaque **lamina dura** and radiolucent **periodontal membrane space** are well illustrated in the second premolar. The **crestal alveolar bone** between the premolars is healthy as it is radiopaque. When the alveolar bone starts to resorb as a result of periodontal disease, the crestal bone (radiopaque line) is lost. The densely radiopaque material in the second premolar and molar crowns is **amalgam**. Notice that the gingival margins of the restorations are smooth and continuous with the remaining tooth structure in the interproximal areas, which helps to maintain proper periodontal health. In this view, the buccal cusps are slightly higher than the lingual cusps owing to excess negative vertical angulation of the BID during film exposure.

Buccal Aspect Molar Region (Fig. 5.6) The external and internal oblique ridges are densely radiopaque structures that sometimes parallel each other. The external oblique ridge is above and posterior to the internal oblique ridge. The smooth, round radiopaque area at the bifurcation of the first molar is frequently mistaken for an enamel pearl or pulp stone. Actually, it is an anatomic artifact (erroneous superimposition of buccal and lingual root structure at the bifurcation) produced by incorrect horizontal angulation of the BID. The artifact disappears when the correct horizontal angulation of the BID is used—in cases in which it does not disappear, an enamel pearl or pulp stone should be suspected.

Lingual Aspect Molar Region (Fig. 5.7) The **submandibular fossa** is a broad radiolucent area immediately beneath the mylohyoid ridge and above the **inferior cortex**. It is seen more often when excessive negative vertical angulation of the BID is used.

Internal Aspect Molar Region (Fig. 5.8) The **inferior alveolar canal** that contains the inferior alveolar nerve and blood vessels appears radiolucent in the molar film. It is outlined superiorly and inferiorly by a radiopaque cortical line representing the canal walls, and may be in close proximity to the molar apices or to developing third molars. This close relationship to third molars is important when considering the removal of the third molars (wisdom teeth). In general, canals are radiolucent and are outlined by a thin radiopaque cortical line. In contrast, foramina are radiolucent without a radiopaque outline. Foramina may appear similar to small cysts; however, cysts usually have a thin radiopaque outline. A **step ladder trabecular pattern** is sometimes seen between the roots of mandibular first molars (and central incisors). This represents a variation of normal. In this instance, the trabeculae are horizontal and more or less parallel to each other. Note the fractured distal surface of the first molar and the subtle occlusal caries in the second molar.

Author comment: We have purposely used no. 2 size film in these radiographic examples to provide as many landmarks as possible in the limited space available. We have omitted some views in the standard full-mouth series because of space limitations. Similar landmarks can be seen in the narrower and popular no. 1 film. Also, some landmarks are seen variably depending on individual patient differences and whether the bisecting angle or paralleling techniques are used or whether excessive vertical or horizontal angulation of the BID is used, either as an error or to better project an anatomic area on the film. We have avoided the placement of arrows as they can obscure adjacent anatomic structures.

Before problems can be identified or assessed the recognition of normal is an absolute prerequisite. As we have often said, "learning should be fun," and we hope this descriptive and illustrative approach helps.

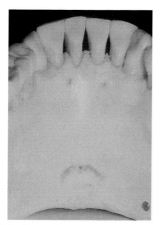

Fig. 5.1. Mandible: lingual aspect incisor–canine region.

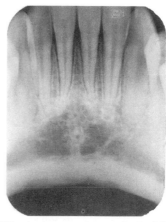

Fig. 5.2. Mandible: incisor–canine periapical film.

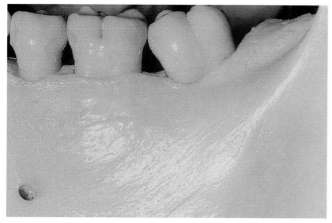

Fig. 5.3. Mandible: buccal aspect premolar–molar region.

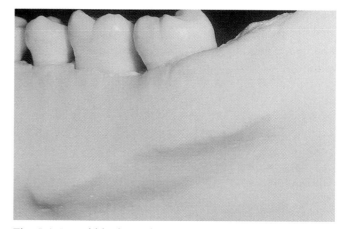

Fig. 5.4. Mandible: lingual aspect premolar–molar region.

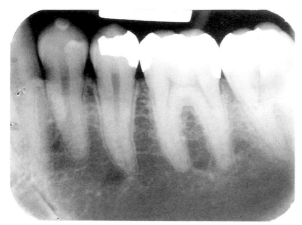

Fig. 5.5. Mandible: premolar periapical film.

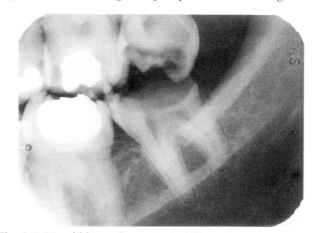

Fig. 5.6. Mandible: molar periapical film.

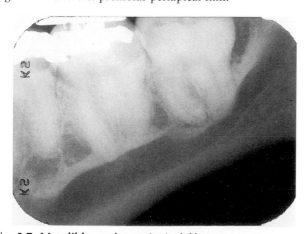

Fig. 5.7. Mandible: molar periapical film.

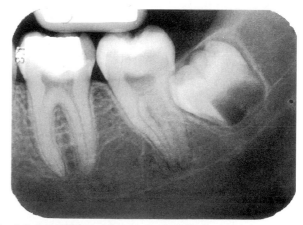

Fig. 5.8. Mandible: molar periapical film.

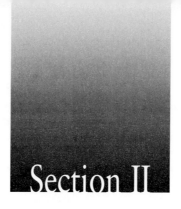

Section II

Diagnostic and Descriptive Terminology

Diagnostic and Descriptive Terminology

Macule (Figs. 6.1 and 6.2) A macule is a circumscribed area of epidermis or mucosa distinguished by color from its surroundings. The macule may appear alone or in groups as a blue, brown, or black stain or spot. The macule is neither elevated nor depressed and may be of any size, although the term is usually reserved for lesions 1 cm or smaller. A macule may represent a normal condition, a variant of normal, or local or systemic disease. The term macule would be used to clinically describe the following conditions: oral melanotic macule, ephelis, amalgam, india ink or pencil tattoos, and focal argyrosis. Conditions that appear as macules are discussed in detail under "Pigmented Lesions" (Figs. 58.1–60.8).

Patch (Figs. 6.3 and 6.4) A patch is a circumscribed area that is larger than the macule and differentiated from the surrounding epidermis by color, texture, or both. Like the macule, the patch is neither elevated nor depressed. Focal argyrosis, lichen planus, mucous patch of secondary syphilis, and snuff dipper's patch represent patchlike lesions that may be seen intraorally. Conditions that appear as patches are discussed in detail under "White Lesions" (Figs. 49.1–51.8), "Pigmented Lesions" (Figs. 58.1–60.8), and "Sexually Transmissible Diseases" (Figs. 72.1–74.8).

Erosion (Figs. 6.5 and 6.6) Erosion is a clinical term that describes a soft tissue lesion in which the epithelium above the basal cell layer is denuded. Erosions are moist and slightly depressed and often result from a broken vesicle, epithelial breakdown or trauma. Healing rarely results in scarring. Pemphigus, erosive lichen planus (desquamative gingivitis), and erythema multiforme are diseases that produce mucocutaneous erosions. Conditions that appear as erosions are discussed in detail under "Vesiculobullous Lesions" (Figs. 64.1–68.8).

Ulcer (Figs. 6.7 and 6.8) An ulcer is an uncovered wound of cutaneous or mucosal tissue that exhibits gradual tissue disintegration and necrosis. Ulcers extend deeper than erosions, from beyond the basal layer of the epithelium into the dermis. Scarring may follow healing of an ulcer. Ulcers may result from trauma, aphthous stomatitis, or infection by such viruses as herpes simplex, variola (smallpox), and varicella-zoster (chickenpox and shingles). Ulcers are usually painful and often require topical or systemic drug therapy for effective management. Conditions that appear as ulcers are discussed in detail under "Vesiculobullous Lesions" (Figs. 64.1–68.8).

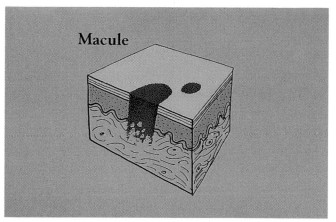

Fig. 6.1. Macule: nonraised area altered in color.

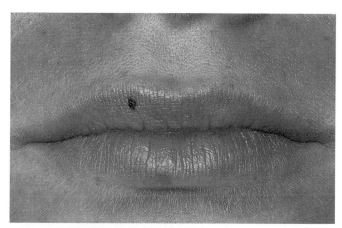

Fig. 6.2. Oral melanotic macule on the lip.

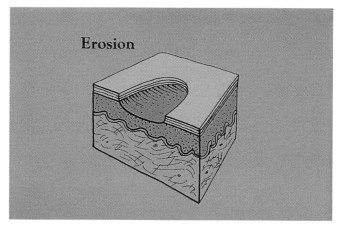

Fig. 6.3. Patch: pigmented area larger than a macule.

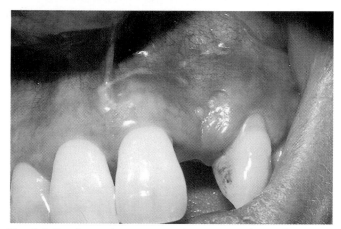

Fig. 6.4. Patch: amalgam tattoo after retrograde amalgam.

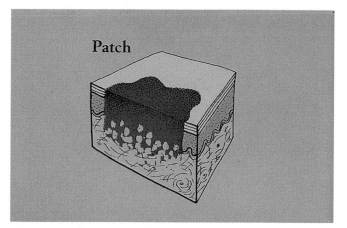

Fig. 6.5. Erosion: denudation above basal layer of epithelium.

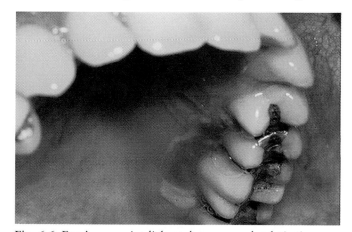

Fig. 6.6. Erosion: erosive lichen planus on palatal gingiva.

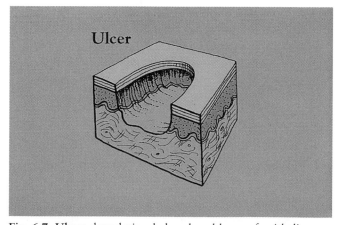

Fig. 6.7. Ulcer: denudation below basal layer of epithelium.

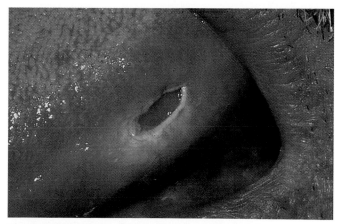

Fig. 6.8. Traumatic ulcer on lateral tongue border.

Diagnostic and Descriptive Terminology

Wheal (Figs. 7.1 and 7.2) A wheal is an edematous papule or plaque that results from acute extravasation of serum into the superficial dermis. Wheals are generally pale red, pruritic, and of short duration. By definition they are only slightly raised. They occur most commonly in persons with allergies. The wheal develops as a result of histamine release from mast cells or activation of the complement cascade. Wheals may be seen after insect bites, an allergic reaction to food, or mechanical irritation (such as that occurring in patients with dermatographia). Conditions that appear as wheals are discussed in detail under "Allergic Reactions and Vesiculobullous Lesions" (Figs. 66.1–66.8).

Scar (Figs. 7.3 and 7.4) A scar is a permanent mark or cicatrix remaining after a wound heals. These lesions are visible signs that indicate a previous disruption in the integrity of the epidermis and dermis and healing of epithelium with collagen connective tissue. Scars are infrequently found in the oral cavity because oral tissue is elastic and less prone to scar formation than skin. When they do occur they may be of any shape or size. The color of an intraoral scar is usually lighter than that of the adjacent mucosa. Histologically, it is more dense than the adjacent epithelium. Oral (i.e., periapical) surgery, burns, or intraoral trauma may result in a scar. Scars are discussed in detail under "White Lesions" (Figs. 50.3–50.6).

Fissure (Figs. 7.5 and 7.6) A fissure is a normal or abnormal linear cleft in the epidermis that affects the tongue, lips, and perioral tissues. The presence of a fissure can indicate a condition representing a variant of normal or disease. Diseased fissures result when pathogenic organisms infect a fissure, causing pain, ulceration, and inflammation. Fissured tongue is an example of a variation of normal that is associated with dry mouth and dehydration. Angular cheilitis and exfoliative cheilitis are examples of disease-associated fissures.

Sinus (Figs. 7.7 and 7.8) The term sinus has two meanings. A common meaning of sinus is a normal recess or cavity such as the frontal or maxillary sinus. The term is also used to describe as an abnormal dilated tract or fistula that leads from a suppurative cavity, cyst, or abscess to the surface of the epidermis. An abscessed tooth often produces a sinus tract together with a clinically evident parulis, which is the terminal end of the tract. In this clinical situation, gutta percha points can be placed into the tract and a radiograph taken. The nonvital tooth is identified by locating the tip of the gutta percha point. Actinomycosis is a condition characterized clinically by several yellow sinus tracts exiting onto the mucosa or skin surface.

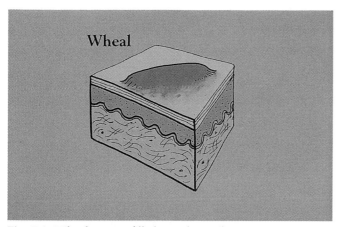

Fig. 7.1. **Wheal:** serum-filled papule or plaque.

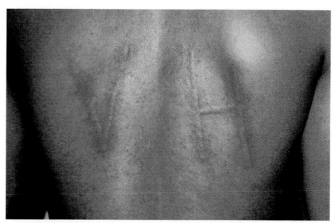

Fig. 7.2. **Wheal:** dermatographism after rubbing the skin.

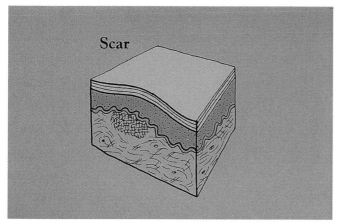

Fig. 7.3. **Scar:** permanent mark from wound.

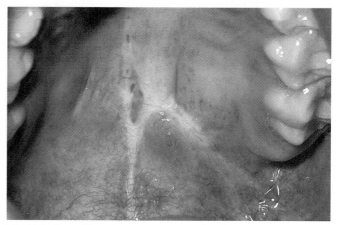

Fig. 7.4. **Scar:** fibrotic tissue as a result of trauma.

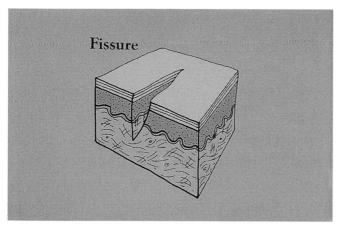

Fig. 7.5. **Fissure:** a linear crack in the epidermis.

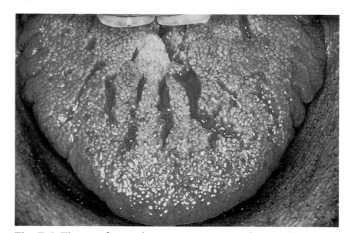

Fig. 7.6. **Fissure:** fissured tongue, a variant of normal.

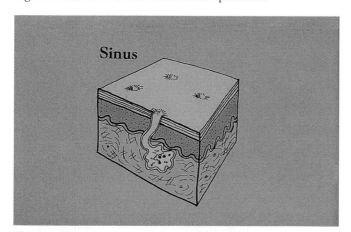

Fig. 7.7. **Sinus:** a recess, cavity, or dilated tract.

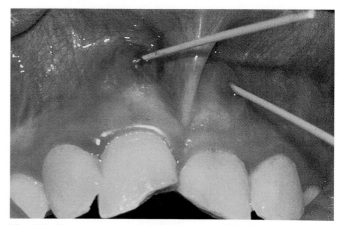

Fig. 7.8. **Sinus tracts** exiting from nonvital incisors.

Diagnostic and Descriptive Terminology

Papule (Figs. 8.1 and 8.2) A papule is a superficial, elevated, solid lesion or structure that is less than 1 cm in diameter. Papules may be of any color and may be attached by a stalk or firm base. A papule often represents a benign or slow-growing lesion such as condyloma acuminatum, parulis, and squamous papilloma. However, basal cell carcinoma can appear as a papule. Conditions that appear as papules are discussed in the section on "Papulonodules" (Figs. 63.1–63.8).

Plaque (Figs. 8.3 and 8.4) A plaque is a flat, solid, raised area that is larger than 1 cm in diameter. Although essentially superficial, plaques may extend deeper into the dermis than papules. The edges may be sloped, and sometimes surface keratin proliferates (a condition known as lichenification). Lichen planus, leukoplakia, or melanoma may initially appear as a plaque. Lichen planus is discussed under "Red and Red/White Lesions" (Figs 55.1–55.8).

Nodule (Figs. 8.5 and 8.6) A nodule is a solid mass of tissue that has the dimension of depth. Like papules, these lesions are less than 1 cm in diameter; however, nodules extend deeper into the dermis. The nodule can be detected by palpation. The overlying epidermis is usually nonfixed and can be easily moved over the lesion. Nodules can be asymptomatic or painful and usually are slow growing. Benign mesenchymal tumors such as fibroma, lipoma, lipofibroma, and neuroma often appear as oral nodules. Other examples of nodules are discussed under "Nodules" (Figs. 61.1–62.8).

Tumor (Figs. 8.7 and 8.8) "Tumor" is a term used to indicate a solid mass of tissue larger than 1 cm in diameter that has the dimension of depth. The term is also used to represent a neoplasm—a new, independent growth of tissue with uncontrolled and progressive multiplication of cells that have no physiologic use. Tumors may be any color and may be located in any intraoral or extraoral soft or hard tissue. Tumors are classified as benign or malignant. **Benign tumors** grow more slowly and are less aggressive than **malignant tumors**. Benign tumors often appear as raised, rounded lesions that have well-defined margins; they do not metastasize. Malignant tumors are comprised of aberrant neoplastic cells that spread rapidly. Clinically, they often have ill-defined margins. Persistent tumors may be umbilicated or ulcerated in the center. The term tumor is often used to describe a benign tissue mass such as a neurofibroma, granular cell tumor, or pregnancy tumor. The term **carcinoma** is reserved for malignant cancers of epithelial tissue. The term **sarcoma** is reserved for a malignant neoplasm of embryonic connective tissue origin, such as osteosarcoma, a malignant neoplasm of bone. Malignancies destroy tissue by direct invasion and extension and by spread to distant sites by metastasis through blood, lymph, or serosal surfaces.

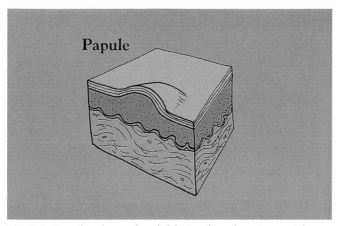

Fig. 8.1. **Papule:** elevated, solid lesion less than 1 cm wide.

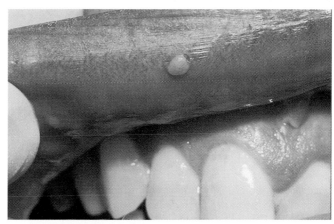

Fig. 8.2. **Papule:** fibroepithelial polyp from chronic irritation.

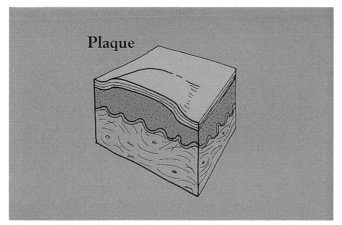

Fig. 8.3. **Plaque:** flat, raised area larger than 1 cm in diameter.

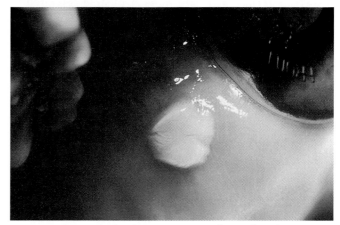

Fig. 8.4. **Plaque:** leukoplakia owing to clasp of appliance.

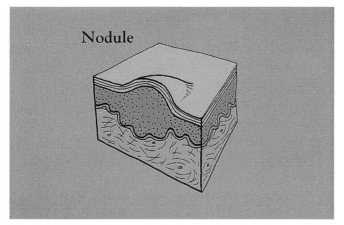

Fig. 8.5. **Nodule:** deep and raised mass less than 1 cm wide.

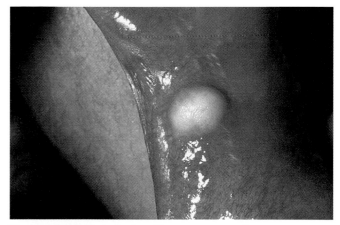

Fig. 8.6. **Nodule:** irritation fibroma at commissure.

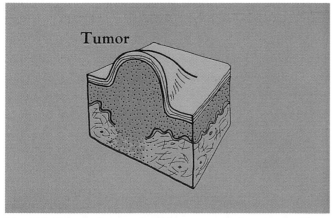

Fig. 8.7. **Tumor:** deep and solid mass more than 1 cm wide.

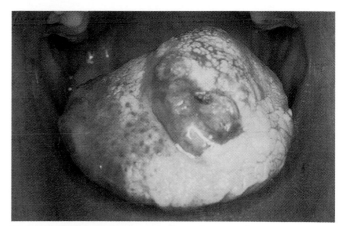

Fig. 8.8. **Tumor:** squamous cell carcinoma of tongue.

Diagnostic and Descriptive Terminology

Vesicle (Figs. 9.1 and 9.2) A vesicle is a circumscribed, fluid-filled elevation in the epidermis that is less than 1 cm in diameter. The fluid of a vesicle generally consists of lymph or serum but may contain blood and infectious agents. The epithelial lining of a vesicle is thin and will eventually break down, thus causing an ulcer and eschar. Vesicles are common in viral infections such as herpes simplex, herpes zoster, chickenpox, and smallpox. In viral infections, the vesicle is laden with virus and is highly infectious. Conditions characterized by vesicles are discussed under "Vesiculobullous Lesions" (Figs. 64.1–68.8).

Pustule (Figs. 9.3 and 9.4) A pustule is a circumscribed elevation filled with purulent exudate resulting from an infection. Pustules are less than 1 cm in diameter and may be preceded by a vesicle or papule. They are creamy white or yellowish and are often associated with an epidermal pore (i.e., pimple). Within the mouth, a pustule is represented by a pointing abscess or parulis. Herpes zoster also produces pustules that eventually ulcerate and cause intense pain. See the discussions under "Localized Gingival Lesions" (Figs. 33.1 and 33.2), "Caries Progression" (Fig. 24.8), and "Vesiculobullous Lesions" (Figs. 65.1–65.4) for examples of diseases that produce pustules.

Bulla (Figs. 9.5 and 9.6) When the diameter of a vesicle exceeds 1 cm, the term "bulla" is used. This condition develops from the accumulation of fluid in the epidermal-dermis junction or a split in the epidermis. Because of their size, bullae represent a more severe disease than do conditions associated with vesicles. Bullae are commonly seen in pemphigus, pemphigoid, burns, frictional trauma, and epidermolysis bullosa. These conditions are discussed under "Vesiculobullous Lesions" (Figs. 68.1–68.8).

Cyst (Figs. 9.7 and 9.8) A cyst is an epithelial-lined mass located in the dermis, subcutaneous tissue, or bone. Cysts result from entrapment of epithelium or remnants of epithelium that grow to produce a cavity. They range in diameter from a few millimeters to several centimeters. Aspiration of a cyst may or may not yield luminal fluid, depending on the nature of the cyst. Cysts that contain clear fluid appear pink to blue, whereas keratin-filled cysts often appear yellow or creamy white. Some of the many types of oral cysts are dermoid cysts, eruption cysts, implantation cysts, incisive canal cysts, lymphoepithelial cysts, mucus retention cysts, nasoalveolar cysts, radicular cysts, odontogenic keratocyst, dentigerous cyst, and the lateral periodontal cyst. Figure 9.8 illustrates the gingival cyst, which is a peripheral variant of the lateral periodontal cyst. Bone cysts are discussed under "Cysts and Tumors of the Jaws" (Figs. 25.1–25.8).

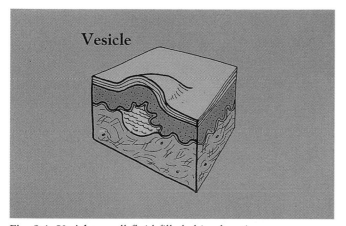

Fig. 9.1. **Vesicle:** small fluid-filled skin elevation.

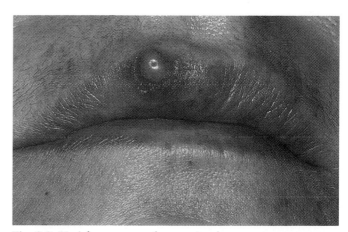

Fig. 9.2. **Vesicle:** recurrent herpes simplex.

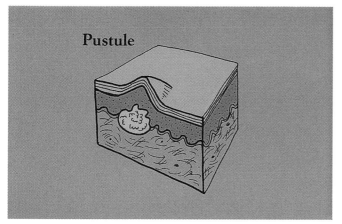

Fig. 9.3. **Pustule:** vesicle filled with purulent exudate.

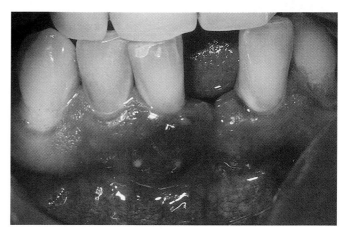

Fig. 9.4. **Pustule:** pointing periodontal abscess.

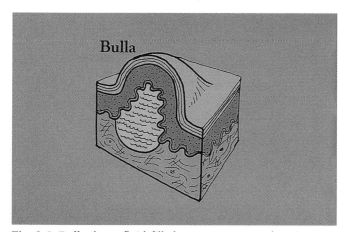

Fig. 9.5. **Bulla:** large fluid-filled mucocutaneous elevation.

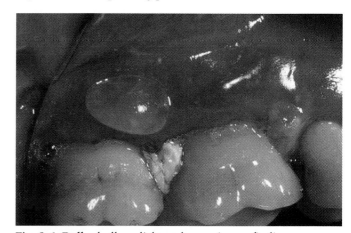

Fig. 9.6. **Bulla:** bullous lichen planus. A rare finding.

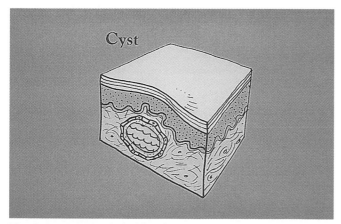

Fig. 9.7. **Cyst:** epithelial-lined cavity.

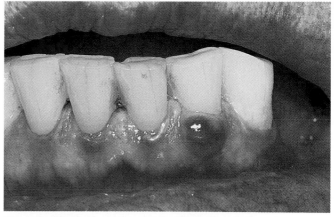

Fig. 9.8. **Gingival cyst:** variant of lateral periodontal cyst.

Oral Conditions Affecting Infants and Children

Oral Conditions Affecting Infants and Children

Commissural Lip Pits (Fig. 10.1) Commissural lip pits are dimplelike invaginations of the corner of the lips. They may be unilateral or bilateral but tend to occur on the vermilion portion of the lip. They are generally less than 4 mm in diameter, and exploration of the pits yields a sealed depression. Commissural lip pits represent failure of fusion of the embryonic maxillary and mandibular processes. The pits occur more frequently in males than in females, and prevalence differs between adults and children. For example, lip pits have been documented in less than 1% of children but in up to 10% of adults. These prevalence figures indicate that the invaginations may be developmental and not congenital. However, an autosomal dominant pattern of transmission has been reported in some families. No treatment is required.

Paramedian Lip Pits (Fig. 10.2) Paramedian lip pits are congenital depressions that occur in the mandibular lip, most often on either side of the midline. They probably develop from the lateral sulci of the embryonic mandibular arch that fail to regress during the sixth week in utero. Paramedian lip pits are more often bilateral, symmetric depressions with raised, rounded borders. However, single pits and unilateral pits have been described. Inspection reveals a sealed depression that may express mucinous saliva. Paramedian lip pits are often inherited as an autosomal dominant trait in combination with cleft lip or cleft palate. When these features occur together, the condition is called **van der Woude's syndrome**. The gene responsible for lip pits shows variable penetrance; some patients who carry the gene may have a minor or submucosal cleft palate or no cleft yet pass the full syndrome on to their children. By themselves, paramedian lip pits require no treatment unless they are of esthetic concern. The clinician should inquire about affected family members and examine them for cleft lip and palate.

Cleft Lip (Figs. 10.3 and 10.4) Cleft lip is the result of a disturbance of lip development in utero. The maxillary lip is most commonly affected. Cleft lip results when the medial nasal process fails to fuse with the lateral portions of the maxillary process of the first branchial arch. Fusion normally occurs during the sixth and seventh weeks of embryonic development.

Cleft lip occurs in about 1 in 900 births and more often in Asian and Native American persons than in Caucasians. The condition occurs more often in males than in females and is more severe in males than in females. About 85% of cleft lips are unilateral and non-midline; 15% are bilateral. Midline cleft lip, resulting from failure of fusion of the right and left medial nasal processes, is rare.

The severity of cleft lips varies. A small cleft that does not involve the nose is called an incomplete cleft; these sometimes appear as a small notch in the lip. A complete cleft lip involves the nasal structures in 45% of cases and is often associated with cleft palate. Cleft lip and cleft palate can be caused by abnormal patterning genes that are transmitted by autosomal dominant and recessive inheritance, as well as X-linked inheritance. Certain drugs taken during pregnancy, such as nicotine and antiepileptic agents, also appear to be causative.

Cleft Palate (Figs. 10.5–10.8) The palate develops from the primary and secondary palate. The primary palate is formed by fusion of the right and left medial nasal processes. It is a small triangular mass that encompasses bone, connective tissue, labial and palatal epithelium, and the four incisor tooth buds. The secondary palate is formed by fusion of the palatine processes (shelves) of the maxillary process. Palatal fusion is initiated during the eighth week in utero by expansion of the mandible; this permits the tongue to drop down and allows the palatal processes to grow inward. The palatal shelves merge with the primary palate, and fusion progresses posteriorly. Except for the posterior soft palate and uvula, fusion of the palate is generally completed by the twelfth week of gestation.

Disruption in palatal fusion leads to clefting. A cleft palate can involve the soft palate only; the hard palate only; the hard and soft palates; or the hard and soft palates, alveolus, and lip. Cleft palate without lip involvement occurs in about 30% of cases.

Bifid uvula is a minor cleft of the posterior soft palate. It occurs most commonly in Asian and Native American persons; the overall incidence is about 1 in 250 people. A **submucosal palatal cleft** may occur with bifid uvula. It develops when the muscles of the soft palate are clefted but the surface mucosa is intact. The clefted region is palpably notched. An **incomplete cleft palate** is a small break in the hard or soft palate that permits communication between the oral and nasal cavities. A **complete cleft palate** extends forward to include the incisive foramen. The triad of cleft palate, micrognathia and retrognathia of the mandible, and glossoptosis (posterior displacement of the tongue) is called **Pierre Robin's syndrome** (anomalad). This condition is characterized by respiratory difficulty.

Cleft lip and palate are often associated with cleft alveolus, missing teeth (most commonly the lateral incisor), malpositioned teeth, and occasionally supernumerary teeth. Cleft palate causes feeding and speech impairment and prominent malocclusion. Treatment involves a multidisciplinary team consisting of a pediatrician, pediatric dentist, oral and plastic surgeon, orthodontist, and speech therapist. Surgical lip closure is generally accomplished early in the infant's life, whereas cleft palate may require several surgical procedures because of growth plate considerations.

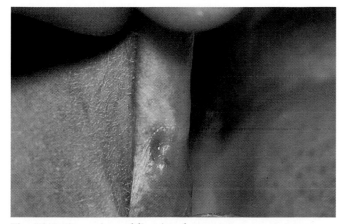

Fig. 10.1. Commissural lip pits: depression at commissure.

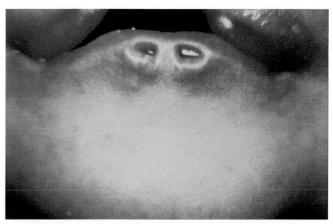

Fig. 10.2. Paramedian lip pits: with cleft lip and palate.

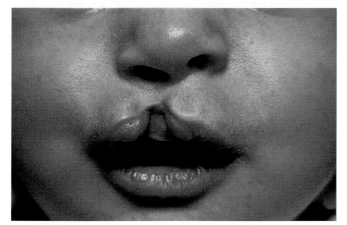

Fig. 10.3. Incomplete cleft lip: rare midline type.

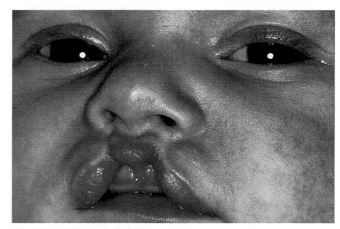

Fig. 10.4. Bilateral cleft lip.

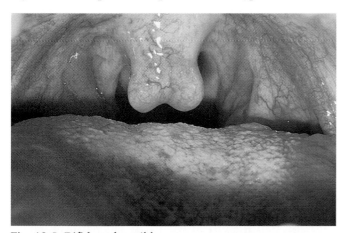

Fig. 10.5. Bifid uvula: mild case.

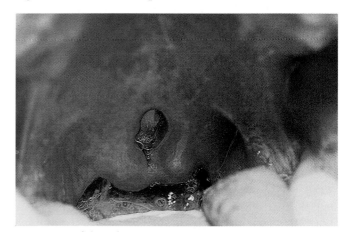

Fig. 10.6. Bifid uvula: more severe case.

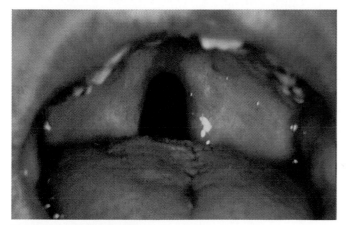

Fig. 10.7. Cleft soft palate.

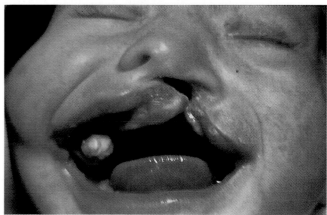

Fig. 10.8. Cleft lip and cleft palate.

25

Oral Conditions Affecting Infants and Children

Congenital Epulis (Fig. 11.1) The congenital epulis of the newborn is a benign, soft tissue polypoid growth arising from the edentulous alveolar ridge. It usually occurs in the anterior maxilla and is 10 times more likely to occur in females than in males. The lesion is pink, soft, and compressible. The surface shows prominent telangiectasis and is attached to the alveolar ridge by a pedunculated stalk or broad base. Lesions can be several centimeters in diameter. It is treated by excision, and recurrence is unlikely. Histologic examination shows granular cells. Multiple lesions are present in 1 in 10 cases.

Melanotic Neuroectodermal Tumor of Infancy (Fig. 11.2) The melanotic neuroectodermal tumor of infancy is a benign, rapidly growing neuroblastic neoplasm commonly located in the anterior maxilla. The tumor shows no sex predilection and begins as a small pink or red-purple nodule that resembles an eruption cyst. Radiography usually shows localized and irregular destruction of underlying alveolar bone and a primary tooth bud floating in a soft tissue mass. Urinary levels of vanyllmandelic acid are elevated in conjunction with this tumor. Treatment is conservative excision. Histologic examination often shows pigmentation. Recurrence and metastasis are rarely documented complications.

Dental Lamina Cysts (Fig. 11.3) Remnants of the dental lamina that do not develop into a tooth bud may degenerate to form dental lamina cysts. These cysts are classified according to clinical location. **Gingival cysts of the newborn** are tiny keratin-filled cysts. They are often multiple and whitish and usually resolve when the tooth erupts. **Palatal cysts of the newborn** can be either Epstein's pearls or Bohn's nodules. **Epstein's pearls** arise from epithelial inclusions that become entrapped at the median palatal raphe during fusion of opposing embryonic palatal shelves; **Bohn's nodules** arise from minor salivary glands. The pearls and nodules are usually small, firm, and whitish and may occur in small groups anywhere in the hard palate. Dental lamina cysts may be incised if they do not resolve spontaneously.

Natal Teeth (Fig. 11.4) Natal teeth are teeth that are present at birth or erupt within 30 days of birth. Some natal teeth have been referred to as "supernumerary" or as "predeciduous" and consist only of cornified and calcific material; the teeth are mobile and do not have roots. However, most natal teeth simply represent premature eruption of the primary teeth. The most common natal teeth are the incisors; the mandible is affected 10 times more often than the maxilla. Natal teeth have been reported to cause ulcers of the ventral tongue (Riga-Fede's disease) that result from irritation during nursing. In this case, extraction may be needed. However, a radiograph should be taken to determine whether the tooth is predeciduous or deciduous.

Eruption Cyst (Gingival Eruption Cyst, Eruption Hematoma) (Fig. 11.5) The eruption cyst is a soft tissue variant of the dentigerous cyst that forms around an erupting tooth crown. Children younger than 10 years of age are most commonly affected. It appears as a small, dome-shaped, translucent swelling overlying an erupting primary tooth. The cyst is lined by odontogenic epithelium and is filled with blood or serum. The presence of blood casts a blue-gray appearance to the cyst. No treatment is necessary because the erupting tooth eventually breaks the cystic membrane. Incising the lesion and allowing the fluid to drain can relieve symptoms.

Congenital Lymphangioma (Fig. 11.6) The congenital lymphangioma is a benign hamartoma of dilated lymphatic channels that may present in the mouth of infants. The tongue, alveolar ridge, and labial mucosa are common locations. There is a 2:1 predilection for males. In 1 in 20 African American neonates, one or more alveolar lymphangiomas may be seen. The lymphangioma typically produces a swelling that is asymptomatic, compressible, and negative on diascopy. When superficial, the swelling is composed of single or multiple discrete papulonodules that may be pink to dark blue. Deepseated tumors produce diffuse swellings with no alteration of the color of the overlying tissue. Large lymphangiomas of the neck are called cystic hygromas. Intraoral lymphangiomas may regress spontaneously, but persistent lesions should be excised.

Thrush (Candidiasis, Moniliasis) (Fig. 11.7) Thrush, or acute pseudomembranous candidiasis, one of four subtypes of candidiasis, is a fungal infection of mucosal membranes caused by *Candida albicans*. It is primarily seen in infants as a surface infection that produces milky-white curds on the oral mucosa. These curds are easily wiped off, leaving a red, raw, painful surface. The buccal mucosa, palate, and tongue are common locations. Newborns often acquire the infection from the mother's birth canal during parturition and show clinical signs of infection within the first few weeks of life. Fever and gastrointestinal irritation may accompany the disorder. Treatment consists of topically applied antifungal agents.

Parulis (Gum Boil) (Fig. 11.8) The parulis is an inflammatory response to a chronic bacterial infection of a nonvital tooth draining through a sinus tract. It most commonly occurs in children when pulpal infection spreads beyond the furcal area of a posterior tooth. The parulis appears as a small, raised, fluctuant yellow-to-red boil that is located near the mucogingival junction adjacent to the affected tooth. Pressure to the area and the resulting discharge of pus are pathognomonic. Spontaneous pain is not a feature, although palpation of the lesion, tooth, or surrounding structures may elicit pain. The condition resolves when the odontogenic infection is eliminated. Failure to eliminate the infection in a primary tooth can affect the development of the succedaneous tooth.

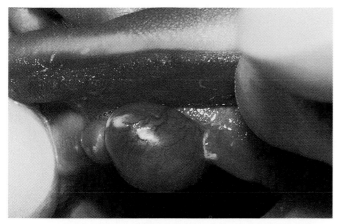

Fig. 11.1. Congenital epulis of the newborn: a pink nodule.

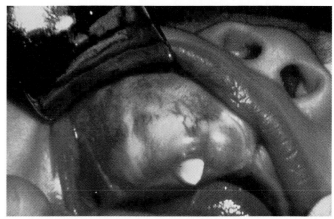

Fig. 11.2. Melanotic neuroectodermal tumor of infancy.

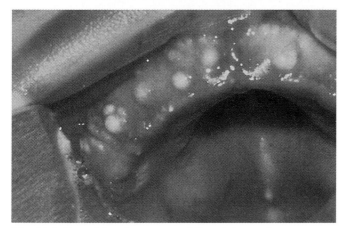

Fig. 11.3. Dental lamina cysts and Epstein's pearl.

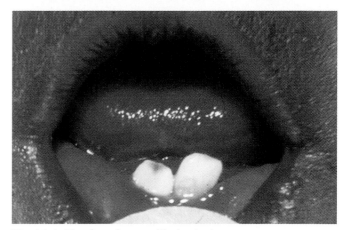

Fig. 11.4. Natal teeth: mandibular incisors.

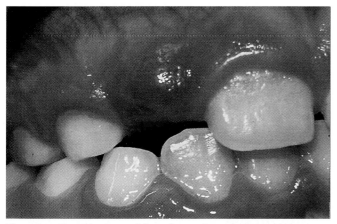

Fig. 11.5. Eruption cyst: blue, dome-shaped cyst nodule.

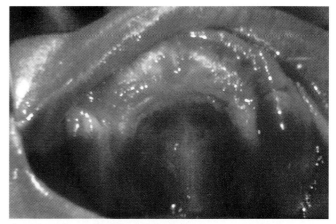

Fig. 11.6. Congenital lymphangioma.

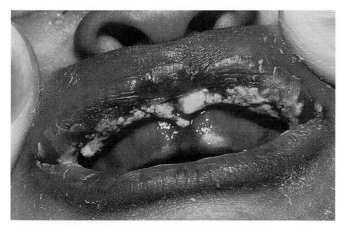

Fig. 11.7. Thrush caused by *Candida albicans*.

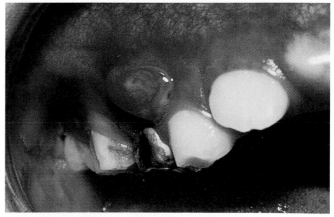

Fig. 11.8. Parulis: nonvital primary first molar.

Dental Anomalies

Alterations in Tooth Morphology

Microdontia (Figs. 12.1 and 12.2) Microdontia refers to teeth that are considerably smaller than normal. The condition is usually seen bilaterally and is often a familial trait. It may occur as an isolated finding, a relative condition, or in a generalized pattern. The most common form occurs as an isolated finding involving one permanent tooth, usually the permanent maxillary lateral incisor. The term "peg lateral" is often used to describe this variant because the tooth is cone-shaped or peg-shaped. Third molars are the second most frequently affected teeth. When microdontia occurs in a generalized pattern it may be relative to the size of the jaws. That is to say, the teeth are normal in size but the jaws are larger than normal. True generalized microdontia is rare and occurs when the jaws are normal in size and the actual tooth size is small. Generalized microdontia may be associated with pituitary dwarfism. Cancer treatments such as chemotherapy and radiation therapy during tooth development are also causative. True microdonts should be distinguished from retained primary teeth.

Macrodontia (Fig. 12.3) Macrodontia is the opposite of microdontia and refers to an abnormal increase in tooth size. This condition may affect one, several, or rarely all teeth. It is usually a relative phenomenon. It is often seen in incisors and mandibular third molars and in a developmental condition known as hemihypertyrophy in which the affected side including the teeth is larger than the unaffected side. Some single or even paired enlarged teeth are affected by fusion or gemination and may be referred to clinically as macrodonts until a more specific condition is discovered with the radiographs. True generalized macrodontia is rare and may be seen in pituitary gigantism.

Dens Invaginatus (Dens in Dente) (Fig. 12.4) Dens in dente is a common developmental anomaly seen in 1% of the population. It is so named because radiographically it resembles a "tooth within a tooth." The enamel and usually dentin of the crown grow inward (invaginate) into the coronal pulp chamber at the site of a lingual pit and extend in an apical direction. The condition is usually bilateral and may be relatively mild or severe with several invaginations in one tooth. The maxillary lateral incisors are the most frequently affected followed by the maxillary central incisors, mesiodens, cuspids, mandibular lateral incisors, and rarely a posterior tooth. The associated lingual pit is more prone to caries leading to early pulpitis and periapical inflammation. These pits require the prophylactic placement of sealants. Radiographically tear drop or bulb-shaped layers of enamel and dentin and sometimes pulp present in the pulp chamber of the crown. The presence of caries may not be evident; however, a periapical radiolucency alerts the practitioner to the loss of tooth vitality and the need for root canal therapy.

Accessory Cusp: Cusp of Carabelli (see Figs. 45.4 and 59.6) The cusp of Carabelli is an extra cusp located about halfway down the palatal aspect of the mesial palatal cusp of maxillary molars, usually the first permanent molar; primary molars may rarely be affected. It is usually bilateral. It is common in Caucasians and rare in Asians. There is often an associated groove between the cusp of Carabelli and the lingual surface of the tooth. This groove is prone to the development of stain and caries in susceptible individuals. When oral hygiene is fair and the diet is high in sugar, sealants are recommended.

Accessory Cusp: Dens Evaginatus (Leong's Tubercle) (Fig. 12.5) Dens evaginatus is less common than dens invaginatus and is usually classified as an accessory cusp. It consists of a small dome-shaped excrescence emanating from either the central groove of the occlusal surface or the lingual ridge of a buccal cusp, or rarely the lingual incline of the buccal cusp of a permanent posterior tooth. The condition occurs almost exclusively in mandibular premolars. It is especially common in persons of Asian decent. It is a feature of the shovel-shaped incisor syndrome common in Native Americans (see Fig. 14.8). The evaginated tubercle consists of enamel, dentin, and a prominent pulp chamber. Pathologic pulp exposure may occur with attrition whereas iatrogenic pulp exposure may occur during tooth preparation.

Accessory Cusp: Protostylid (Fig. 12.6) The protostylid is an accessory cusp on the buccal surface of a tooth. When canines are affected the term "premolarization" is used to describe the appearance; "molarization" is used for affected premolars; and on molars the accessory cusp is sometimes termed a "paramolar cusp." This should be distinguished from the term "paramolar" that is used to describe a small supernumerary tooth that develops lingual or buccal to a molar.

Accessory Cusp: Talon Cusp (Figs. 12.7 and 12.8) The talon cusp is a markedly enlarged lingual cingulum of a maxillary incisor tooth. Its name originates from the resemblance to an "eagle's talon." The talon cusp can interfere with occlusion, and a deep developmental groove may be present at the junction with the lingual surface of the tooth in which case caries can develop. Accordingly, the fissure should be prophylactically treated with a sealant. This condition may be an incidental finding or may be seen in association with the Rubenstein-Taybi syndrome characterized by mental retardation, broad thumbs and great toes, characteristic facial features, delayed or incomplete descent of the testes, and bone age below the 50th percentile.

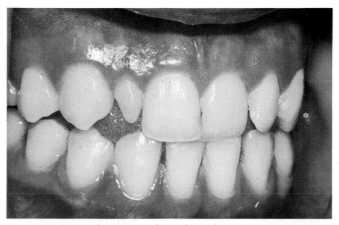

Fig. 12.1. **Microdontia:** peg lateral incisor.

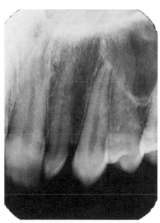

Fig. 12.2. **Microdontia:** radiograph of peg lateral incisor.

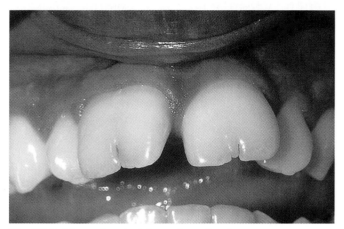

Fig. 12.3. **Macrodontia:** bilateral gemination.

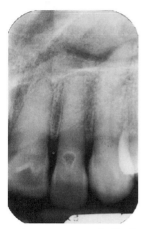

Fig. 12.4. **Dens invaginatus:** tear or bulb-shaped.

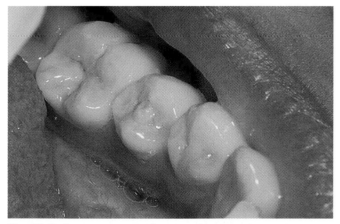

Fig. 12.5. **Accessory cusp:** dens evaginatus.

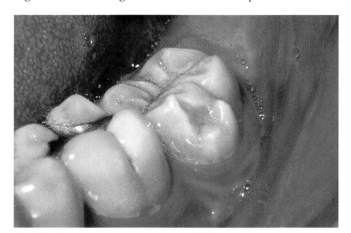

Fig. 12.6. **Accessory cusp:** protostylid.

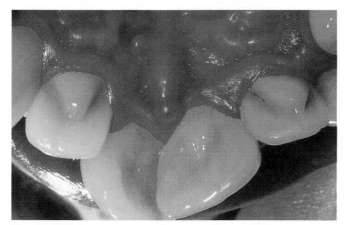

Fig. 12.7. **Accessory cusp:** talon cusps.*

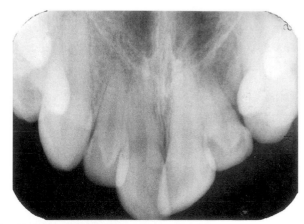

Fig. 12.8. **Accessory cusp:** talon cusps.*

Alterations in Tooth Morphology

Introduction (Fig. 13.1) The differences between gemination, twinning, fusion, and concrescence are explained on this page. Figure 13.1 illustrates the essential differences among these similar conditions. It is important to note that sometimes gemination and fusion are clinically indistinguishable as can be seen in the variety of presentations illustrated. Serial radiographs may be necessary to distinguish these conditions from supernumerary teeth.

Fusion (Figs. 13.3 and 13.5) In fusion two separate tooth buds attempt to join. The fused portion usually consists of dentin and, rarely, enamel. Fusionlike gemination is seen in less than 1% of the population and may be familial. The primary teeth are affected about 5 times more frequently than the permanent teeth. Bilateral presentations are about 10 times less common than unilateral examples. The incisors are the most commonly involved teeth. One distinguishing feature is the number of teeth; there will be an apparent missing tooth as two teeth have fused into one. An exception occurs when a tooth from the normal complement fuses with an adjacent supernumerary tooth creating the appearance of gemination. Fused teeth often resemble geminated teeth with a notch at the incisal edge and a groove along the labial or lingual surface. Radiographically, fused teeth are said to be more likely to have two pulp chambers and root canal spaces. However, variations much like gemination occur depending on the degree of fusion present. Fusion of primary teeth is often followed by hypodontia of the succeeding permanent teeth.

Gemination (Figs. 13.2, 13.4, and 13.5) In gemination a single tooth bud attempts to divide into two teeth; however the division is incomplete. It is seen in less than 1% of the population and may be familial. Involvement of primary teeth is about 5 times more common than the permanent teeth. The most commonly involved teeth are the primary mandibular incisors and the permanent maxillary incisors. Bilateral gemination is rare. Clinically, the most difficult problem is to distinguish gemination and fusion. Because gemination involves a single tooth bud, the patient will have a normal complement of teeth; however, one tooth will appear to be enlarged (macrodont). The crown may be normal in appearance, or it may have a notch at the incisal edge or a groove on the labial or lingual surface. Radiographically, a geminated tooth is said to have a single enlarged pulp chamber and an associated enlarged root. However, other variations are possible, as seen in Figure 13.2.

Twinning (Figs. 13.6 and 16.2) Twinning is the complete division of a single tooth bud. The condition is considered very rare. The divided teeth are seen as completely separate with no connection to each other except each tends to be a mirror image of the other. They are often smaller than usual and could thus be described as microdonts. When the teeth are counted, an extra tooth is present and there may be crowding of the remaining teeth. To add to the confusion, this condition is difficult if not impossible to distinguish from the circumstance in which there is a microdont such as a peg lateral and a microdontic supernumerary incisor, a situation involving two separate tooth buds. In the clinical example illustrated in Figure 16.2, it would be difficult to know whether the supernumerary lateral incisor is the result of twinning of a single tooth bud or whether it developed from an extra tooth bud that erupted.

Concrescence (Fig. 13.7) Concrescence is the union between two teeth by cementum alone after the crown has formed. This condition is thought to be more environmental than developmental. That is to say, it is caused by crowding during tooth development or trauma in which the interdental alveolar bone is resorbed thus allowing two adjacent teeth to approximate each other, a condition necessary for concrescence. It may occur between two normal teeth, between a normal tooth and a supernumerary tooth, or between two supernumeraries. **True concrescence** occurs before the completion of tooth development and is seen most commonly between the second and third molars in the maxilla owing to lack of space. **Acquired concrescence** occurs after the teeth have completed development but are joined by hypercementosis associated with chronic inflammation in the region. Concrescence is important in tooth extraction. For example, when concrescence affects a third and second molar, luxating the wisdom tooth can result in movement of the concrescenced second molar. It may or may not be possible to surgically separate such teeth.

Palato-Gingival Groove (Fig. 13.8) This condition is difficult to illustrate either clinically or radiographically because of its location but is included because of its importance. It occurs most commonly in persons of Chinese or East Indian descent although it can be detected in other populations such as Hispanics. It is located almost exclusively in maxillary incisors on the palatal root surface. The groove begins at the junction of the cingulum and one of the lateral marginal ridges and extends onto the root. This groove is a frequent site of an unsuspected periodontal defect because cementum fails to cover the groove and the periodontal ligament fails to attach to the root. The periodontal defect is detected with a periodontal probe as part of the routine periodontal examination; then the groove is found by probing the palatal aspect of the root adjacent to the defect. Thus, periodontal defects in this location should be further evaluated for the presence of the palato-gingival groove. When present the periodontal prognosis is diminished.

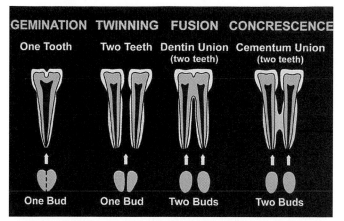

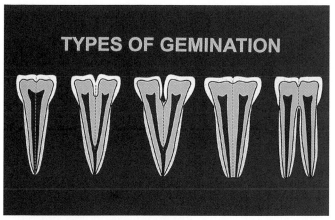

Fig. 13.1. Gemination, twinning, fusion, and concrescence.

Fig. 13.2. Variants of gemination.

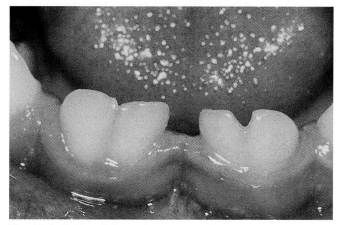

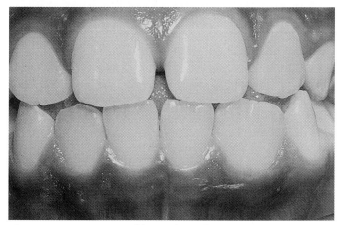

Fig. 13.3. Fusion: bilateral.

Fig. 13.4. Gemination of lower lateral incisor.

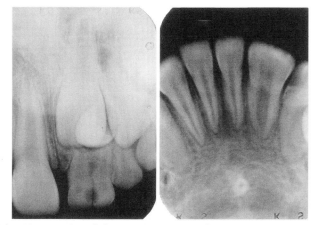

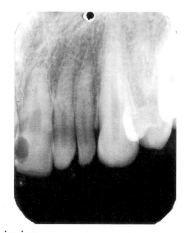

Fig. 13.5. Fusion (left), gemination (right).

Fig. 13.6. Twinning.

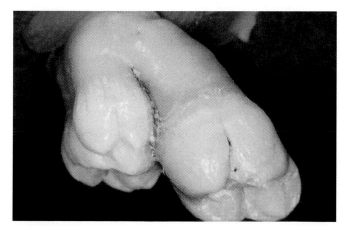

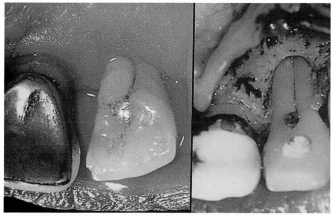

Fig. 13.7. Concrescence.

Fig. 13.8. Palato-gingival groove.

Alterations in Tooth Morphology

Supernumerary Roots (Fig. 14.1) These are developmental extra roots. Any tooth may be affected. The normal number of roots is one in incisors, canines, mandibular premolars, and maxillary second premolars; two in maxillary first premolars and mandibular molars, and three in maxillary molars. Supernumerary roots occur more frequently in permanent third molars, mandibular canines, and premolars. Mandibular molars are affected in 1% of Caucasians, 20% of persons of Mongolian extraction, and up to 44% among Aleuts. Radiographically, extra roots can be suspected when the root canal space abruptly diminishes in size and bifurcates into two separate canals. This entity is important in root canal therapy, extraction, prosthetics and orthodontics.

Ectopic Enamel: Enamel Pearl (Figs. 14.2 and 14.3) Enamel pearls are pearl-like deposits of enamel at the furcation of molars. They are more common in Mongoloids and Asians. On upper molars they locate on the mesial or distal surface whereas in mandibular molars they occur on the buccal or lingual surface. They are seven times more common in maxillary molars. Enamel pearls are 1 to 2 mm in size and rarely are multiple. There is no pulp in enamel pearls. Radiologically, false pearls occur in lower molars (see Figs. 5.6 and 5.7). They may be associated with chronic periodontal infection, and may hinder scaling and root planning and home care. In Figure 14.3, the pearl moves opposite to the x-ray beam location; thus, the pearl is on the palatal surface of the tooth.

Ectopic Enamel: Cervical Enamel Extensions (Fig. 14.4) Cervical enamel extensions occur at the mid-cervical line and consist of a V-shaped, smooth or roughened extension of the buccal enamel with the point of the V extending toward the furcation of a lower first molar. They are more common in persons of Mongoloid or Asian descent and are less frequently seen in Caucasians. Mandibular molars are involved more often than maxillary molars with the first, second, and third molars affected in descending order of frequency. The cervical extension is difficult to see in radiographs but may be detected with an explorer or periodontal probe, especially when there is a roughened projection on an otherwise smooth cementoenamel junction. Cervical enamel extensions are associated with chronic periodontal infection in furcal areas and an inflammatory cyst known as the **buccal bifurcation cyst** (Fig. 25.7). The cyst is a radiolucent area delineated by a thin radiopaque line superimposed on the buccal root surface of the tooth, sometimes extending to the distal. Cystic complications tend to develop in children and adolescents.

Dilaceration (Fig. 14.5) Dilaceration is a sharp bend in a root or crown of a tooth usually greater than 20 degrees. Interference with the path of eruption as a result of crowding, trauma, or orthodontic traction is the usual cause. Dilaceration is common in third molar and maxillary lateral incisor roots. The bend is often toward the distal or distobuccal distolingual surface. When the dilaceration is buccal or lingual, radiographically it appears as a bull's-eye with the center representing the pulp canal. Dilaceration is important in root canal therapy and exodontia.

Bulbous Root (Figs. 14.5 and 27.4) Bulbous root refers to a developmental variation in root morphology whereby the normal apical taper is replaced by localized widening of the root. This phenomenon is genetically determined rather than a response to local factors. The bulbous appearance is the result of increased amount of dentin—not cementum. Affected teeth are more difficult to extract.

Hypercementosis (Fig. 14.6) Hypercementosis is the excessive deposition of secondary cementum on the roots. It is associated with supraeruption, apical periodontal infection, occlusal trauma, and Paget's disease, toxic thyroid goiter, acromegaly, and pituitary gigantism. In a German study of 22,000 patients the incidence was 2%; any tooth may be involved; mandibular molars, second premolars, and first premolars were the most commonly affected in descending order of frequency; and mandibular teeth were affected twice as often as maxillary. Radiologically, the root outline is enlarged and delineated by the periodontal membrane space, with the dentinal root outline seen within the excess cementum. Hypercementosis occurs more often at the apical root region; it affects exodontia.

Taurodontism (Fig. 14.7) Taurodontism (bull-like with large body and short legs) is a condition affecting multirooted teeth whereby the pulp chamber extends apically, the roots are disproportionately short, and the cementoenamel junction lacks typical constriction. Primary and permanent dentitions are affected involving one or more teeth. The incidence ranges from 0.5% in Japanese to 2.5% in Caucasian and 5% in Israeli populations. It is most common in molars and premolars. Severity is classified as **hypotaurodont** (mild), **mesotaurodont** (moderate), and **hypertaurodont** (severe). It is seen in some cases of amelogenesis imperfecta as well as Down's, Mohr's, Klinefelter's, and trichodento-osseous syndromes. Taurodonts are treated as normal, although the bifurcation is deeper and the pulp space affects root canal therapy.

Shovel-Shaped Incisor Syndrome (Fig. 14.8) This syndrome is seen in Native Americans and Canadians, Eskimos, and Hispanics. The main features are prominent marginal (shovel-shaped) ridges, accentuated lingual pits in maxillary incisors and markedly shortened roots, especially the premolars; dens evaginatus in the lower premolars; and class VI caries at cusp tips. Patients are prone to class III and lingual pit caries in maxillary incisors.

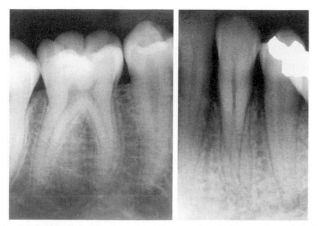

Fig. 14.1. **Supernumerary root:** first molar (left), canine (right).

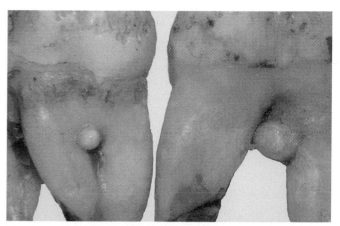

Fig. 14.2. **Ectopic enamel:** enamel pearl.

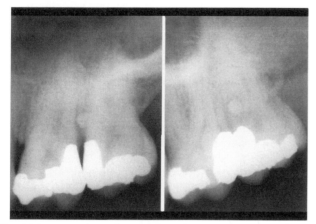

Fig. 14.3. **Enamel pearl:** palatal surface.

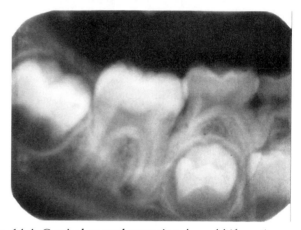

Fig. 14.4. **Cervical enamel extension:** buccal bifurcation cyst.

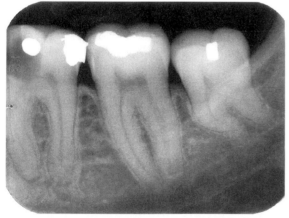

Fig. 14.5. **Dilaceration third molar; bulbous root first molar.**

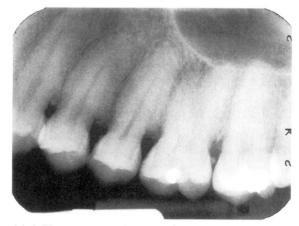

Fig. 14.6. **Hypercementosis:** premolars.

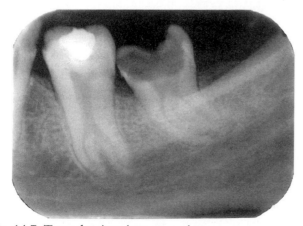

Fig. 14.7. **Taurodontism:** hypertaurodont.

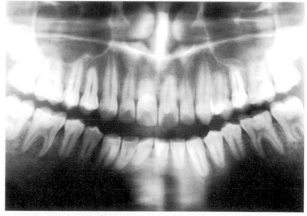

Fig. 14.8. **Shovel-shaped incisor syndrome.**

Alterations in Tooth Numbers: Hypodontia

Hypodontia (Figs. 15.1–15.3) Hypodontia is the congenital absence of one or a few teeth because of agenesis. Similar in meaning is the term **oligodontia**, which is used to refer to *numerous* congenitally missing teeth. The term **anodontia** is reserved for the rare condition in which no teeth develop. When missing teeth are discovered, the patient must be carefully questioned to determine the reason for hypodontia. If teeth are missing for reasons such as previous removal or lack of eruption, the use of the term hypodontia is inappropriate.

Hypodontia may involve either sex, any race, and the primary or permanent teeth; however, it is most common in the permanent dentition. About 5% of the population is affected, and a familial tendency is common. The most frequent congenitally missing teeth are the third molars, followed by the mandibular second premolars, the maxillary second premolars, and the maxillary lateral incisors. Visible space or overretained primary teeth are often the clinical signs of a missing tooth. Counting the teeth together with radiographs confirms the condition.

Many syndromes are associated with congenitally missing teeth, including Böök's syndrome, chondroectodermal dysplasia, ectodermal dysplasia, Hajdu-Cheney (acroosteolysis) syndrome, incontinentia pigmenti, otodental dysplasia, and Rieger's syndrome. Radiation therapy to the head and neck of infants or children and rubella (measles) during pregnancy have been implicated in the failure of teeth to develop.

Acquired Hypodontia (Partial and Complete Edentulism) (Fig. 15.4) Acquired hypodontia is the loss of teeth as a result of trauma or extractions. Sport and motor vehicle accidents are the source of most traumatic cases, whereas periodontal disease, caries, and space requirements for orthodontia contribute to dental extraction. Tooth loss produces excess space that may result in drifting, tipping, rotation, and supraeruption of adjacent or opposing teeth. In particular, splaying and spacing of the anterior teeth is an indirect result of loss of a posterior tooth because of distribution of the occlusal load onto the remaining anterior teeth. The single-rooted anterior teeth are less able to handle the load and tilt anteriorly when the periodontal support is poor. Acquired hypodontia can produce alterations in occlusion that require surgical, orthodontic, periodontic, and prosthodontic therapy to restore function and esthetics. When all the teeth have been extracted the condition is referred to as complete **edentulism**. In contrast, the term **anodontia** is used when all teeth are congenitally absent.

Ankylosis (Figs. 15.5 and 15.6) Ankylosis, a term meaning tooth fused to bone, is associated with hypodontia. It occurs when a primary molar fails to exfoliate, usually as a result of a missing permanent tooth. Ankylosis is associated with loss of the periodontal ligament and fusion of the cementum of the roots with the bone. The most commonly ankylosed tooth is the primary second molar; the permanent second premolar is the tooth that usually fails to develop and erupt. The ankylosed tooth is typically submerged several millimeters below the marginal ridges of adjacent teeth; the adjacent teeth are slightly or severely tipped toward the ankylosed tooth. The opposing maxillary tooth may be supraerupted. Percussion of the ankylosed tooth produces a dull sound. Ankylosed teeth often remain in the arch for many years but may exfoliate and create a small edentulous space. Exfoliation is often preceded by tooth mobility and pocket formation. Treatment can involve a crown to restore occlusion and marginal ridge height.

Ectodermal Dysplasia (Figs. 15.7 and 15.8) Ectodermal dysplasia is a group of more than 150 inherited diseases characterized by hypoplasia or aplasia of ectodermal structures, such as the hair, nails, skin, sebaceous glands, and teeth. In its best-known **hypohidrotic form**, it demonstrates an X-linked recessive inheritance. This means that the defective gene located on the X chromosome is carried by the female and manifested in the male. Less common forms of ectodermal dysplasia have been reported in females and can be caused by autosomal dominant and autosomal recessive transmission. One in 50,000 persons are affected. These patients have fine, smooth dry skin; hypodontia; hypotrichosis (sparse hair); and hypohidrosis (partial or complete absence of sweat glands). Other signs include a depressed bridge of the nose, pronounced supraorbital ridges, periorbital hyperpigmentation, ruddy complexion, thin sparse hair and eyebrows, protuberant lips, indistinct vermilion border, and varying degrees of xerostomia. Most patients have many missing teeth, and the teeth that are present often are conical and tapered. The canine is the most commonly present tooth, whereas incisors are generally missing. When present, molars show reduced coronal diameter. Anodontia sometimes occurs. Most patients do not perspire and consequently suffer from heat intolerance. Treatment involves several health care workers, genetic counseling, and the avoidance of heat. Partial dentures, full dentures, overdentures, and implants can be fabricated and placed for functional and esthetic purposes. Patients do well with prostheses even at a young age. However, new dentures must be reconstructed periodically as the jaws grow.

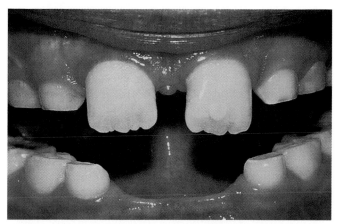

Fig. 15.1. **Hypodontia:** congenitally missing incisors.

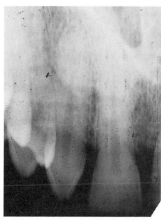

Fig. 15.2. **Hypodontia:** congenitally missing lateral incisor.*

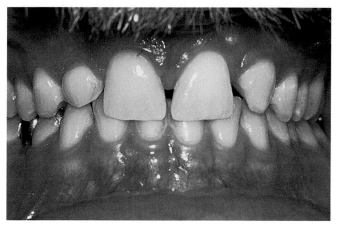

Fig. 15.3. **Hypodontia:** missing maxillary lateral incisor.*

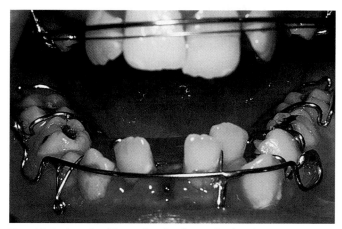

Fig. 15.4. **Acquired hypodontia:** for orthodontic space.

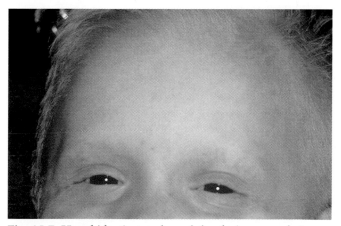

Fig. 15.5. **Ankylosis:** second primary molar.

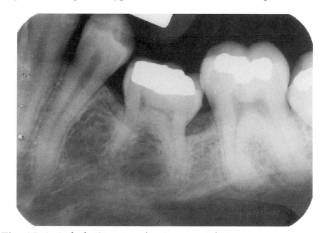

Fig. 15.6. **Ankylosis:** second primary molar.

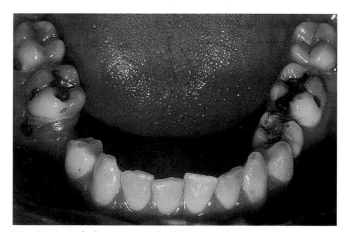

Fig. 15.7. **Hypohidrotic ectodermal dysplasia:** sparse hair.

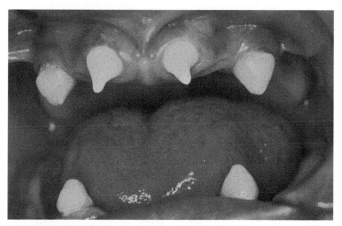

Fig. 15.8. **Hypohidrotic ectodermal dysplasia.**

Alterations in Tooth Numbers: Hyperdontia

Hyperdontia (Figs. 16.1–16.4) Hyperdontia is an extra or supernumerary deciduous or permanent tooth. The condition results from focal overproliferation of the developing dental lamina. It occurs more often in the maxilla than in the mandible (8:1), more often in males than females (2:1), more often in the permanent dentition than the primary dentition (1.0% of the population compared with 0.5%), and more often unilaterally than bilaterally. The most common supernumerary tooth is the mesiodens; this tooth is located, either erupted or impacted, near the midline between the maxillary central incisors. It may be of normal size and shape but is usually a small tooth with a short root and conically shaped crown that tapers toward the incisal surface.

The second most common supernumerary tooth is the maxillary fourth molar, which can be fully developed or microdontic in size. If the fourth molar is buccal or lingual to the erupted third molar, the term "paramolar" is used. When the fourth molar is positioned behind the third molar, the term "distomolar" is correct. Mandibular premolars are the third most common supernumerary tooth. They are usually malpositioned (ectopic eruption) because of late eruption into the arch.

Supernumerary teeth may fail to erupt or may erupt improperly. Those impacted in the jaw have the propensity to develop dentigerous cysts. Other supernumerary teeth have been reported to erupt into the gingiva, palate, tuberosity, nasal cavity, and orbital rim. Space limitations in the arch often force the supernumerary tooth to erupt buccally or lingually. Such teeth are often nonfunctional and may cause inflammation; food impaction; interference with tooth eruption; esthetic and masticatory problems. In general, supernumerary teeth should be extracted to permit proper growth, development, and occlusion.

One supernumerary tooth may represent an isolated occurrence, but it more commonly affects several family members. Familial hyperdontia is probably related to a common defective gene that has not yet been identified. The presence of several supernumerary teeth is commonly associated with specific syndromes such as cleidocranial dysplasia and Gardner's syndrome and less commonly with Hallermann-Streiff and orofaciodigital syndromes. These syndromes should be ruled out when supernumerary teeth are present.

Cleidocranial Dysplasia (Figs. 16.5 and 16.6) Cleidocranial dysplasia is an autosomal dominant disturbance linked to a defect in the *CBFA1* gene on chromosome 6. Most cases are inherited; however, up to 40% of cases result from spontaneous mutation. The syndrome affects women and men equally and is usually discovered during childhood or early adolescence.

The developmental disorder is characterized by defective ossification of the clavicles and cranium together with oral and sometimes long bone disturbances. Prominent features include delayed closure of the frontal, parietal, and occipital fontanelles of the skull; short stature; prominent frontal eminences with bossing; small paranasal sinuses; an underdeveloped maxilla with a high narrow palate; and relative prognathism of the mandible. The head appears large compared with the short body, the neck appears long, and the shoulders appear narrow and drooping. The clavicles may be absent or underdeveloped, permitting hypermobility of the shoulders whereby patients can bring their shoulders together in front of the chest.

The oral changes are dramatic, particularly as seen on the panoramic radiograph, which can lead to early diagnosis of the condition. The palate is usually high, arched, narrow, and sometimes clefted. There is prolonged retention of the primary dentition; numerous unerupted supernumerary teeth, especially in the premolar and molar areas; and delayed eruption of the permanent teeth. The permanent teeth are often short-rooted and lack cellular (secondary) cementum, which may be the cause of the defective eruption pattern. Treatment is complex, involving surgical exposure of unerupted teeth and orthodontic and possibly prosthodontic therapy to produce a functional and esthetic occlusion.

Gardner's Syndrome (Figs. 16.7 and 16.8) Gardner's syndrome is an autosomal dominant condition caused by a mutation in the adenomatous polyposis coli (*APC*) gene on chromosome 5. The syndrome has prominent orofacial features characterized by hyperdontia, impacted supernumerary teeth, odontomas, and jaw osteomas. In addition, patients have several epidermal cysts, many dermoid tumors, and many intestinal polyps. The osteomas occur most frequently in the craniofacial skeleton, especially in the mandible, mandibular angle, and paranasal sinuses; however, osteomas of the long bones are possible. Radiographs often demonstrate several supernumerary teeth, many odontomas, numerous round osteomas, and multiple diffuse enostoses that impart a cotton-wool appearance to the jaws. When superficial in the skin, these slow-growing tumors are clinically detectable as rock-hard nodules. The skin cysts (epidermoid, dermoid, or sebaceous) are smooth-surfaced lumps. Lipomas, fibromas, leiomyomas, or desmoid tumors may accompany this disorder.

The most serious consideration of Gardner's syndrome is the presence of multiple polyps that affect the colorectal mucosa. These intestinal polyps have an extremely high potential for malignant transformation, resulting in adenocarcinoma of the colon in nearly 100% of patients by the age of 40 years. Early recognition of the orofacial manifestations necessitates prompt referral to a gastroenterologist and genetic counseling. Close annual colorectal examination is required; prophylactic colectomy is usually recommended. Facial osteoma may be surgically removed for esthetic reasons.

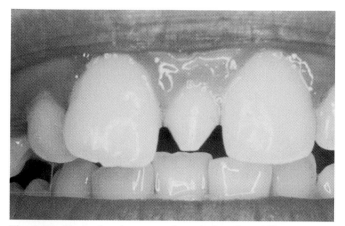

Fig. 16.1. Hyperdontia: erupted mesiodens in midline.

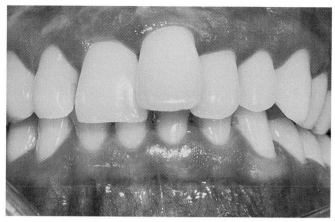

Fig. 16.2. Hyperdontia: extra maxillary lateral incisor.

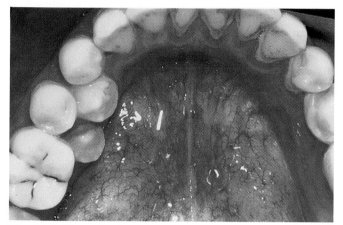

Fig. 16.3. Hyperdontia: supernumerary premolars.

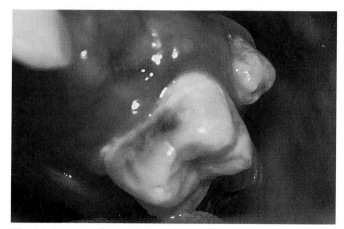

Fig. 16.4. Hyperdontia: buccal erupted paramolar.

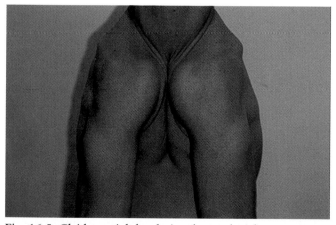

Fig. 16.5. Cleidocranial dysplasia: absent clavicles.

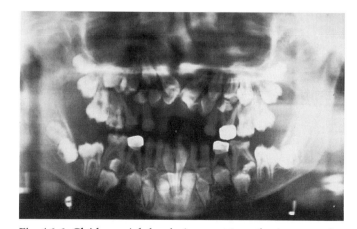

Fig. 16.6. Cleidocranial dysplasia: retention of primary teeth.

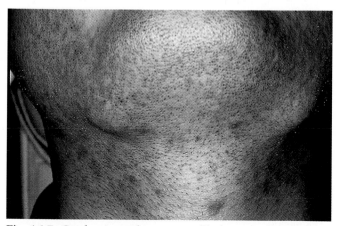

Fig. 16.7. Gardner's syndrome: mandibular osteomas.

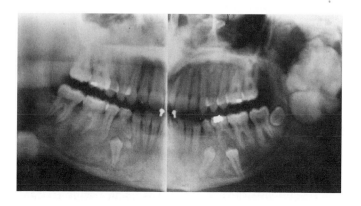

Fig. 16.8. Gardner's syndrome: osteomas, supernumerary teeth.

Alterations in Tooth Structure and Color

Enamel Hypoplasia Enamel hypoplasia is incomplete or defective formation of the organic enamel matrix of primary or permanent teeth. Two types exist: one caused by environmental factors and the other being a hereditary factors termed **amelogenesis imperfecta**.

Enamel Hypoplasia: Environmental Type (Figs. 17.1–17.3) Etiologic factors that can cause environmental enamel hypoplasia include nutritional deficiencies of vitamins A, C, and D; exanthematous infections that result in fever (i.e., measles, chickenpox, scarlet fever); congenital syphilis; hypocalcemia; birth injury; congenital Rh hemolytic disease; local infection or trauma; ingestion of chemicals (excessive fluoride); therapeutic radiation to the jaws at a young age; and idiopathic causes. The location of the enamel defect dates the disturbance as seen in Figure 17.1. Enamel formation starts incisally and proceeds cervically; thus, the defects in Figure 17.2 occurred around age 3 years.

Fever-related enamel hypoplasia occurs in all teeth undergoing mineralization during the fever. Defects vary from a horizontal white line, pits, or a groove on the crown to severe malformations owing to lack of enamel. Mildly affected areas appear whitish; more severe cases are darker yellow to brown (Fig. 17.2).

Congenital syphilis results in clinical abnormalities such as **Hutchinson's triad** consisting of interstitial keratitis of the cornea resulting in blurred vision; inner ear defects resulting in hearing deficiencies; and enamel hypoplasia of the central incisors called Hutchison's incisors. Affected incisors taper like a screwdriver with a notch on the incisal edge. Affected molars have supernumerary cusps and resemble mulberries (mulberry molars).

Turner's (tooth) environmental enamel hypoplasia (Fig. 17.3) is caused by inflammation or trauma to a primary tooth that overlies a developing permanent tooth. The insult damages the developing ameloblasts of the permanent enamel organ resulting in a malformed Turner's tooth. Turner's teeth are limited to the permanent dentition developing beneath primary teeth. The premolars are most often damaged by an abscessed primary molar (Fig. 11.8). This abscess is located at the furcation immediately over the developing permanent premolar crown causing occlusal hypoplastic enamel. When permanent maxillary incisors are affected, common causes include abscess or traumatized primary maxillary incisors (as in a fall) that intrude causing damage to the underlying developing central incisor. Affected teeth may have a white spot or a more severe enamel defect.

Fluorosis or mottled enamel (see Fig. 19.4) is caused by ingestion of excessive prescribed or natural fluoride in the drinking water during tooth development. The ideal concentration in the water is about 0.7 to 1 part per million (ppm). Levels greater than 1.5 ppm can induce fluorosis. Severity increases with increasing concentrations of fluoride. Fluorosis occurs symmetrically in both arches ranging from chalky white to pale yellow or dark brown spots. The most common and severely involved teeth are premolars followed by second molars, maxillary incisors, canines, and first molars. The mandibular incisors are least affected. Discoloration increases posteruption and can be removed by prophylaxis and bleaching.

Enamel Hypoplasia: Hereditary Type (Amelogenesis Imperfecta) (Figs. 17.4–17.8) Amelogenesis imperfecta is a group of inherited disorders characterized by a generalized defect in enamel formation of the primary or permanent dentition. The condition is divided into four main types (hypoplastic, hypomature, hypocalcified, and hypomaturation or hypoplasia with taurodontism) and 15 subtypes according to clinical, histologic, radiographic, and genetic features. A subset of the X-linked recessive forms is linked to mutations in the gene encoding amelogenin. Autosomal dominant forms have been linked to defects in enamelin and a gene on chromosome 4.

Hypoplastic amelogenesis imperfecta (type I), the most common form, is the result of deficient enamel matrix. The enamel that forms is well mineralized and does not chip. There are seven subtypes referred to alphabetically as type I A through G; four are autosomal dominant, two autosomal recessive, and one X-linked dominant. Clinically, the enamel demonstrates generalized or localized pitting or roughness.

Hypomaturation amelogenesis imperfecta (type II) has quantitatively normal amounts of enamel, but the matrix is immature so the enamel is soft and poorly mineralized; thus, a dental explorer under pressure will pit the enamel surface. In this type, the enamel appears chalky, rough, grooved, and discolored. Fracturing of the enamel is common. Some teeth resemble crown preparations, with excessive interdental spacing. There are four subtypes II A through D, with autosomal and X-linked recessive inheritance.

Hypocalcified amelogenesis imperfecta (type III) has normal enamel matrix, but little calcification occurs. There are two subtypes III A (autosomal dominant) and III B (autosomal recessive). Developing and erupting teeth are normal in shape; radiographically the enamel has a density similar to dentin. On eruption, the enamel is honey-brownish. Soon after eruption severe enamel chipping occurs, leaving a roughened, brown dentinal surface with some enamel remaining, especially at the gingival margin. An anterior open bite is often present as a result of loss of posterior vertical dimension.

Hypomaturation or hypoplastic amelogenesis imperfecta with taurodontism (type IV) has predominantly hypomature or predominantly hypoplastic subtypes IV A and IV B. The teeth are yellowish with opaque mottling, cervical pitting, and attrition, and exhibit taurodontism. Both subtypes are seen in the trichodento-osseous syndrome (brittle nails and sclerotic bone).

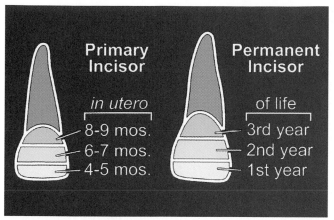

Fig. 17.1. Enamel formation in teeth.

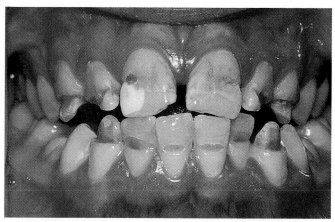

Fig. 17.2. Enamel hypoplasia: white and brown defects.

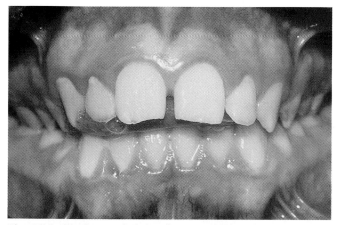

Fig. 17.3. Turner's teeth: maxillary first premolars.

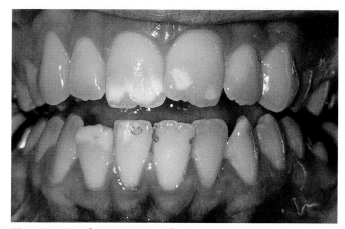

Fig. 17.4. Amelogenesis imperfecta type II-C: snow capped.

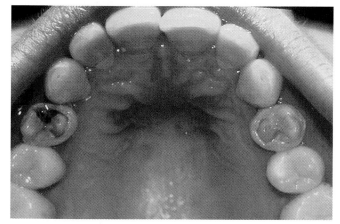

Fig. 17.5. Amelogenesis imperfecta, type I-D.

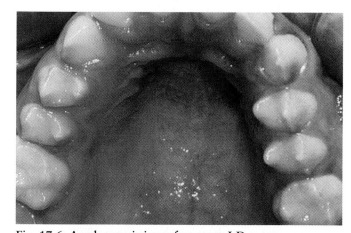

Fig. 17.6. Amelogenesis imperfecta type I-D.

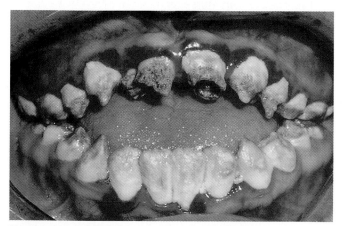

Fig. 17.7. Amelogenesis imperfecta type III-B.*

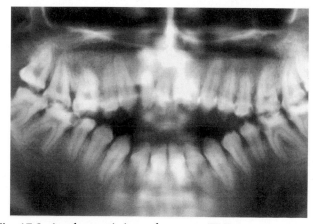

Fig. 17.8. Amelogenesis imperfecta type III-B.*

Alterations in Tooth Structure and Color

Dentinogenesis Imperfecta (Figs. 18.1–18.3)

Dentinogenesis imperfecta, a hereditary disorder, involves abnormal dentin development of the primary and permanent teeth. It occurs in about 1 in 8,000 newborns. Three types have been classified according to systemic involvement, clinical features, and histologic findings: Shields type I, Shields type II (hereditary opalescent dentin), and Shields type III.

Shields type I is a manifestation of osteogenesis imperfecta, a systemic condition involving bone fragility, blue sclerae, joint laxity, and hearing impairment. It is caused by a defect in (type I collagen alpha 1 gene) collagen formation. **Shields type II** appears to result from a gene defect on chromosome 4 that regulates dentin phosphoprotein production. It has the same dentinal features as type I but has no osteogenic component. **Shields type III**, also known as **Brandywine isolate**, occurs in isolated triracial groups originally from southern Maryland. Its genetic defect maps to chromosome 4 in a region that overlaps the type II critical region. Teeth affected by type III are opalescent (as in types I and II) but have a shell-like appearance.

Dentinogenesis imperfecta affects the primary teeth more severely than permanent teeth. Affected teeth look clinically normal when they first erupt but shortly thereafter become discolored, amber to gray-brown or opalescent. Incisal and occlusal surfaces chip and flake away, resulting in fissuring and significant attrition. Radiographs show bulbous crowns, exaggerated cervical constrictions, short tapered roots, and progressive obliteration of the root canal. Affected teeth are more susceptible to root fractures.

Dentin Dysplasia (Figs. 18.4–18.7)

Dentin dysplasia is a hereditary disorder of dentin characterized by alterations in pulp configuration, pulp stones, shortened roots, and idiopathic periapical radiolucencies. There are two types: type 1 radicular dentin dysplasia and type 2 coronal dentin dysplasia. Both are inherited in an autosomal dominant pattern. The distinction between types 1 and 2 is based on radiographic and histopathologic findings. Histologically the crowns are normal; however, the roots have central whorls of dentin with normal dentin at the edges resembling a "stream flowing around boulders."

Type 1 or radicular dentin dysplasia affects the primary and permanent dentitions. Affected teeth appear normal in size, consistency, and shape but may display a slight amber translucency. Although the eruption pattern is normal, delayed eruption sometimes occurs. The teeth may be malaligned, exhibit mild to severe mobility, and be exfoliated with minor trauma owing to extremely short roots. O'Carroll's classification describes the degree to which teeth are affected (Fig. 18.4). Dentin dysplasia type 1 is divided into four subgroups depending on the degree of root shortening. The earlier the condition occurs during tooth development, the more severe are the pulpal obliteration and root stunting. In type 1a the roots are almost nonexistent (Fig. 18.5A). In types 1b and 1c there is progressively more root formation; the pulp chambers are nearly obliterated and exhibit one or several thin horizontal radiolucent lines (Fig. 18.4). In type 1d root length is normal; however, the presence of large pulp stones within the root canal spaces is a prominent feature (Fig. 18.5B). The development of spontaneous periapical radiolucencies mainly affects types 1a, 1b, and 1c. They are inflammatory and may develop from ingress of bacteria from caries through microscopic threads of pulpal remnants or from a periodontal defect near the apical pulp whereby shortened roots, tooth mobility, and proximity of the apical pulp to periodontal inflammation may play a role.

Type 2 or coronal dentin dysplasia affects the primary and permanent teeth although the involvement of each dentition is different histologically, clinically, and radiographically. Histologically and clinically, the primary teeth demonstrate changes similar to dentinogenesis imperfecta; thus, they have an amber, translucent appearance. Radiographically, the crowns are bulbous, the roots are thin and tapered, and there is early obliteration of the pulp spaces, exactly as in dentinogenesis imperfecta. Histologically, the permanent teeth demonstrate interglobular dentin in the crown with stones in the pulp chamber and abnormal radicular dentin with no dentinal tubules. Although the permanent teeth are usually normal in coloration but bigger in size, our patient (Fig. 18.7) demonstrates a slight amber opalescent hue resembling dentinogenesis imperfecta, especially in the mandibular teeth, and the maxillary central incisors seem a little enlarged. The patient's radiograph (Fig. 18.6) is typical with the altered pulp chamber shape and pulp stones and nontapering thin root canal spaces resembling a thistle tube (Fig. 18.4). Tooth loss is less likely as there is no tendency for the formation of so-called spontaneous idiopathic inflammatory periapical lesions.

Regional Odontodysplasia (Ghost Teeth) (Fig. 18.8)

Regional odontodysplasia is a rare developmental anomaly characterized by defective (thinned) enamel and dentin formation and calcifications within the pulp and dental follicle. Although most cases occur idiopathically, some are associated with syndromes and vascular or growth abnormalities. Microscopically, the dentin is interglobular and diminished in amount, the enamel is abnormal, and pulp stones are present. Clinically, ghost teeth are often carious and painful, and are usually extracted. Occasionally they remain impacted. Affected teeth have reduced radiographic density producing a ghostlike appearance. The normal demarcation between enamel and dentin is absent, the pulp chambers appear abnormally large, and root formation is minimal. One or several adjacent teeth can be affected, thus the term regional. Figure 18.8 is typical and from a patient with focal dermal hypoplasia (Goltz-Gorlin syndrome).

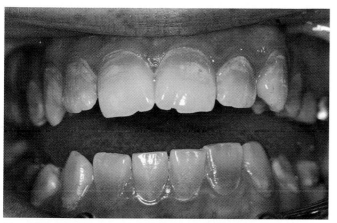

Fig. 18.1. Dentinogenesis imperfecta Shields type I.

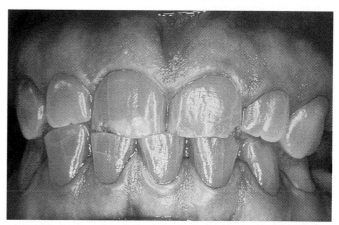

Fig. 18.2. Dentinogenesis imperfecta Shields type II.

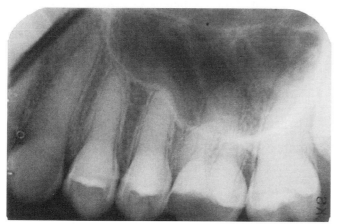

Fig. 18.3. Dentinogenesis imperfecta: radiographic features.

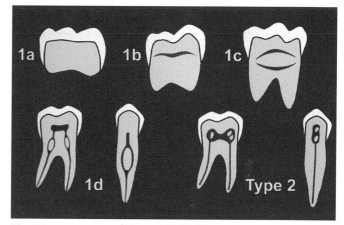

Fig. 18.4. Features of dentin dysplasia types 1 and 2.

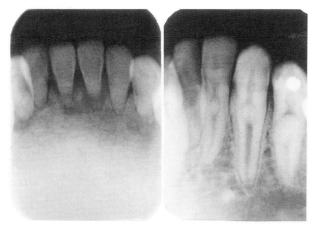

Fig. 18.5. Dentin dysplasia types 1a (left A) and 1d (right B).

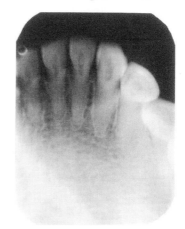

Fig. 18.6. Dentin dysplasia type 2: radiographic features.*

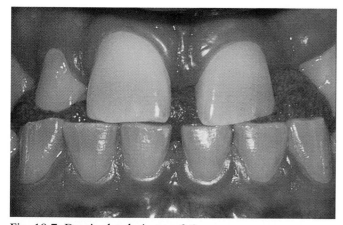

Fig. 18.7. Dentin dysplasia type 2.*

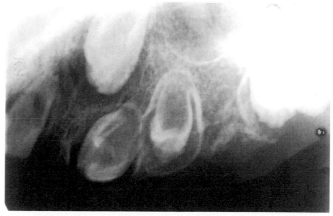

Fig. 18.8. Regional odontodysplasia (ghost teeth).

Alterations in Tooth Color

Intrinsic Staining (Figs. 19.1–19.4) A change in tooth color from the usual whitish appearance indicates a genetic or acquired abnormality. Genetic processes that alter tooth color include amelogenesis and dentinogenesis imperfecta and dentin dysplasia. Acquired alterations in tooth color result from intrinsic or extrinsic processes. Intrinsically stained teeth are caused by loss of tooth vitality, intake of drugs (such as tetracycline) and chemicals (such as excess fluoride), and certain disease states (hepatitis, biliary disease, erythroblastosis fetalis, and porphyria) that occur during periods of tooth development. Extrinsic staining results from adherence of dark substances to the external tooth surface.

Nonvital Teeth (Figs. 19.1 and 19.2) A nonvital tooth can be discolored (yellow-brown to gray-purple) because of loss of pulpal fluids and the darkening of dentin. These teeth often have concurrent signs of caries, restorations, fractured incisal edges, or vertical fracture lines. A large amalgam restoration may contribute to the gray-blue hue seen. Nonvital teeth also darken from the extravasation of pulpal blood into the dentin as the result of trauma. This situation usually produces a pink to purple tooth in which the neck of the crown is more discolored than the incisal edge. A pink, discolored nonvital tooth has been called the **"pink tooth of Mummery."** Lepromatous leprosy has also been reported to cause rupture of pulpal blood vessels and pink teeth.

Tetracycline Staining (Fig. 19.3) The tetracyclines are a group of bacteriostatic antibiotics that inhibit protein synthesis of certain bacteria. The drug is used to treat skin and periodontal infections as well as chlamydial, certain rickettsial, and penicillin-resistant gonococcal infections. Embryos, infants, and children who receive tetracyclines are prone to develop varying degrees of permanent tooth discoloration. This is more likely to occur during long-term use and repeated short-term courses and is directly related to the quantity of drug absorbed during embryogenesis and tooth development. Presence of tetracycline in the bloodstream promotes deposition of the drug in the developing enamel and dentin of teeth and bones in the form of tetracycline–calcium orthophosphate. This complex causes teeth to become discolored when they erupt and are exposed to sunlight (i.e., ultraviolet light). The discoloration is generalized and bandlike if the drug was administered in courses; prolonged use produces a more homogeneous appearance. The discoloration appears light yellow with oxytetracycline (Terramycin); yellow with tetracycline (Achromycin); or green to dark gray with the synthetic tetracycline, minocycline. Chlortetracycline (Aureomycin), which is no longer available in oral form, was best known for its ability to produce gray-brown staining. Doxycycline and oxytetracycline appear to be the least discoloring. The diagnosis is confirmed by using an ultraviolet light, which makes the teeth fluoresce.

Adults receiving long-term tetracycline therapy have been reported to acquire tetracycline staining. Accordingly, alternative antibiotics should be selected in children younger than 8 years of age, and long-term tetracycline treatment should be avoided in adults if possible.

Fluorosis (Fig. 19.4) Fluoride is a caries-preventive chemical that has greatest benefit when used at the appropriate concentration. The optimal fluoride concentration in drinking water is between 0.7 and 1 ppm. At this level, fluoride is incorporated into the enamel matrix and adds hardness and caries resistance. At levels between 1.2 and 4 ppm there is a increased risk for mild to severe fluorosis, respectively. Fluorosis is a disturbance of the developing enamel that is caused by excess levels of fluoride in the blood and plasma. Blood levels are directly related to the level of fluoride ingested in water; excess levels can be acquired from drinking well water (endemic fluorosis) or from excessive treatment with and ingestion of fluoride. At elevated fluoride levels, ameloblasts are affected during the apposition of enamel and produce deficient organic matrix. At high levels, interference of the calcification process occurs. Mild fluorosis produces isolated, lusterless, whitish-opaque spots in enamel. These spots occurring near the incisal edge are called "snow-caps." Moderate fluorosis is characterized by more-generalized yellow to brown spots, whereas severe fluorosis has many symmetrically and bilaterally affected teeth with mottled and pitted enamel and brown-white spots. In severe form, crown morphology can be grossly altered.

Extrinsic Staining (Figs. 19.5–19.8) Extrinsic stains result from the adherence of colored material or bacteria to the enamel of teeth. Most extrinsic stains tend to localize in the gingival third of the tooth above the gingival collar, where bacteria accumulate and absorb stain. Chromogenic bacteria produce green to brown stains in this region; these stains result from the interaction of bacteria with ferric sulfide and iron in the saliva and gingival crevicular fluid. Colored fluids, such as coffee, tea, and chlorhexidine, and inhaled tobacco smoke can cause brown to black stains. These stains appear darkest in the gingival third of the tooth and develop from frequent oral contact and enhanced contact by bacterial absorption. Amalgam restorations that leak into dentin produce blue-gray to black stains. This is most often apparent in the facial aspect of maxillary premolars that have a large class II restoration or a central incisor that has a lingually placed amalgam restoration. Along the gingival margin, the stain should be distinguished from calculus and caries. Calculus adheres to the external surface of the tooth and appears greenish-black when subgingival or tan when supragingival. Like stains, caries can be dark; unlike stains, caries causes loss of tooth structure.

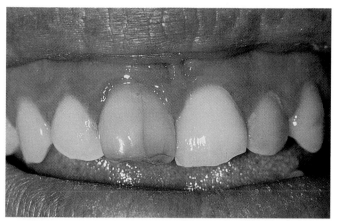

Fig. 19.1. **Intrinsic staining:** nonvital right central.

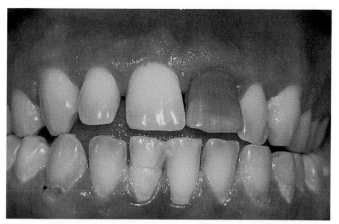

Fig. 19.2. **Intrinsic staining:** pink tooth of Mummery.

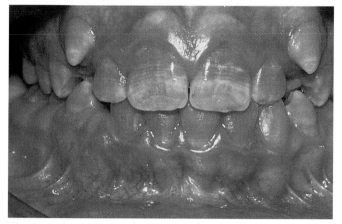

Fig. 19.3. **Intrinsic staining:** tetracycline staining.

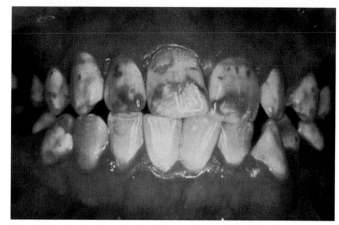

Fig. 19.4. **Intrinsic staining:** fluorosis.

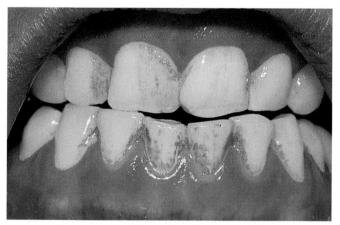

Fig. 19.5. **Extrinsic staining:** chlorhexidine staining.

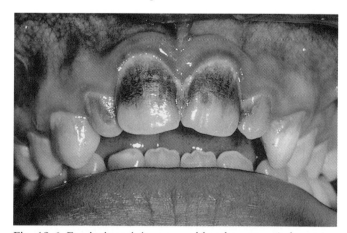

Fig. 19.6. **Extrinsic staining:** caused by chromogenic bacteria.

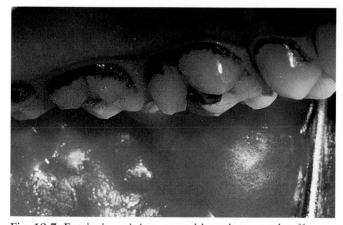

Fig. 19.7. **Extrinsic staining:** caused by tobacco and coffee.

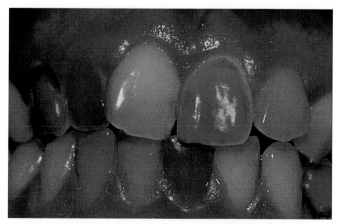

Fig. 19.8. **Extrinsic staining:** applied with holiday spirit.

Alterations in Tooth Position

Rotated Teeth (Fig. 20.1) A rotated tooth is one that is altered in orientation or position in the dental arch. Teeth may be rotated any amount, with severe cases reversing the buccal-lingual aspect of the tooth. Slightly rotated teeth are associated with crowding and malocclusion, such as rotated (tilted) maxillary laterals in the class II division 2 malocclusion.

Axial Tilting (Fig. 20.1) All teeth have a normal axial inclination, which when altered is a sign of crowding and malocclusion. For example, anterior teeth have a normal slightly outward axial inclination, which contributes to convex lip form and appropriate arch and facial profile. Teeth may be abnormally tilted inward or outward.

Ectopic Eruption (Fig. 20.1) In ectopic eruption one or more teeth erupt into an abnormal location outside of the normal dental arch, usually because of a lack of space. This can result in overlapping or a "double row of teeth" (Fig. 20.1). This frequently occurs when the primary teeth (especially mandibular incisors) are retained and the permanent successors erupt lingually. Similarly one or more supernumerary teeth may erupt adjacent to the normal teeth and compete for the location (Figures 16.1, 16.3, and 16.4). Another cause of ectopic eruption is a cyst or tumor that forces an adjacent developing tooth to erupt in an abnormal place. Some unusual ectopic eruption locations include teeth in the floor of the mouth, nose, sinus, and periocular region. Treatment is orthodontics or extraction.

Orthodontic Tooth Movement (Fig. 20.2) In orthodontic tooth movement abnormally positioned teeth are brought into normal position. Teeth also can be moved into abnormal positions. In Figure 20.2, the first premolar has been extracted, and the canine and lateral have been positioned distally. This method can result in excellent arrangement of the teeth, but the lower face may have a flattened appearance. In Figure 20.2, mild resorption of several root apices has resulted from the orthodontic forces. The thickened lamina dura and prominent periodontal membrane space are suggestive of orthodontic movement and possible hyperocclusion.

Transposition (Fig. 20.3) In transposition two teeth exchange places, each occupying the normal place of the other within the dental arch. This may occur idiopathically or it may be a sign that a barrier to the normal path of eruption may have existed. Such patients should be examined radiographically. In this case, the maxillary canine and lateral incisor are transposed. If the problem is esthetics, porcelain laminate veneers can remedy the situation.

Translocation (Fig. 20.4) Translocation occurs when a tooth erupts into an abnormal location but remains within the dental arch. In this example, the permanent lateral incisor was congenitally missing and the permanent canine did not encounter the root of the permanent lateral incisor to guide it in, so the canine erupted into the position of the lateral incisor and the primary canine was retained. The primary canine roots can resorb and the tooth exfoliate. Alternatively, the retained primary canine may last for many years.

Distal Drift (Fig. 20.5) Distal drift is distal movement of an erupted tooth or teeth within the dental arch as a result of a missing tooth. The normal forces of occlusion usually cause teeth adjacent to missing teeth to drift or tip mesially. Distal drift is more prone to occur in younger persons who have had a first molar extracted. In this case, the mandibular second premolar has drifted distally into the position of the absent first molar; the first premolar and canine have also drifted distally.

Migration (Fig. 20.6) Migration refers to the movement of an unerupted tooth into an abnormal position within the jaw. Migrated teeth may, but usually do not, erupt. Premolars are prone to migration, and some move into the ramus and other distant sites. In our example, a second premolar has migrated to the apical region of the first molar.

Partial Eruption (Fig. 20.6) Partial eruption occurs when a tooth erupts, but not fully into occlusion. This may be caused by an impediment such as insufficient space. To assess eruptive potential, root length is evaluated. For example, when root length is half complete (i.e., exceeds crown length), the tooth should be erupting through the gingiva. When the root is three-fourths formed, the tooth should be entering occlusion. When the apex has closed, eruption should be complete. Eruptive potential is strongest during the first half of root development and diminishes as the apical half of root formation develops. In Figure 20.6, the root length exceeds crown length. Thus, eruption is delayed. However, the apex is open, thus eruption is possible, but the premolar is impeded by the first molar. Interceptive orthodontic traction and tipping can alleviate this condition.

Supraeruption (Extrusion) (Figs. 20.7 and 20.8) In supraeruption one or more teeth erupt passively beyond the occlusal plane owing to the loss of opposing occlusion. Both maxillary and mandibular teeth can supraerupt. Periodontal disease may accelerate the problem, but its absence cannot prevent it. Supraeruption contributes to poor interproximal contact, food impaction, periodontal defects, and root caries. The extruded tooth (Fig. 20.8) can occlude with the opposite edentulous ridge, causing pain, an ulcer, or leukoplakia, and leave little space for a replacement tooth. Extruded teeth may need root canal therapy, crown lengthening, and a crown to reestablish a normal plane of occlusion before replacing its antagonist.

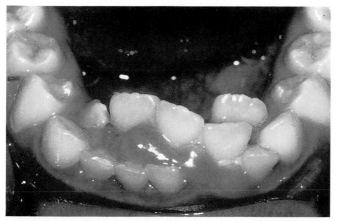

Fig. 20.1. Ectopic eruption, axial tilting, and rotated teeth.

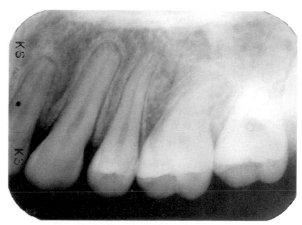

Fig. 20.2. Results of orthodontic tooth movement.

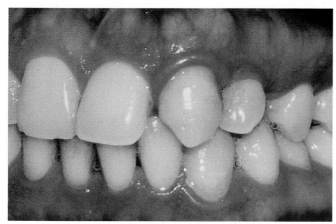

Fig. 20.3. Transposition of maxillary canine and lateral.

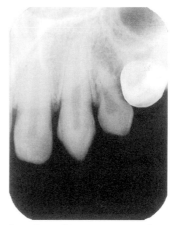

Fig. 20.4. Translocation of permanent canine.

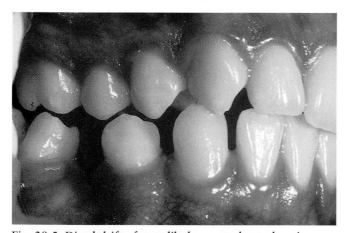

Fig. 20.5. Distal drift of mandibular premolar and canine.

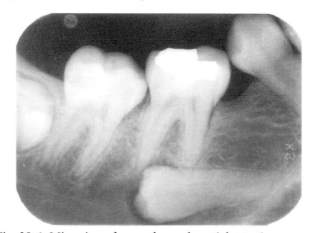

Fig. 20.6. Migration of premolar and partial eruption.

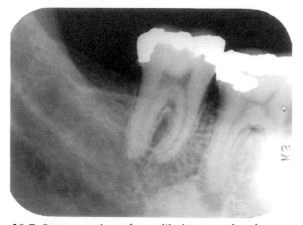

Fig. 20.7. Supraeruption of mandibular second molar.

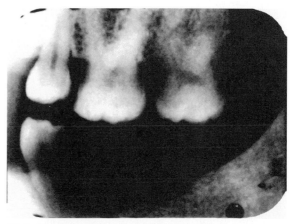

Fig. 20.8. Supraeruption of maxillary molars.

Acquired Defects of Teeth: Noncarious Loss of Tooth Structure

Attrition (Fig. 21.1) Attrition, considered a physiologic process, is the wearing down and loss of occlusal, incisal, and interproximal tooth structure because of chronic tooth-to-tooth frictional contact. Although the condition occurs most frequently in older adults, the primary teeth of young children may also be affected. Attrition is often a generalized condition accelerated by bruxism and abnormal use of selective teeth. Flattening of the incisal and occlusal surfaces, wear facets, and widened interproximal contact areas are common findings. Close examination reveals a smooth and highly polished tooth surface that is broad and angled, loss of the superior interproximal space, the outline of the dentin-enamel junction, and a receded pulp chamber. Pulp exposure is rare, however, because the deposition of secondary dentin and pulpal recession occur concurrently with attrition. Affected teeth are generally not sensitive to hot, cold, or the explorer tine. Restoration of worn teeth may be challenging because of acquired changes in vertical dimension.

Abrasion (Figs. 21.2–21.5) Abrasion is the pathologic loss of tooth structure caused by abnormal and repetitive mechanical wear. Various agents can cause abrasion, but the most common form is **toothbrush abrasion**. It results from abrasive toothpastes being brushed against the teeth too frequently, with improper technique, and with too much vigor. Toothbrush abrasion produces a rounded, saucer-shaped, or V-shaped notch in the cervical portion of the facial aspect of several adjacent teeth. The abraded area is usually shiny or polished and yellow (because of exposed dentin). The dentin is typically firm and noncarious, little plaque accumulation is present, and the marginal gingiva is not inflamed. Premolars opposite to the dominant hand are most often affected. Abraded teeth demonstrate dentinal sensitivity to hot, cold, or the explorer tine and are more susceptible to pulp exposure and tooth fracture.

Abrasive notching of the teeth also can be created by clasps of partial dentures, or by factitial injury: pins or nails habitually held with the teeth, or a pipe stem persistently clamped between the teeth. Inappropriate use of toothpicks and dental floss can also abrade the interproximal regions of teeth. Porcelain restorations placed in occlusion often result in abrasion of the incisal and occlusal surfaces of unrestored teeth in the opposite arch. When the porcelain teeth are maxillary incisors, the mandibular incisors are abraded at an upward and backward angle. Exposure to abrasive substances in the diet; chewing tobacco; powder cocaine; and long-term inhalation of sand, quartz, or silica can also promote abrasion. Abrasion caused by chewing tobacco frequently occurs on the side of the mouth in which the tobacco is most often placed. Cocaine addiction can cause localized abrasion of the maxillary anterior teeth when the drug is chronically rubbed against the gingiva and teeth.

Abrasion is a slow and chronic process, requiring many years before giving rise to signs. Restoration of normal tooth contour may be unsuccessful in the long term, if the patient does not alter the causative behavior.

Abfraction (Stress-Induced Cervical Lesions) (Fig. 21.4) Abfraction means "to break away" and is a term used in dentistry to define the pathologic loss of tooth structure at, or under, the cementoenamel junction caused by abnormal biomechanical loading. Abfraction appears as a sharp, wedge-shaped or V-shaped defect of enamel and dentin along the cervical region of the facial aspect of a tooth. Defects occur as a result of eccentric occlusal loading, which creates tensile and compressive forces, flexure and shearing stresses, and disruption of the chemical bond between enamel and dentin. Invariably, the periodontal support around these teeth is excellent, occlusal wear facets are present, and abrasive and erosive factors are nonidentifiable. Adults older than age 35 years are most often affected. One tooth in a quadrant is typically involved, particularly mandibular premolars. Abfraction may be associated with multiple lesions and with concurrent abrasion and attrition.

Erosion (Figs. 21.6–21.8) Erosion refers to the loss of tooth structure caused by such chemicals as dietary, gastric, or environmental acids that are placed in prolonged contact with the teeth. The condition is exacerbated by hyposalivation and drugs that produce xerostomia, because loss of saliva reduces the buffering capacity of the oral cavity. The most commonly affected tooth surfaces are the labial and buccal surfaces.

The pattern of tooth erosion often indicates the causative agent or a particular habit. For example, sucking on lemons (citric acid) produces characteristic changes of the facial surfaces of the maxillary incisors. Horizontal ridges are initially apparent, followed by smooth, cupped-out, yellowish depressions. Eventually the incisal edges thin and fracture. A similar erosive pattern may be seen in dedicated swimmers whose anterior teeth are chronically exposed to chlorinated swimming pools.

Erosion limited to the lingual surfaces of the maxillary teeth (**perimolysis**, also known as perimylolysis) indicates chronic regurgitation or vomiting caused by bulimia, anorexia, pregnancy, hiatal hernia, gastroesophageal reflux, or alcohol abuse. The occlusal margins of several existing amalgams are often raised above the eroded and adjacent enamel. Sensitivity of the exposed area is an early symptom. Excessive consumption of sweetened beverages and carbonic acid–containing beverages may accelerate the condition. Fluoride treatments for early erosions and restorations that cover exposed dentin for more-extensive lesions are the treatment of choice. Elimination of the causative habit or behavior modification is required for success. In cases of gastroesophageal reflux, the condition can be controlled by medications (antacids, H_2 histamine blockers, proton pump inhibitors). Patients should also be advised to rinse with sodium bicarbonate after vomiting or reflux into the mouth.

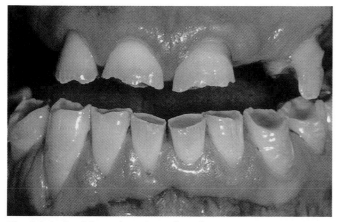

Fig. 21.1. Attrition: along incisal surfaces.

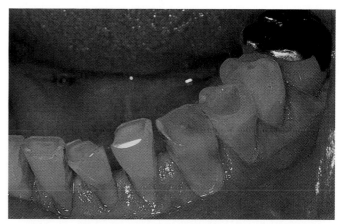

Fig. 21.2. Attrition: polished incisals, abrasion at cervical.

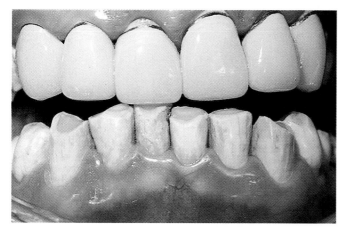

Fig. 21.3. Abrasion: worn by friction against porcelain.

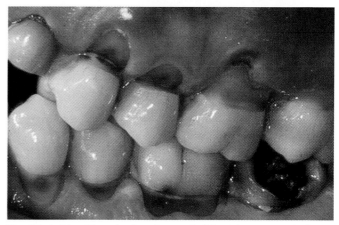

Fig. 21.4. Toothbrush abrasion and **abfraction** at cervical.

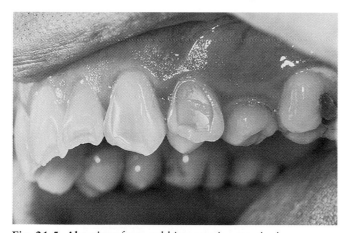

Fig. 21.5. Abrasion: from rubbing cocaine on gingiva.

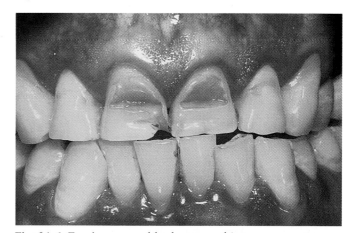

Fig. 21.6. Erosion: caused by lemon sucking.

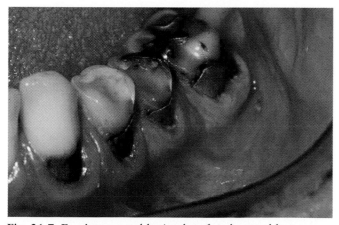

Fig. 21.7. Erosion: caused by intake of carbonated beverages.

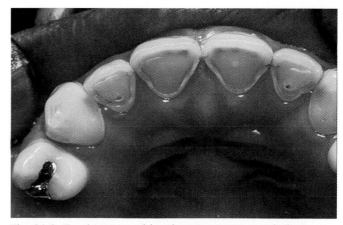

Fig. 21.8. Erosion: caused by chronic vomiting in bulimia.

Dental Caries

Dental Caries

Caries (Figs. 22.1–22.8) Dental caries, one of the most common bacterial infections affecting humans, is characterized by demineralization and destruction of the organic matrix of teeth that results from interaction of bacterial plaque, diet components, altered host responses, and time. Caries results when electrochemical changes produced by acid cause outflow of calcium and phosphate ions from the mineralized portion of the tooth. The primary pathogen, *Streptococcus mutans*, together with *Actinomyces viscosus*, *Lactobacillus* species, and *Streptococcus sanguis* are involved in tooth adherence and the production of lactic acid needed for enamel dissolution.

Caries begins as an enamel decalcification that appears as a chalky white spot, line, or fissure. The initial lesion is termed **incipient**. As the lesion matures, it causes destruction of enamel and lateral spread along the dentinoenamel junction, through the dentin, and eventually toward the pulp. The classic clinical features of a carious lesion are (1) color change (chalky white, brown, or black discoloration), (2) loss of hard tissue (cavitation), and (3) stickiness to the explorer tine. The color change is caused by decalcification of enamel, exposure of dentin, and demineralization and staining of dentin. Classic symptoms of caries are sensitivity to sweets, hot, and cold. These symptoms are generally absent with incipient lesions. Larger lesions permit ingress of fluids into exposed dentinal tubules. The hydrostatic changes are sensed by pulpal nerves that transmit signals to the trigeminal sensory complex, which results in the perception of pain.

There are two types of caries classified according to location: fissural and smooth surface. **Fissural caries** is the most common form. It occurs most often in deep fissures in the chewing surfaces of the posterior teeth. **Smooth surface caries** occurs at places that are protected from plaque removal, such as just below the interproximal contact, at the gingival margin, and along the root surface. Caries is subdivided into six classes according to anatomic location. Class I caries is fissural; the remaining five classes are smooth surface caries.

Management of caries is based on lesion size, location, esthetic requirement and the following risk factors: plaque score (*Streptococcus mutans* level); cariogenic diet; number of initial, prior, and active caries; number of restorations present; level of fluoride exposure and oral hygiene; patient compliance; number of exposed root surfaces; and salivary flow (systemic diseases and medications can influence salivary flow).

Class I Caries (Figs. 22.1 and 22.2) Class I caries is decay affecting the occlusal surface of a posterior tooth. It arises when bacteria invade a central pit, deep occlusal groove, or fissure, remain sheltered for months, and produce acid dissolution of enamel. Destruction of enamel and dentin permits the carious groove to enlarge, darken, and become soft. A small class I carious lesion is the size of a sharp-tip lead pencil and may exist beneath a stained fissure. Larger lesions can encompass the entire occlusal surface, leaving only a shell of facial or lingual enamel and a symptomatic tooth. Current recommendations are to detect these lesions by visual inspection, bitewing radiographs (for a radiolucent shadow in the dentin beneath the occlusal enamel), and minimal probing. Class I caries that are incipient or small are managed by remineralization with fluoride varnish application and sealants. Larger lesions require use of composite materials or amalgam.

Class II Caries (Figs. 22.3 and 22.4) Class II caries is decay that affects the interproximal surface of a posterior tooth. These lesions are often difficult to identify clinically and require an astute eye; a clean, dry tooth surface; and a bitewing radiograph. One feature that may help in the detection of class II caries is decalcification (chalkiness or translucency) along the marginal ridge that is caused by hollowing of the subjacent dentin. The caries can occasionally be seen from the lingual or buccal aspect of the interproximal contact. Class II caries is most easily recognized on bitewing radiographs. The carious lesion appears as a triangular radiolucency in the enamel just below the contact point; the base of the triangle parallels the external aspect of the tooth, and the tip of the triangle points inward toward the dentin. As the lesion reaches dentin, demineralization spreads along the dentinoenamel junction and progresses toward the pulp.

Remineralization procedures (i.e., fluoride varnish applied to demineralized areas) are used for smaller lesions limited to enamel. In moderate caries (radiographic evidence of enamel penetration vertically along the dentinoenamel junction without further penetration into the dentin), remineralization can be used if risk factors are minimal or reduced, and lesions are closely monitored. Custom-made fluoride trays and daily fluoride applications reduce the risk of caries progression. Moderate to large lesions are restored with posterior composites, amalgam, or castings.

Class III Caries (Figs. 22.5–22.8) Class III caries is decay affecting the interproximal surface of an anterior tooth. Like class II interproximal caries, class III caries begins just below the contact point. Invasion results in triangular destruction of enamel and lateral spread into dentin. Interproximal caries (classes II and III) are common in persons who seldom floss their teeth and have a frequent intake of sugar in beverages and candy. Class III caries is seen frequently in Asian and Native American persons who have prominent marginal ridges (shovel-shaped incisors). It can be diagnosed using transillumination. This technique demonstrates caries as dark regions within the enamel (or deeper) located below the interproximal contact point, even when evidence of caries is unclear radiographically (Figs. 22.5 and 22.6). Class III caries in the mandibular incisors indicates high caries risk behavior.

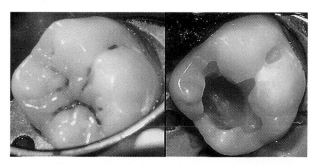

Fig. 22.1. Class I caries: before and after preparation.

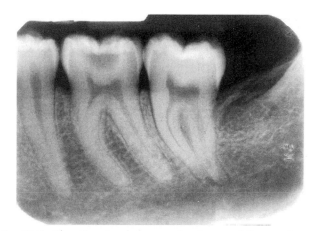

Fig. 22.2. Class I caries: below occlusal enamel first molar.

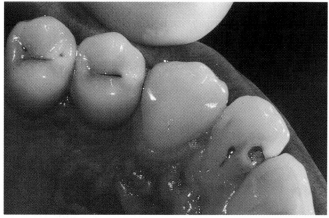

Fig. 22.3. Caries: Class II mesial premolars; **Class III** lateral.*

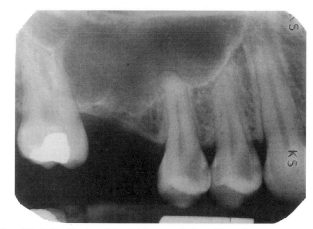

Fig. 22.4. Radiographic evidence of class II caries.*

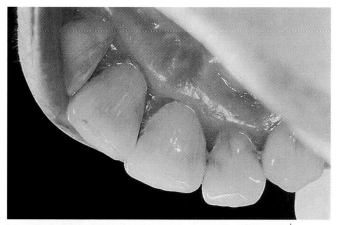

Fig. 22.5. Class III caries: between central and lateral.‡

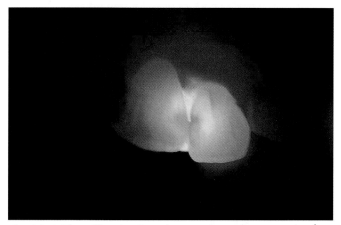

Fig. 22.6. Transillumination: demonstrates class III caries.‡

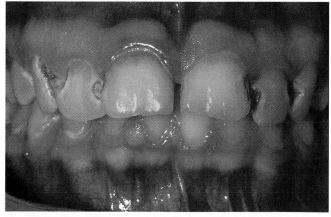

Fig. 22.7. Class III caries: centrals, laterals, and canines.

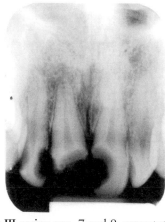

Fig. 22.8. Class III caries: nos. 7 and 9; amputation caries no. 8.

Dental Caries

Class IV Caries (Figs. 23.1 and 23.2) Class IV caries affects the incisal line angle of an anterior tooth. It usually results when class III caries remains untreated, allowing the lesion to progress and undermine the dentin that supports the incisal line angle. Subsequently, loss of the enamel at the line angle occurs when the undermined enamel is impacted by occlusion or trauma. Class IV carious lesions are restored with bonded composite resins providing excellent esthetics. Porcelain laminate veneers are also useful in select cases.

Class V Caries (Figs. 23.3 and 23.4) Class V caries is characterized by decay along the gingival margin of a posterior or anterior tooth. Early signs of class V caries are chalky, white decalcification lines traversing cervical tooth structure parallel to and just above the gingiva. Any plaque covering the lesion must be removed for adequate detection of the caries. With time, the lesions enlarge mesially and distally at a rate faster than gingival-incisal spread, thereby producing an oval defect. As class V caries reach interproximal regions, spread toward the contact point occurs and the lesion becomes L-shaped. Patients with class V caries usually consume large amounts of sugary carbonated drinks, sip on such drinks for several hours during the day, or produce low amounts of saliva. Radiographically, class V caries should be distinguished from cervical burnout and toothbrush abrasion. In Figure 23.4, a typical class V lesion is present on the first premolar; the second premolar has recurrent decay beneath the amalgam restoration, and toothbrush abrasion is evident by a tipped V–shaped radiolucent area. Smaller class V lesions can be treated with disking and fluoride varnish to remove either whitish or brownish stains without further treatment. Cavitated lesions require composite resins or amalgam. Esthetic situations can require the use of porcelain bonded-laminate veneers.

Class VI Caries (Fig. 23.5) Class VI caries is characterized by decay of the incisal edge or cusp tip. This type of caries is seldom seen, but is more common in persons who frequently chew sugary gums or consume sticky candy bars. Patients with low salivary flow are also predisposed to this type of caries. Class VI caries (along with the class III caries and class I lingual pit caries) is seen in the shovel-shaped incisor syndrome.

Root Caries (Fig. 23.6) Root caries, also known as cemental caries, radicular caries, and senile caries, is decay that occurs on exposed root surfaces. This form of decay is detected more often on posterior teeth in older patients. The elderly are more commonly affected because they have (1) increased prevalence of gingival recession; (2) increased prevalence of periodontal disease, altered interproximal contacts, and food impaction; and (3) increased prevalence of hyposalivation. Root caries starts at the cementoenamel junction. Although it often occurs on the interproximal surface below the contact point, it may be seen on any surface. Early on it appears as a shallow, ill-defined, softened and discolored area that tends to extend more circumferentially than in depth. Probing detects a soft rubbery consistency. As it progresses, the decay surrounds the root, leading to the crown fracturing off; this is called **amputation caries** (Fig. 22.8). Radiographically, root caries is seen in the interproximal areas below the cementoenamel junction, and although neither the contact point nor the enamel is involved, the caries may spread coronally under the enamel. Root caries often recurs when root surfaces remain exposed, salivary flow remains low, and oral hygiene does not improve. Frequent prophylaxis and home daily applications of fluoride are often needed.

Recurrent Caries (Secondary Caries, Redecay) (Figs. 23.7 and 23.8) Recurrent caries is defined as decay within the immediate vicinity of a restoration. It may be a sign of a high caries risk, poor oral hygiene, or a defective restoration. Recurrent caries begins at a failing margin of any restoration. It appears dark and is soft to probing. Radiographically, this caries presents in two diametrically opposite ways: first, the decay may be seen as a radiolucent area beneath a restoration with or without a visibly defective margin as seen in Figure 23.8 beneath the distal amalgam of the mandibular second premolar. Second, the decay may be seen as one or several flame-shaped or arrow-shaped radiopaque areas occurring uniquely beneath an amalgam-type restorative material, with the point of the arrow directed toward or encroaching on the pulp or pulp horn. In Figure 23.8, this phenomenon is seen beneath the mesial amalgam of the mandibular first molar. An associated radiolucent area is sometimes present as in this case. Spectroscopy studies have shown the radiopaque material represents softened dentin into which radiopaque zinc from the adjacent amalgam restoration has been leached. Replacing the restoration treats recurrent caries.

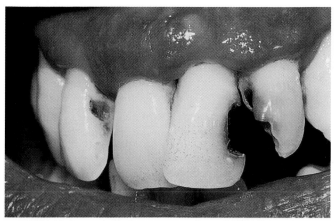

Fig. 23.1. Class IV caries: mesial of lateral incisor.

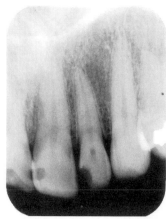

Fig. 23.2. Class IV caries: mesial of lateral; lingual caries.

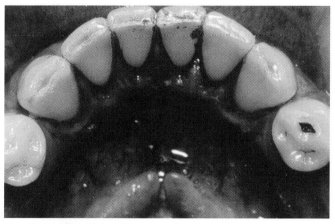

Fig. 23.3. Class V caries: maxillary anteriors.

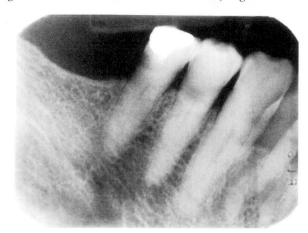

Fig. 23.4. Class V caries: first premolar.

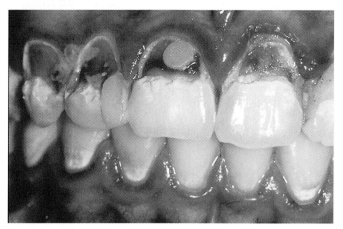

Fig. 23.5. Class VI caries: premolar cusp tip.

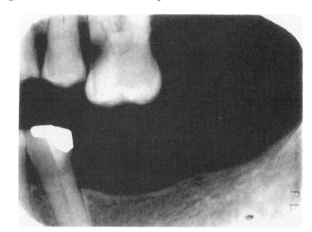

Fig. 23.6. Root caries: on extruded molar.

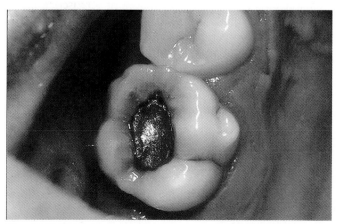

Fig. 23.7. Recurrent caries: evident around restoration.

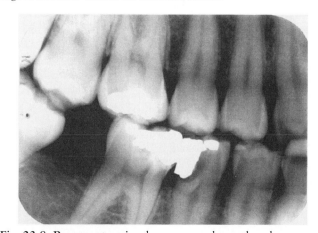

Fig. 23.8. Recurrent caries: lower premolar and molar.

Dental Caries and Sequelae

Progression of Caries (Figs. 24.1–24.8) The invasion of caries may be a slow or fast process and may involve the pulp before the patient is aware of the carious lesion. In most cases, it takes several years for caries to reach the pulp. Some caries are particularly aggressive or have a unique cause. These caries have received descriptive definitions. For example, **rampant caries** is a type of caries that develops at an extremely rapid pace in some children and young adults. **Radiation, or amputation, caries** is another form of caries that occurs and progresses rapidly in patients receiving radiotherapy who lack the protective action of saliva. This caries appears along the gingival margin of teeth and can weaken teeth so severely that the crown fractures. **Root caries** has an appearance similar to that of radiation caries but is not associated with a history of radiation therapy; rather, affected patients usually have a history of xerostomia or drug-induced xerostomia. Root caries progresses more slowly than radiation caries because xerostomia is less severe. **Nursing bottle caries** results from prolonged contact of primary teeth with sugar-containing liquids (e.g., in the baby bottle) in infants.

If caries is left untreated, the bacterial infection can progress through tooth dentin and produce pulpal inflammation. The initial stage of pulpal involvement, **reversible pulpitis**, is characterized by pulpal hyperemia and tooth sensitivity to hot and cold that dissipates when the temperature source is removed. Persistent pulpal inflammation produces irreversible changes, or **irreversible pulpitis**, in which the patient experiences spontaneous and persistent pain in the tooth after removal of the temperature source. Severe destruction of pulpal tissue from bacterial infection or interruption of the blood supply to the pulp produces a nonvital pulp and subsequent periapical changes (chronic periapical inflammation).

Prevention is the best way to reduce the incidence and progression of caries. Clinical examinations should be provided at least twice a year to minimize the sequelae of caries. Bitewing radiographs should be taken at 6-month intervals in children if clinical caries are detected or the patient has a high risk for caries. Adults at high risk should receive bitewing radiography annually. Composite resin sealants should be placed over deep fissures of posterior teeth in caries-susceptible children and adolescents. Remineralization products such as fluoride and certain sugarless gums are advocated to prevent caries. Pulp vitality should be tested when a carious lesion has invaded to, or beyond, 50% of the space between the dentinoenamel junction and pulp margin.

Pulp Polyp (Fig. 24.2) The pulp polyp is an inflammatory and hyperplastic response of a wide-open pulp chamber to a chronic bacterial infection. Extensively carious primary molars and 6-year molars of young children are most frequently affected. On clinical examination, the soft, red, nonpainful, pedunculated mass is seen projecting up from the pulp chamber beyond the broken-down occlusal surface of the tooth. Although the tooth is initially vital, the condition eventually erodes and results in nonvitality. Treatment is extraction or root canal therapy.

Periapical Inflammation (Apical Periodontitis) (Figs. 24.4–24.6) Periapical inflammation or apical periodontitis are clinical terms used to describe the radiographic changes and clinical findings associated with inflammation that involves the periodontal ligament at the periapex of a chronically inflamed tooth. The condition is most commonly associated with a pulpal degeneration (nonvital tooth) but may occur in vital teeth from occlusal trauma or constant and repetitive pressure placed on a tooth. Radiographs show a widening of the apical periodontal ligament space. The condition may be symptomatic or asymptomatic, acute or chronic. Chronic periapical inflammation has chronic inflammatory cells at the periapex and often shows greater periradicular destruction of alveolar bone than acute periapical inflammation. The chronic form may be symptomatic or asymptomatic. In contrast, acute periapical inflammation is painful. Both conditions cause the apical periodontal ligament to be sensitive to percussion.

In response to the degradation products of a nonvital pulp, the periapical tissue produces two usual reactions: either a periapical granuloma or periapical cyst. Histologically, the **periapical granuloma** is an accumulation of granulation tissue, lymphocytes, plasma cells, histiocytes, and polymorphonuclear leukocytes as an early periapical reaction. The **periapical cyst** arises from a preexisting periapical granuloma as the inflammation stimulates proliferation of periapical epithelial rests of Malassez. Both the periapical granuloma and periapical cyst originate from a nonvital tooth and both have a similar appearance radiographically. The distinction is made histologically. Regression follows root canal therapy in most cases.

Periapical Abscess (Figs. 24.7 and 24.8) A periapical abscess is the acute phase of an infection that spreads from a nonvital tooth through the alveolar bone into the adjacent soft tissue. The abscess is composed of polymorphonuclear leukocytes and necrotic debris. Clinical examination shows a red or reddish yellow, swelled nodule that is warm and fluctuant to the touch. The affected tooth is tender to percussion and responds abnormally or not at all to heat, cold, and electric pulp testing. Abscesses can be drained by opening into the pulp chamber or incising the soft tissue swelling. An alternate treatment is extraction, which provides an avenue for drainage. Antibiotics are used when the abscess is large and spreading, lymphadenopathy and fever are present, and drainage is not established. Penicillin VK is the antibiotic of choice. If the infection is unresponsive to penicillin, a bacterial culture and sensitivity should be obtained. Antibiotics are generally not needed if the affected tooth is extracted and adequate drainage is established.

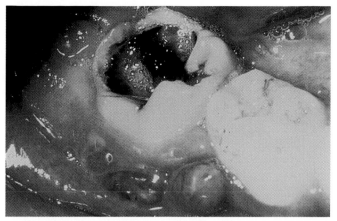

Fig. 24.1. **Extensive caries:** mandibular molar with parulis.

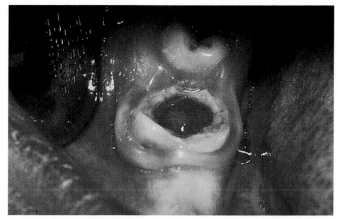

Fig. 24.2. **Pulp polyp:** red, exuberant mass arising from pulp.

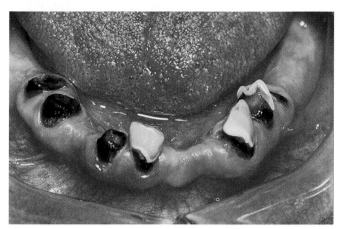

Fig. 24.3. **Rampant caries:** associated with xerostomia.

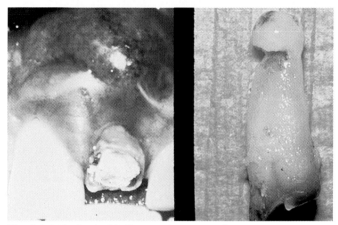

Fig. 24.4. **Periapical inflammation:** granuloma at apex.

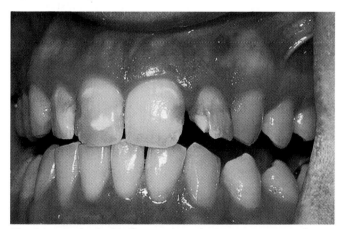

Fig. 24.5. **Periapical inflammation:** draining at periapical parulis.*

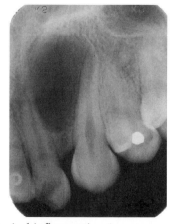

Fig. 24.6. **Periapical inflammation.***

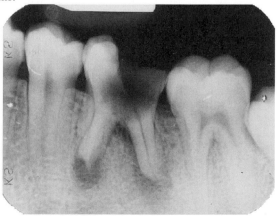

Fig. 24.7. **Caries and chronic periapical inflammation:** first molar.‡

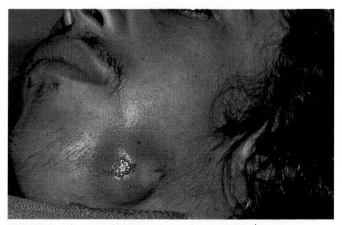

Fig. 24.8. **Abscess:** draining through mandible.‡

Section VI

Cysts and Tumors
of the Jaws

Cysts and Tumors of the Jaws: Cysts

Cysts of the Jaws (Figs. 25.1–25.8) Cysts are epithelial-lined cavities that occur within tissue. They develop commonly in jaws when epithelial remnants of developing and erupted teeth undergo cystic degeneration within bone. Jaw cysts are classified as developmental, odontogenic, inflammatory, and pseudocysts (those not epithelium-lined). Radiographically, jaw cysts appear as unilocular or multilocular radiolucencies. Multilocular types tend to be aggressive and are more likely to recur.

Nasopalatine Duct Cyst (Incisive Canal Cyst) (Fig. 25.1) This developmental cyst arises from entrapped epithelium in the incisive canal. Radiographically, it produces a classic heart-shaped radiolucency between the roots of vital maxillary central incisors. It is discussed under "Swellings of the Palate" (see Figs. 44.3 and 44.4). The **cyst of the incisive papilla** (Fig. 25.1) is a developmental soft tissue variant of the incisive canal cyst. It occurs within the incisive papilla as a slow-growing swelling. Occlusion against the lesion can cause it to appear red or ulcerated. Mastication-associated pain may be a complaint. Excision is the treatment of choice. Recurrence is rare.

Lateral Periodontal Cyst (Fig. 25.2) This cyst is a developmental nonkeratinizing odontogenic cyst that develops adjacent or lateral to a tooth root, commonly in the mandibular premolar region. It arises from proliferation of epithelial rests of dental lamina and occurs mostly in males between 40 and 70 years. It appears as a small (less than 5 mm) corticated interdental radiolucency. The adjacent teeth are vital. It has two variants: the **gingival cyst of the adult** and the **botryoid lateral periodontal cyst.** The gingival cyst is found entirely within soft tissue (Fig. 9.8). Gingival and lateral periodontal cysts rarely recur after excision.

Botryoid Lateral Periodontal Cyst (Fig. 25.3) The botryoid lateral periodontal cyst is a multilocular variant of the lateral periodontal cyst. Unilocular variants occasionally occur. Grossly the botryoid cyst appears grape-like (botryoid). The average age at occurrence is 46 years, and it occurs slightly more often in men. The most frequent complaint is swelling or pain in the area. Most are found in the mandibular canine, premolar, and incisor areas. Radiographically, one of the locules occupies the usual location of a simple lateral periodontal cyst, whereas the remaining smaller locules are apically located. About 10 years after removal, 30 to 50% recur.

Dentigerous Cyst (Fig. 25.4) By definition this odontogenic cyst associates with the crown of an erupting or impacted tooth. It arises from proliferation of remnants of the enamel organ or reduced enamel epithelium (the follicular sac). It is the most common pathologic pericoronal radiolucency and the second most common jaw cyst after the periapical cyst. It occurs usually before the age of 20 years and more often in males. Radiographically, the cyst is a well-corticated pericoronal radiolucency that must be distinguished from the normal follicular space. Both are identical histologically; the difference is based on radiographic size. The normal follicular space is less than 2.5 mm in intraoral radiographs and 3.0 mm on panoramic radiographs; larger spaces are considered cystic. The most common location is the mandibular third molar region (56%). They can give rise to an **ameloblastoma, squamous cell carcinoma,** or **mucoepidermoid carcinoma;** thus, excision is essential.

Odontogenic Keratocyst (OKC) (Figs. 25.5 and 25.6) This jaw cyst arises from remnants of the dental lamina and is defined by its histologic appearance. It frequently appears as a primordial cyst when a tooth (e.g., third molar) fails to develop. It is seen mostly in the second and third decades, more often in men. Often it is asymptomatic. Radiographically, it can be unilocular but is more often multilocular. The margins are radiopaque and scalloped and may demonstrate bony expansion. Internally some septa and a cloudy lumen (representing desquamated keratin) are seen. Histologically, the cystic epithelium is uniform, 8 to 10 cell layers thick, and **parakeratinized.** After excision, recurrence is up to 50% within 10 years.

Jaw Cyst–Basal Cell Nevus Syndrome (Gorlin-Goltz Syndrome) (Fig. 25.6) This syndrome is characterized by multiple jaw OKCs, basal cell nevi on the skin, skeletal anomalies (bifid and other rib anomalies), and soft tissue anomalies like prominent finger pads and palmar pitting of the hands. These OKCs have a recurrence rate of up to 80%.

Buccal Bifurcation Cyst (Inflammatory Paradental Cyst) (Fig. 25.7) The buccal bifurcation cyst is an inflammatory cyst that develops as bacteria are entrapped below buccal cervical enamel extensions of lower first, second, and third molars in descending order of frequency. Most occur in young males before age 20 years. Radiographically, these pericoronal radiolucencies develop adjacent (buccally) to the involved tooth and are bounded by a thin or thick dense cortical line. Treatment is cystectomy, enameloplasty, and correction of the associated periodontal defect. Involved third molars are usually extracted.

Traumatic (Simple) Bone Cyst (Fig. 25.8) This entity is an intrabony cavitation that affects the jaws or long bones. It is a pseudocyst as it lacks an epithelial lining. It arises after trauma, although many patients do not provide a history of trauma. Females are affected almost as often as males. The average age of detection is 18 years. Most are asymptomatic, and most occur in the mandible in the molar–premolar area. Radiographically, the traumatic cyst appears as a radiolucency with a scalloping superior radiopaque margin extending between roots and a rounded inferior margin. The mesiodistal dimension is usually wider than the superior-inferior. The cyst regresses spontaneously or after currettage.

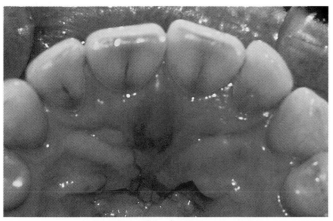

Fig. 25.1. **Cyst of the incisive papilla:** entirely in soft tissue.

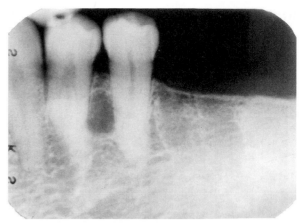

Fig. 25.2. **Lateral periodontal cyst:** common location and size.

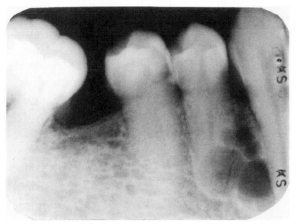

Fig. 25.3. **Botryoid lateral periodontal cyst:** often multilocular.

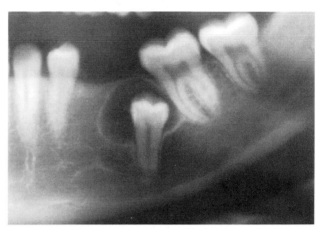

Fig. 25.4. **Dentigerous cyst:** in mandibular premolar location.

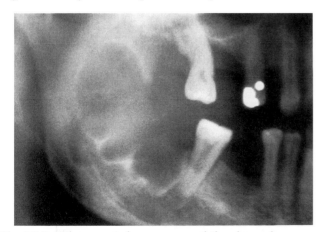

Fig. 25.5. **Odontogenic keratocyst:** multilocular and recurs.

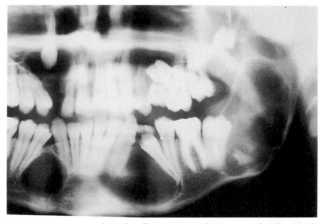

Fig. 25.6. **Jaw cyst–basal cell nevus syndrome:** multiple OKCs.

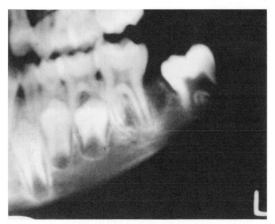

Fig. 25.7. **Buccal bifurcation cyst:** most common location.

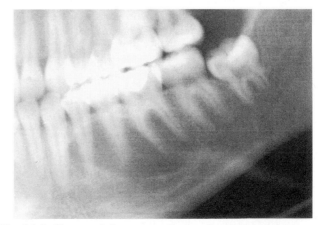

Fig. 25.8. **Traumatic bone cyst:** interradicular extension.

Cysts and Tumors of the Jaws: Radiolucent Lesions

Unicystic (Mural) Ameloblastoma (Fig. 26.1)
This odontogenic tumor develops de novo from epithelium that forms teeth or from a preexisting cyst. The average age at development is 27 years, and there is a male predilection. These tumors are detected on routine radiographs or because of a complaint of a painless swelling. Most unicystic ameloblastomas occur in the mandibular molar region. Radiologically, this pericoronal radiolucency is often associated with a displaced third molar, buccal and lingual expansion, occasional perforation, and root resorption of adjacent erupted molars. Internally, there are locules or septa. They can perforate the cortical plate. Recurrence rate after treatment is about 15%.

Adenomatoid Odontogenic Tumor (Fig. 26.2)
The adenomatoid odontogenic tumor is composed of polyhedral epithelial cells that produce ductlike structures within bone. The majority occur in young females (13 to 14 years). Rarely symptoms or swelling occurs. Radiographically, the tumor produces a radiolucent lesion in the maxillary canine area. This unique location aids in the diagnosis. In about 65% of cases radiopaque flecks occur within the central part of the lesion. The margin of the tumor is radiopaque and may be thick, thin, or absent focally as a result of infection. An unerupted permanent tooth (e.g., canine) is associated with these lesions in 75% of cases. The lesion enucleates easily and does not tend to recur.

Calcifying Epithelial Odontogenic (Pindborg) Tumor (Fig. 26.3) This tumor is composed of large polyhedral, neoplastic, epithelial cells. The cause of growth is unknown. The tumor occurs around age 40 years and equally in males and females. Patients usually present with an asymptomatic swelling. The most common location is the mandibular molar area. There is an associated unerupted tooth in 60% of cases and often tumor-induced migration of a molar into the inferior cortex of the mandible. Smooth radiopaque flecks within the lesion cluster at the occlusal aspect of the tumor and form a linear pattern as the impacted tooth is pushed inferiorly, leaving a trail of radiopaque flecks described as "driven snow." After excision, recurrence occurs in about 20% of patients.

Ameloblastic Fibro-Odontoma (Fig. 26.4) This mixed odontogenic tumor is composed of neoplastic epithelium and mesenchyme. It occurs almost exclusively in tooth development years (i.e., younger than 20 years). Males are affected slightly more often. The most frequent complaint is the noneruption of one or several teeth. Most cases occur in the posterior jaws, with an equal distribution between the jaws. It appears radiographically as a pericoronal radiolucency with internal radiopacities and an unerupted tooth. The radiopacities may resemble a compound (toothlike) or complex odontoma with a radiolucent rim and radiopaque peripheral boundary. Expansion is present in larger lesions. They have little tendency to recur after excision.

Odontoameloblastoma (Ameloblastic Odontoma) (Fig. 26.5) The ameloblastic odontoma is a rare variant ameloblastoma that demonstrates focal odontoma differentiation. Most occur in the first two decades of life with an equal sex distribution. Radiographically, more occur in anterior regions as expansive pericoronal radiolucency with opacities. Often they are associated with one or more impacted or unerupted teeth. This lesion is prone to recurrence after treatment.

Ameloblastoma (Fig. 26.6) This aggressive tumor arising from odontogenic epithelium is the second most common odontogenic tumor. The average age at detection is about 34 years, and men and women are equally affected. The tumor is characterized by slow growth and painless swelling that may reach huge proportions if untreated. The majority occur in the mandibular molar region, with some 63% extending into the ramus. The lesion is usually multilocular with bilocular, soap-bubble, and honeycomb variants; smaller lesions may be unilocular. Typically both buccal and lingual expansion of the cortex is present in larger lesions, and perforation is possible. An impacted or displaced unerupted tooth is seen in about 40% of patients. Knife-edge resorption of adjacent teeth is characteristic. With multiple recurrences and treatments the **histologically benign** ameloblastoma may metastasize; hence, it is referred to as **malignant ameloblastoma.**

Odontogenic Myxoma (Fig. 26.7) The myxoma arises from follicular connective tissue resembling pulp tissue. The mean age at occurrence is 25 to 35 years with an equal male to female ratio. Most cause a painless swelling and cortical expansion of the posterior mandible. Maxillary lesions can involve the sinus and produce exophthalmos and nasal obstruction. Rare cases develop in the upper ramus and base of the condyle. Early lesions are unilocular, and advanced lesions are multilocular radiolucencies that have internal septa that intersect at right angles forming geometric shapes. Perforation of the outer cortex and invasion of local soft tissue produces fine or coarse septa directed at right angles to and outside the cortex, producing a comb appearance. About 30% recur after treatment.

Central Giant Cell Granuloma (Fig. 26.8) This unique granuloma is composed of spindle-shaped mesenchymal cells and aggregates of multinucleated giant cells. More occur in women younger than 30 years. There are two variants: aggressive and nonaggressive forms. The aggressive variant produces pain, rapid growth, swelling, radiographic resorption of root apices, perforation of the expanded cortex, and has a diameter exceeding 2 cm. Nonaggressive lesions tend to be asymptomatic and exhibit slow growth and smaller size. Most are seen in the mandible anterior to the first molars and may cross the midline. The typical lesion is multilocular with wispy trabeculae or crenations at the periphery. About 20% recur, especially the aggressive form.

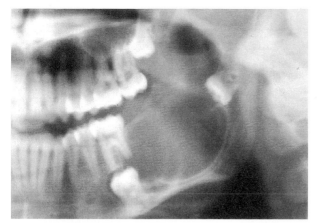

Fig. 26.1. Unicystic ameloblastoma: cystlike with locules.

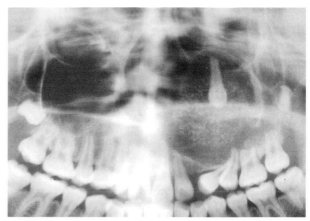

Fig. 26.2. Adenomatoid odontogenic tumor: with flecks.

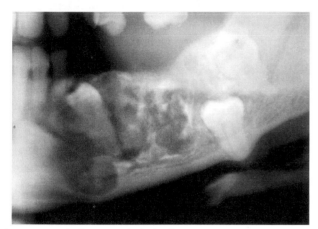

Fig. 26.3. Calcifying epithelial odontogenic tumor.

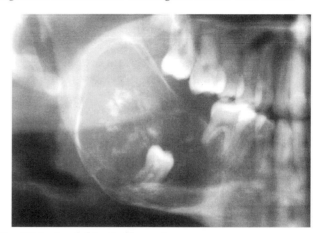

Fig. 26.4. Ameloblastic fibro-odontoma.

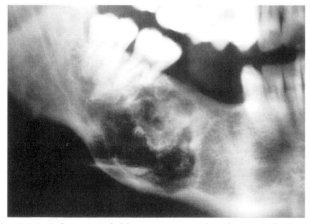

Fig. 26.5. Odontoameloblastoma: some locules with flecks.

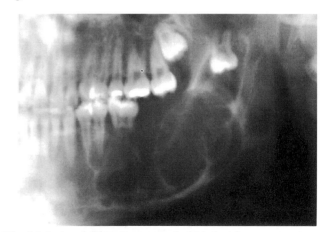

Fig. 26.6. Ameloblastoma: soap-bubble locules.

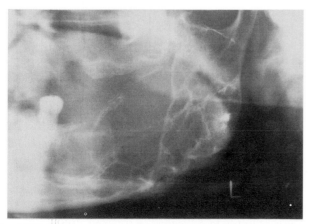

Fig. 26.7. Myxoma: septa shaped like letters X, Y, and V.

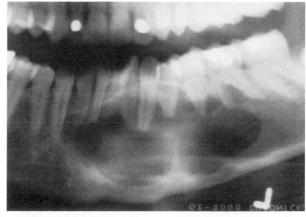

Fig. 26.8. Central giant cell granuloma: peripheral crenations.

Cysts and Tumors of the Jaws: Radiopaque Lesions

Exostosis (Figs. 27.1, 27.2, and 61.5) Exostoses are asymptomatic, bony outgrowths of the outer cortex of the mandible and maxilla. Specific types include mandibular tori, palatal tori, and reactive subpontine exostosis. The clinical and histologic features are discussed under "Nodules" (see Fig. 61.5). All have a shell of cortical bone with various amounts of inner spongy bone. They occur on buccal or lingual alveolar bone as rounded bony nodules; radiographically, they appear as dense round radiopacities.

Mandibular Tori (Fig. 27.1) Mandibular tori are exostoses on the lingual alveolar bone adjacent to the premolars and canines, and sometimes molar region. They are developmental outgrowths. Most show a hereditary pattern. Sizes range from 0.5 to 1.5 cm in diameter. (see "Nodules," Fig. 61.5). They appear as focal, uniformly dense radiopacities with single or multiple lobes in the mandibular anterior and premolar periapical radiographs and occlusal and panoramic views. The bosseleated types appear as separate rounded or ovoid radiopacities with a smooth outline.

Palatal Tori (Fig. 27.2) Palatal tori are bony hard masses that arise from the midline of the hard palate. These developmental and usually hereditary exostoses occur in at least 10% of the population. Most appear as dome-shaped midline protruberances, but flat, nodular, and lobular variants exist (see Fig. 44.1 description and clinical example). Radiographically, they appear as a focal, homogeneously dense radiopacity in the palatal region of maxillary anterior or posterior periapical radiographs and panoramic views. No treatment of tori is required, unless desired for prosthetic reasons.

Reactive Subpontine (Hyperostosis) Exostosis (Fig. 27.3) Subpontic hyperostosis is a reaction of crestal alveolar bone to the presence of a mandibular fixed partial denture pontic. They occur in men twice as often as women, most after 40 years of age most in the mandibular molar premolar region within 10 years of prosthesis placement. They have mild growth potential and can enlarge beneath the pontic causing the tissue to become red or inflamed, or even to dislodge the bridge. Radiographically, they appear as a conelike radiopacity or broad-based opacity that completely fills the space. Regression occurs when the bridge is removed.

Socket Sclerosis (Fig. 27.4) Socket sclerosis is an asymptomatic, reactive lesion that occurs with systemic disorders (i.e., gastrointestinal and kidney disease) after tooth extraction. It is a permanent marker of systemic disease even after the problem resolves. Most cases occur after 40 years of age, males and females are affected equally, and there is no racial predilection. Radiographically, the lesion is characterized by (1) lack of resorption of the lamina dura, which usually resorbs between 6 and 16 weeks after tooth extraction, and (2) deposition of sclerotic bone within the confines of the socket. Socket sclerosis requires no treatment.

Idiopathic Osteosclerosis (Enostosis) (Fig. 27.5) Idiopathic osteosclerosis (enostosis) is dense bone deposition within marrow spaces of the jaws. There is no racial or sex predilection and no inflammatory or infectious cause. Most lesions are in the mandible in the premolar molar area. They appear as radiopaque densities or foci (55% of cases) at or near the apex of a tooth, in interradicular areas (28%), and distant to teeth (17%). When associated with teeth, the teeth are always vital (confirmed by vitality testing), and the apical periodontal membrane space is normal or rarely obliterated by the opaque bone. No treatment is required.

Condensing Osteitis (Fig. 27.6) Condensing osteitis is a proliferative reaction of dense bone deposited within marrow spaces of the jaws in response to pulpal inflammation. It is more common in persons younger than 20 years. Affected teeth are usually asymptomatic. Most lesions are in the mandibular molar region. The lesion consists of a densely radiopaque area at the apex of a tooth, with widening of the apical periodontal membrane space. Often there is carious involvement of the pulp, or a large restoration or crown. Although the radiographic appearance is similar to periapical idiopathic osteosclerosis, the associated tooth is nonvital. Root canal therapy is recommended for the nonvital tooth.

Periapical Cemento-Osseous Dysplasia (Periapical Cemental Dysplasia, Cementoma) (Fig. 27.7) Periapical cemento-osseous dysplasia is an asymptomatic fibro-osseous disorder belonging to a subclass known as the cemento-osseous dysplasias. It is seen almost uniquely in women of African origin in the mandibular anterior region in association with vital teeth. Three distinct stages occur. In stage one, the alveolar bone demonstrates periapical osteoporotic change. Stage two demonstrates a frank radiolucency resembling a periapical radiolucency. In stage three, calcific spherules develop within the radiolucencies and coalesce to form a central radiopaque mass. Stage three lesions have a "target" appearance. After pulp testing, no treatment is required.

Odontoma (Fig. 27.8) The odontoma, usually classified as an odontogenic tumor, is now believed to be a hamartoma of enamel and dentin that exhibits defective architecture. Two forms exist: **compound odontomas** whose components assemble to resemble teeth and **complex odontomas** amorphous radiopaque masses that do not resemble teeth. Most are identified within the first two decades on routine radiographs or when a permanent tooth fails to erupt. The most common location is the anterior maxilla with about two thirds occurring in the anterior jaws. Radiographically, the compound odontoma resembles a conglomeration of little teeth. The complex odontoma appears as gnarled densities of enamel, dentin, and pulp. Odontomas have little growth potential unless they are associated with dentigerous cysts. Removal is curative.

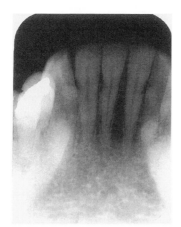

Fig. 27.1. Mandibular tori and small facial exostoses.

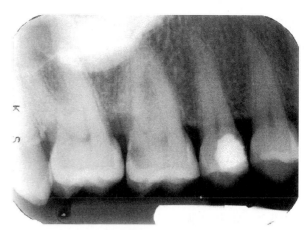

Fig. 27.2. Palatal torus: large rounded radiopacity.

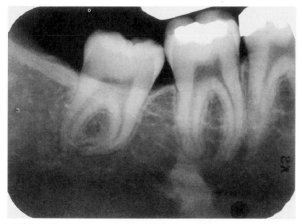

Fig. 27.3. Reactive subpontine exostosis: under pontic.

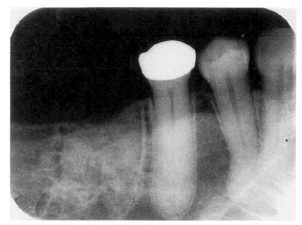

Fig. 27.4. Socket sclerosis: molar area.

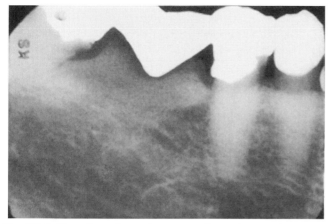

Fig. 27.5. Idiopathic osteosclerosis: vital second molar.

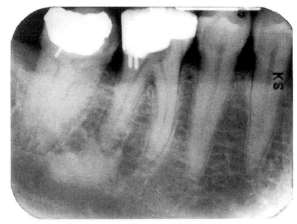

Fig. 27.6. Condensing osteitis: nonvital first molar.

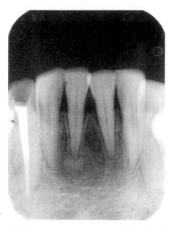

Fig. 27.7. Periapical cemento-osseous dysplasia: vital incisor.

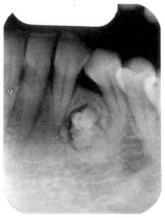

Fig. 27.8. Odontoma: compound type and dilaceration.

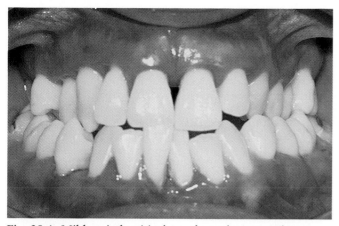

Fig. 30.1. **Mild periodontitis:** loss of attachment evident.

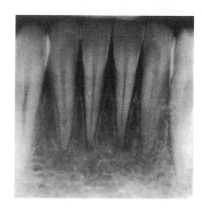

Fig. 30.2. **Mild periodontitis:** loss of crestal alveolar bone.

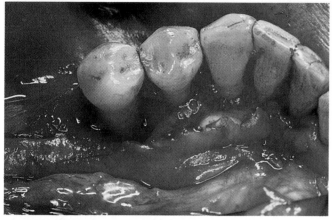

Fig. 30.3. **Moderate periodontitis:** 4-mm moat defect.

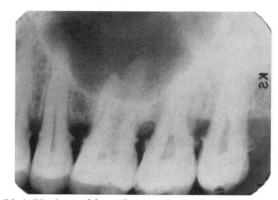

Fig. 30.4. **Horizontal bone loss:** and calculus.

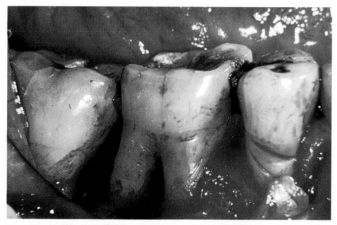

Fig. 30.5. **Class II furcation:** a sign of moderate periodontitis.

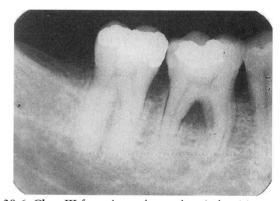

Fig. 30.6. **Class III furcation:** advanced periodontitis.

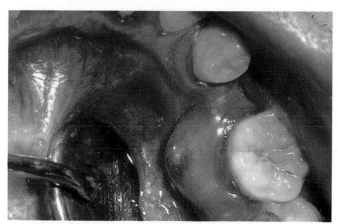

Fig. 30.7. **Periodontal abscess:** fluctuant and pointing.

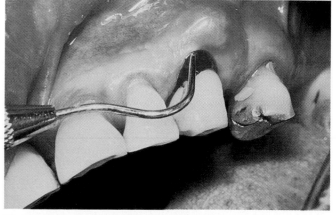

Fig. 30.8. **Periodontal abscess:** with 12-mm pocket.

Radiographic Features of Periodontal Disease

There are several radiographic features associated with periodontal disease—the most prominent being alveolar bone loss. This basic finding, although suggestive of periodontitis, is a nonspecific radiographic finding. It suggests inflammatory and resorptive processes have been active. However, bone loss only provides historical reference; it is not indicative of whether the loss occurred years ago or recently.

Local Factors: Overhang (Fig. 31.1) Local factors can contribute indirectly to the development of periodontal disease. Examples include calculus (Fig. 30.4), crowding (Fig. 30.1), traumatic occlusion (Fig. 20.2), supraeruption (Figs. 20.7 and 20.8), and restoration overhangs. An **overhang** is a specific portion of restoration that extends beyond the gingival preparation margin into the interproximal space. It is usually caused by inadequate banding and wedging of a prepared tooth before placement of the final restoration. Overhangs are seen with class II amalgams, as well as with composites and castings. Overhangs are iatrogenic because they are caused by a dental procedure. In Figure 31.1, a bone defect is associated with the mesial overhang of the second molar. There is also a small overhang on the mesial of the second premolar; however, it is associated only with a mild crestal irregularity. Overhangs should be removed and the margins smoothed either during periodontal procedures or as a new restoration.

Local Factors: Open Contact and Poor Restoration Contour (Fig. 31.2) These factors can contribute to food impaction, the accumulation of plaque, and the development of periodontitis. An open contact is an area between teeth where interproximal contact is absent. A poor restoration contact can be rough, or have inappropriate width, length, height or contour. Poor and open contacts can result from tooth mobility caused by malocclusion or periodontal disease, supraeruption, drifting of erupted teeth, attrition and flattening of the interproximal contacts, and iatrogenic dentistry (when a contact is improperly restored). In Figure 31.2, both factors are present between the first and second molars, a bone defect is present, and the under-contoured restoration needs replacement.

Bone Loss: Localized (Figs. 31.1, 31.3, and 30.2) Healthy crestal alveolar bone is superiorly convex, densely radiopaque, continuous with the lamina dura on both sides, and located 1 to 1.5 mm apical to the cementoenamel junction. Localized bone loss occurs when inflammatory cytokines cause bone resorption. Radiographically, one sees crestal irregularities, triangulation (bone defect formation), loss of bone density, and interseptal bone changes. These changes may be localized to one or more areas. Triangulation is a wedge-shaped radiolucent defect on the mesial or distal of the crestal interalveolar bone. Interseptal bone changes consist of prominent nutrient canals especially in the mandibular anterior region (Fig. 30.2). These canals appear as vertical radiolucent lines and indicate increased vascularity to the region and susceptibility to bone loss if treatment is not provided.

Bone Loss: Generalized (Figs. 31.4 and 30.4) Generalized bone loss indicates resorption of alveolar bone in multiple, often continuous sites. It occurs most frequently as **horizontal bone loss**; however, there may be areas of **vertical (or angular) bone loss** suggestive of continuing disease. In our example, there is generalized horizontal bone loss; areas of vertical bone loss distal to the second premolar and mesial to the first molar; contact flattening caused by attrition, especially of the premolars; extrusion of the first molar with root caries; calculus, class III furcal involvement of the first molar; and furcal involvement of the second molar. The level of the soft tissue outline of the gingiva indicates deep periodontal pockets are present.

Bone (Infrabony) Defects Angular or vertical bone defects are classified by the number of walls remaining after destruction of alveolar bone by periodontal disease. Although radiographs are suggestive of an infrabony defect and its severity, defects are best delineated by careful probing or surgical exploration. A **crater** is simply a scooped out area of alveolar bone anywhere about the circumference of a tooth and is not classified as a walled defect.

One-Wall Infrabony Defect (Figs. 31.3 and 31.5) This defect has only one wall of interseptal bone (hemiseptum) remaining. The wall may slope mesio-distally as seen distal to the second premolar in Figure 31.3 or ramp buccal or lingually as seen in Figure 31.5 between the molars. This defect is difficult to treat.

Two-Wall Infrabony Defect (Fig. 31.6) A two-wall bony defect has two walls of interseptal bone remaining. Radiographically, there is a combination of the ramping as seen in Figure 31.5 and the vertical defect as seen in Figure 31.3. The result is a combination of bony walls creating an osseous defect in the interseptal bone at the mesial or distal of a tooth. This defect makes up 35% of all defects and 62% of mandibular defects. In our example the crater is mesial alongside the lower second molar.

Three-Wall Infrabony Defect (Fig. 31.7) and Moat Defect (Fig. 31.8) This infrabony defect has bone on three sides with the tooth root forming the fourth wall. The defect surrounds only a portion of the root. When it involves the buccal or lingual surface or completely surrounds the root it is referred to as a **circumferential** or **moat** defect. In the case in which the defect involves the periapex, inflammation and vascular compromise can result in necrosis of the pulp. This is known as an endo-perio lesion.

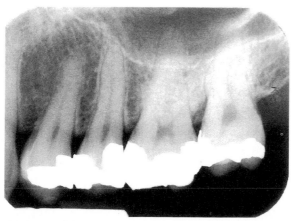

Fig. 31.1. **Local factors:** overhang and crestal defects.

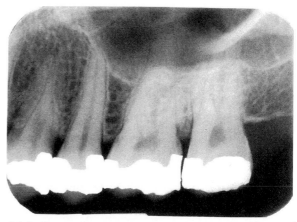

Fig. 31.2. **Open contact, poor restoration contour:** first molar.

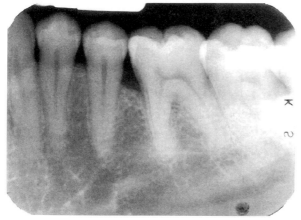

Fig. 31.3. **Vertical one wall defect:** distal to premolar.

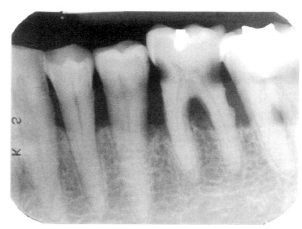

Fig. 31.4. **Bone loss:** generalized; extrusion and root caries.

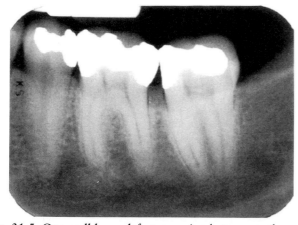

Fig. 31.5. **One-wall bone defect:** ramping between molars.

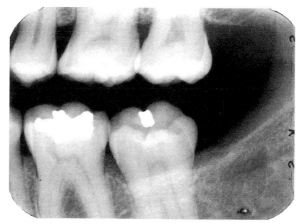

Fig. 31.6. **Two-wall cratering defect:** around lower 2nd molar.

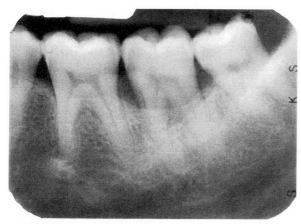

Fig. 31.7. **Three-wall bone defect:** second molar area.

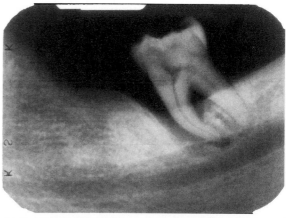

Fig. 31.8. **Circumferential (moat) defect and nonvital tooth.**

Localized Gingival Lesions

Pyogenic Granuloma (Figs. 32.1 and 32.2)
Pyogenic granuloma (a misnomer because the condition is neither pus-filled nor a granuloma) is a form of inflammatory hyperplasia rich in neocapillaries and immature fibrous connective tissue. The growth is an exaggerated response to irritation and appears bright red, fleshy, and soft. The surface is glossy and ulcerated. The base is polypoid or pedunculated. Although the condition is usually asymptomatic, minor manipulation induces bleeding because of the thinned epithelium and highly vascular tissue. Maturation of the lesion results in increased fibrosis, decreased vascularity, and pinker color.

Pyogenic granulomas develop in patients who have poor oral hygiene or a chronic oral irritant such as overhanging restorations or calculus. Women are more susceptible to the condition because of hormonal imbalances that occur during puberty, pregnancy, or menopause; in such cases, the granulomas are called hormonal or pregnancy tumors. About 1% of pregnant women develop this lesion.

Pyogenic granulomas most frequently arise from the interdental papilla and can enlarge from the labial and lingual aspects to several centimeters. Other sites of development include the tongue, lips, buccal mucosa, and edentulous ridge. Treatment is surgical excision that, in the gravid female, should be delayed until after parturition. Recurrence is possible, if excision and local debridement are incomplete or plaque control is inadequate.

Peripheral Giant Cell Granuloma (Figs. 32.3 and 32.4)
The peripheral giant cell granuloma is a reactive epulis-like growth that develops exclusively on the gingiva. It is generally associated with a history of trauma or irritation and is thought to originate from the mucoperiosteum or periodontal ligament. Therefore, the peripheral giant cell granuloma demonstrates a restricted area of development—the dentulous or edentulous ridge. The mandibular gingiva anterior to the molars is particularly affected, especially in women between the ages of 40 and 60. Histologic examination shows multinucleated giant cells and numerous fibroblasts.

The peripheral giant cell granuloma is a well-defined, firm swelling that seldom ulcerates. The base is sessile, the surface is smooth or slightly granular, and the color is pink to dark red-purple. The nodule is usually a few millimeters to 1 cm in diameter, although rapid enlargement may produce a large growth that encroaches on adjacent teeth. The lesion is generally asymptomatic; however, because of its aggressive nature, the underlying alveolar bone is often involved, producing a pathognomonic superficial peripheral-cuff radiolucency. Treatment is surgical excision that includes the base of the lesion and curettage of the underlying bone. Incomplete removal may result in recurrence. On histologic examination, this lesion cannot be distinguished from the central giant cell granuloma and the brown tumor of hyperparathyroidism.

Peripheral Ossifying Fibroma (Figs. 32.5 and 32.6)
The peripheral ossifying fibroma is a reactive growth that is especially prone to occur in the anterior region of the maxilla of young females in the second decade of life. The cause of the peripheral ossifying fibroma is uncertain, but inflammatory hyperplasia of superficial periodontal ligament origin has been suggested. The condition arises exclusively from the gingiva, usually the interdental papillae. When calcifications are present, they may consist of bone, cementum, or dystrophic calcification. Peripheral ossifying fibroma is unrelated to the central ossifying fibroma. The salient clinical features of this solitary swelling are firmness, red or pink color, possible ulceration, and sessile attachment. An important diagnostic clue is the marked tendency of the condition to cause displacement of adjacent teeth. The chief sign is often an asymptomatic, slow-growing round or nodular swelling. Immature lesions are soft and bleed easily, whereas older lesions become firm and fibrotic. Radiographs may reveal central radiopaque foci and mild resorption of the crest of the ridge at its base. Treatment is excision. The recurrence rate is about 15%.

Irritation Fibroma
The irritation fibroma is a common benign oral lesion that occasionally develops on gingival tissues. It is more typically seen on moveable mucosa and is discussed in Section X (Fig. 62.1).

Peripheral Odontogenic Fibroma (Fig. 32.7)
The peripheral odontogenic fibroma is clinically similar to the irritation fibroma but is characterized by its unique location and tissue of origin. In most cases, the peripheral odontogenic fibroma is found as a circumscribed swelling in the region of the interdental papilla, generally located anterior to the molar teeth. A cuplike erosion of the underlying alveolar bone may be seen radiographically. It probably arises from cellular components of the periodontal ligament (PDL). Microscopic examination shows clusters of odontogenic epithelium among dense collagenous tissue.

Desmoplastic Fibroma (Fig. 32.8)
The desmoplastic fibroma is a rare tumor composed of fibroblasts and abundant collagen that most frequently affects the metaphyseal regions of the long bones of the arms and legs. The fourth most commonly affected site is the mandible. Most cases occur in adults younger than age 30; the posterior jaw is the most common intraoral location. These tumors begin as painless firm swellings within bone that appear unilocular radiographically. Erosion of the cortical bone results in root resorption and a pink, firm soft tissue mass of the alveolar ridge or gingiva. The tumor is locally aggressive and recurs in about 30% of patients who receive surgical treatment. Resection is recommended for recurrent lesions.

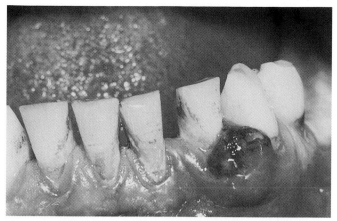

Fig. 32.1. **Pyogenic granuloma:** at interdental papilla.

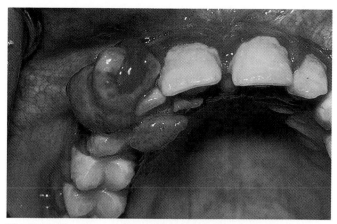

Fig. 32.2. **Pregnancy tumor:** 3 days after parturition.

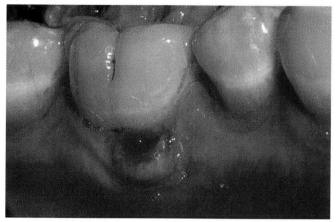

Fig. 32.3. **Peripheral giant cell granuloma:** on gingival margin.

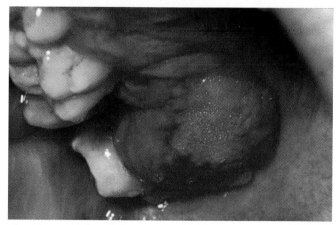

Fig. 32.4. **Peripheral giant cell granuloma:** maxilla.

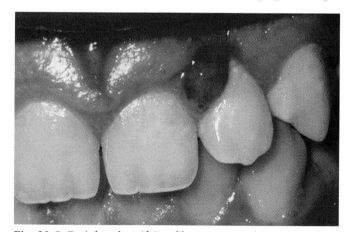

Fig. 32.5. **Peripheral ossifying fibroma:** typical location.

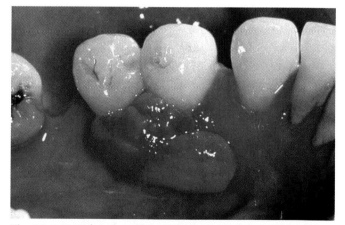

Fig. 32.6. **Peripheral ossifying fibroma:** pink and firm.

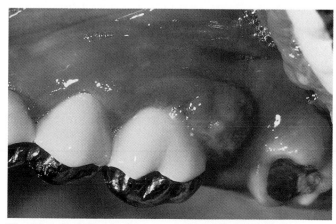

Fig. 32.7. **Peripheral odontogenic fibroma:** from PDL.

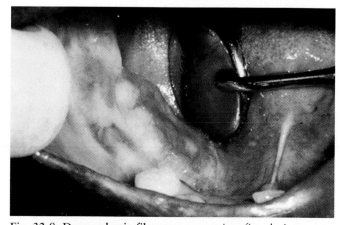

Fig. 32.8. **Desmoplastic fibroma:** aggressive, firm lesion.

Localized Gingival Lesions

Parulis (Gumboil) (Figs. 33.1 and 33.2) The parulis, or gumboil—the latter term being reserved for children (Fig. 11.8)—is a localized area of inflammatory hyperplasia that occurs at the end point of a draining dental sinus tract. It appears as a soft, solitary reddish papule, located apical and facial to a chronically abscessed tooth, usually on or near the labial mucogingival junction. Occasionally the parulis is slightly yellow in the center and emits a purulent yellowish exudate on palpation. Acute swelling and pain may accompany the condition if the sinus tract is obstructed.

To locate the nonvital tooth from which the parulis arises, a sterile gutta-percha point may be inserted into the sinus tract. Periapical radiographs are then taken to demonstrate the proximity of the gutta-percha point to the apex of the offending tooth. After the nonvital tooth is diagnosed, the treatment of choice is root canal therapy. After treatment the parulis usually regresses. If the problematic tooth is left untreated, the parulis may persist for years. A persistent lesion may mature into a pink-colored fibroma.

Pericoronitis (Operculitis) (Figs. 33.3 and 33.4) Pericoronitis is inflammation of the soft tissue surrounding the crown of a partially erupted or impacted tooth. Pericoronitis may develop at any age but most frequently occurs in children and young adults whose teeth are erupting. Generally, it is associated with an erupting mandibular third molar that is in good alignment but is limited in its eruption by insufficient space. Radiographs of the region reveal a flame-shaped radiolucency in the alveolar bone distal to the tooth, with the cortical outline either absent or distinctly thickened because of infection, deposition of reactive bone, or inflammatory cyst formation.

Pericoronitis develops from bacterial contamination beneath the operculum, resulting in gingival swelling, redness, and halitosis. Pain varies and may be extreme, but the discomfort usually resembles that of gingivitis, a periodontal abscess, or tonsillitis. Regional lymphadenopathy, malaise, and low-grade fever are common. If edema or cellulitis extends to involve the masseter muscle, trismus often accompanies the condition. Pericoronitis is frequently complicated by pain induced by trauma from the opposing tooth during closure.

Pericoronitis is best managed by entering the follicular space, flushing the purulent material from the gingival sulcus with saline solution, and eliminating any occlusal trauma to the operculum from the opposing third molar. Definitive treatment is usually extraction of the involved tooth. Antibiotic coverage is recommended when constitutional symptoms are present and the spread of infection is likely. Recurrences and chronicity are likely if the condition is managed only with antibiotics.

Periodontal Abscess The periodontal abscess produces a localized gingival swelling. It is previously discussed (Fig. 30.7).

Epulis Fissuratum (Irritation Hyperplasia) (Figs. 33.5 and 33.6) The epulis fissuratum is a reactive inflammatory fibrous hyperplasia caused by a chronic irritant, usually the flange area of an old, poorly fitting complete or partial denture. The overextended denture margin initially produces an ulcer that heals incompletely because of repeated trauma. Hyperplastic healing results in a pink-red, fleshy exuberance of mature granulation tissue. The hyperplastic lesion, located where the denture flange rests, is found mostly in older women. It is nonpainful, grows slowly on either side of the denture flange, and causes the patient little concern.

The epulis fissuratum in the early stages consists of a single fold of smooth soft tissue. As the swelling grows, a central cleft or several clefts become apparent, the boundaries of which may drape over the denture flange. The mucolabial fold of the anterior region of the maxilla is the most common location, followed by the mandibular alveolar ridge and the mandibular lingual sulcus. Adjustment of the denture, a reline, or construction of a new denture may reduce the trauma and inflammation but will not cause the underlying fibrous tissue to regress. Likewise, surgical excision without alteration of the dentures promotes recurrence. Successful treatment usually requires surgical removal of the redundant tissue, microscopic examination of the excised tissue, and correction or reconstruction of the denture.

Gingival Carcinoma (Figs. 33.7 and 33.8) The gingiva is the site of approximately 5 to 10% of all cases of oral squamous cell carcinoma. Generally, at the time of diagnosis the disease is advanced because of its asymptomatic nature, posterior location, and delay of examination.

Gingival carcinoma varies in appearance. It usually appears as a reddish proliferative mass with focal white areas arising from the gingiva. It may also mimic benign inflammatory gingival conditions, erythroplakia, leukoplakia, or a simple ulceration. Carcinoma should be suspected when close examination reveals a pebbly surface, many small blood vessels in the overlying epithelium, and surface ulceration. Etiologic factors include tobacco use, alcoholism, and poor oral hygiene. Elderly men are especially susceptible, and the condition seems to have a slight predilection for the alveolar ridge of the posterior mandible. Completely dentate persons rarely have this disease.

Gingival carcinoma may extend onto the floor of the mouth or mucobuccal fold, or it may invade the underlying bone. Radiographs may reveal a cupping out of the alveolar crest. Metastasis to regional lymph nodes occurs frequently. Metastatic nodes are firm, rubbery, matted, nonmovable, and nonpainful. Treatment consists of surgery and radiotherapy.

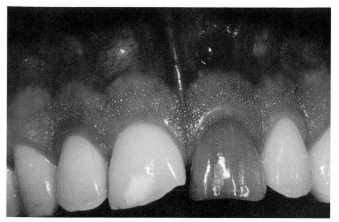

Fig. 33.1. Parulis: reddish papule above nonvital central.

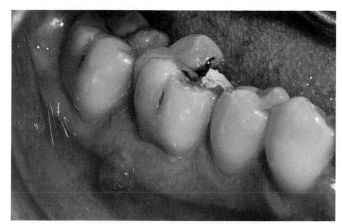

Fig. 33.2. Parulis: adjacent to nonvital first molar.

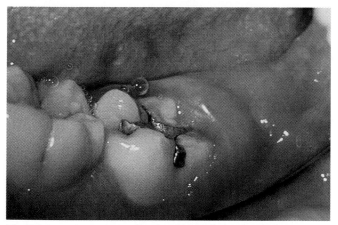

Fig. 33.3. Pericoronitis: distal to partially erupted molar.

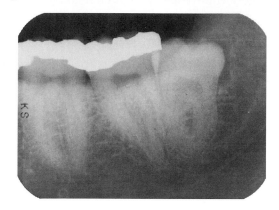

Fig. 33.4. Pericoronitis: flame-shaped radiolucency.

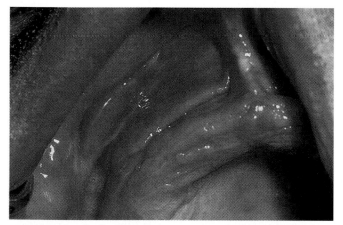

Fig. 33.5. Epulis fissuratum: in maxillary labial fornix.

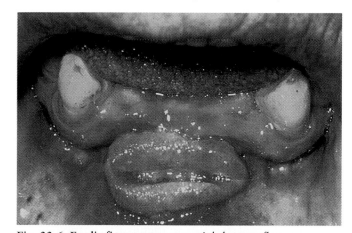

Fig. 33.6. Epulis fissuratum: at partial denture flange.

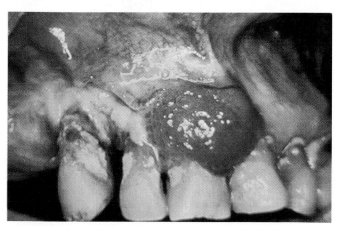

Fig. 33.7. Gingival carcinoma: poor oral hygiene.

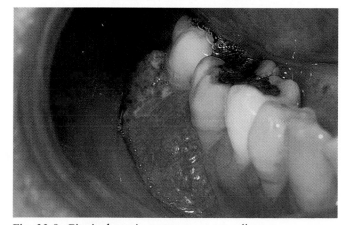

Fig. 33.8. Gingival carcinoma: squamous cell type.

Generalized Gingival Enlargements

Fibromatosis Gingivae (Figs. 34.1 and 34.2)

Fibromatosis gingivae is a rare progressive fibrous enlargement of the gingiva that is usually inherited as an autosomal dominant trait. The fibromatosis tissues contain fibroblasts that have low growth activity but produce greater amounts of collagen and other extracellular substances compared with normal fibroblasts. The condition begins with tooth eruption and becomes more prominent with age. The enlargement is usually generalized and noninflammatory, affecting the buccal and lingual surfaces of one or both jaws. The free, interproximal, and marginal gingiva are enlarged, uniformly pink, firm, nonhemorrhagic, and often nodular.

There are two varieties of fibromatosis gingivae: generalized and localized. The generalized type is nodular and diffuse, exhibiting several coalesced areas of globular gingival overgrowths that encroach on and eventually cover the crowns of the teeth. In the occasionally seen localized variety, solitary overgrowths are limited to the palatal vault of the maxillary tuberosity or the lingual gingiva of the mandibular arch. These gingival overgrowths appear smooth, firm, and symmetrically round. The localized involvement may be unilateral or bilateral, and the term **focal gingival fibromatosis** has been suggested for this variant.

Fibromatosis gingivae may interfere with tooth eruption, mastication, and oral hygiene. In severe cases, noneruption of the primary or permanent teeth may be the chief symptom. Regression in dentate patients is not a feature of this disease, even with effective oral hygiene measures. However, in areas of tooth loss gingival size tends to decrease. Gingivectomy, with either a blade or a carbon dioxide laser, is the usual treatment of choice. Continued growth may require several operations. The condition may be accompanied by acromegalic facial features, hypertrichosis, mental deficits, deafness, and seizures.

Drug-Induced Gingival Overgrowth (Figs. 34.3–34.7)

Gingival overgrowth is an adverse effect associated with use of specific prescription drugs. It occurs in 25 to 50% of patients taking phenytoin (Dilantin) and cyclosporine (Sandimmune). Phenytoin is taken to prevent seizures (antiepileptic properties). It stabilizes the threshold against hyperexcitability in motor neurons. Cyclosporine is taken by organ transplant patients because it inhibits T-cell proliferation and prevents transplant rejection.

Gingival overgrowth also occurs in 1 to 10% of patients who take calcium-channel blocker drugs (such as nifedipine [Procardia], diltiazem [Cardizem], verapamil [Calan], felodipine [Plendil], and amlodipine [Norvasc]). Sodium valproate (Depakene) and estrogen (in birth control pills and Premarin) have also been associated with gingival overgrowth, generally at high doses. Although the mechanism of drug-induced gingival overgrowth remains unknown, many of these drugs affect calcium ion flux in gingival fibroblasts that appear to alter normal homeostasis, collagenase activity, and the local immune response. Estrogen may work separately by increasing the blood supply and inflammatory mediators to the gingiva.

Drug-induced gingival hyperplasia can occur at any age and in either sex. Although the overgrowth results from a hyperplastic response, an inflammatory component induced by dental bacterial plaque often coexists and tends to exacerbate the condition. The gingival overgrowth is usually generalized and begins at the interdental papillae. It appears most exaggerated on the labial aspects of the anterior teeth. The overgrowths form soft red lumpy nodules that bleed easily. Progressive growth results in fibrotic changes: the interdental tissue becomes enlarged, pink, firm, and resilient to palpation. With time the condition can completely engulf the crowns of the teeth; this aggravates home care, limits mastication, and compromises esthetics.

Treatment may involve changing drug therapy (e.g., changing cyclosporine to tacrolimus, an alternative immunosuppressant) or minimizing the overgrowth with meticulous and frequent plaque control measures. The gingival swelling may completely regress by discontinuing drug use. However, excess fibrotic tissue unresponsive to changes in drug therapy must be surgically removed.

Primary Herpetic Gingivostomatitis (Fig. 34.8)

Herpes simplex virus is a large DNA virus with a propensity to infect human epithelium. Transmission is by contact with infected secretions such as saliva. The initial infection is usually subclinical (not readily visible) but can be prominent depending on the amount of initial inoculum, location, integrity of the epithelium, and the host response. Herpetic gingivostomatitis is the prominent manifestation of the primary oral infection. Replication of the virus in gingival epithelium causes generalized swelling, redness, and pain of the marginal gingiva. The interdental papillae become bulbous and bleed easily about 4 days after infection. Several oral vesicles and ulcers also develop. Virus can spread throughout oral mucosa and invade peripheral nerve endings. Infected nerve endings allow virus to travel intraaxonally to the trigeminal ganglion where it enters into a latent state. Thus, systemic antiviral agents such as acyclovir (Zovirax), famciclovir (Famvir), or valacyclovir (Valtrex) are recommended early during the herpetic infection. Antimicrobial mouthrinses with chlorhexidine gluconate 0.12% (Peridex, Periogard) also help to reduce oral sepsis. Systemic antibiotics are occasionally needed when patients become septic and their temperature is persistently elevated above 101°F. Healing normally takes about 14 to 21 days. Thereafter, 30 to 40% of latently infected patients develop recurrent herpes simplex virus infections that reappear at sites previously infected (see Figs. 64.1–64.6 for more information).

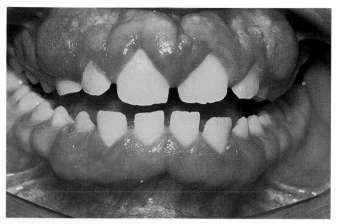

Fig. 34.1. Fibromatosis gingivae: generalized.

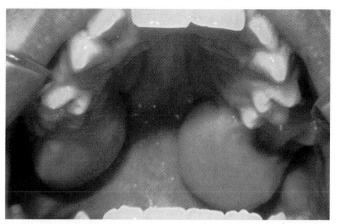

Fig. 34.2. Fibromatosis gingivae: localized variant.

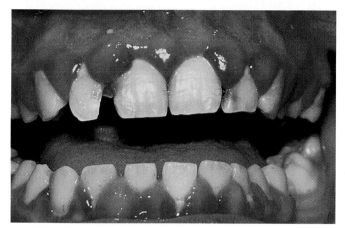

Fig. 34.3. Dilantin-induced gingival overgrowth.

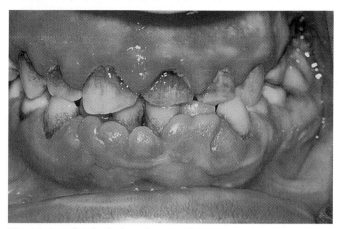

Fig. 34.4. Dilantin-induced gingival overgrowth.

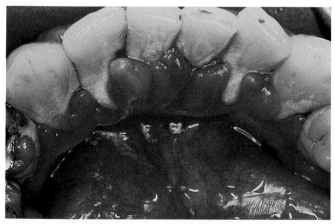

Fig. 34.5. Nifedipine-induced gingival overgrowth.

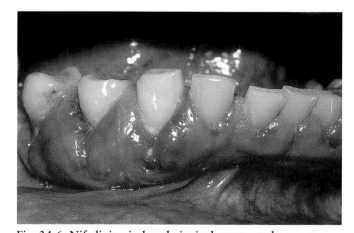

Fig. 34.6. Nifedipine-induced gingival overgrowth.

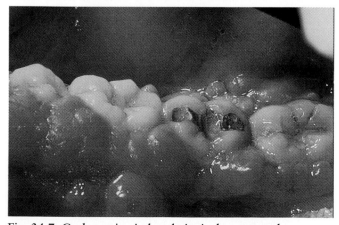

Fig. 34.7. Cyclosporine-induced gingival overgrowth.

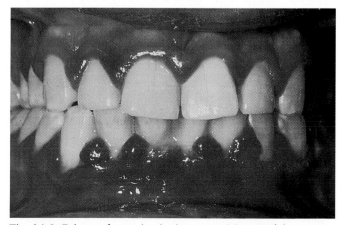

Fig. 34.8. Primary herpetic gingivostomatitis: painful.

Endocrine-Associated Gingival Enlargements

Hormonal Gingivitis (Pregnancy Gingivitis) (Figs. 35.1–35.3) Hormonal gingivitis is a hyperplastic reaction to microbial plaque that affects a large percentage of women during pregnancy, and to a lesser extent during puberty and menopause. Elevated estrogen or progesterone levels resulting from hormonal shifts and use of (previously marketed versions of) birth control pills have been implicated. These hormones enhance tissue vascularity, which permits an exaggerated inflammatory reaction to plaque.

Hormonal gingivitis begins at the marginal and interdental gingiva; usually in the second month of pregnancy. It produces fiery red, swollen, and tender marginal gingiva and compressible and swollen interdental papillae. The tissue is tender to palpation and bleeds easily on probing. The severity is related to microbial accumulation and poor oral hygiene. This is often the case with the gravid female because toothbrushing may precipitate nausea.

Hormonal gingivitis is usually transitory and responds to meticulous home care, oral prophylaxis, and a decrease in hormone levels—which occurs after parturition or with a change of hormone medication. Persistence can result in fibrosis and pinker, firmer, and lumpy tissues. In a small percentage of pregnant women, the hyperplastic response may exacerbate in a localized area resulting in a pyogenic granuloma or pregnancy tumor (Fig. 32.2). Gingivectomy is used to reduce fibrotic gingivae and excise tumorous growths.

Diabetic Gingivitis (Figs. 35.4–35.6) Diabetes mellitus is a common metabolic disease, affecting approximately 1 to 3% of the U.S. population and a high percentage of Hispanic Americans (15–20%). It is characterized by diminished insulin production (type 1) or diminished insulin utilization (type 2) that results in poor control of blood glucose levels. Before diagnosis, patients present with hyperglycemia, glucosuria, polyuria, polydipsia, pruritis, weight gain or loss, loss of strength, visual problems, and loss of peripheral nerve sensation. Because diabetes is a progressive disorder affecting large and small blood vessels, complications include many vascular-related problems, renal disease, risk for infection, dry mouth, burning tongue, and persistent gingivitis.

The severity of diabetic gingivitis is disease dependent. In the patient with uncontrolled or poorly controlled diabetes, peculiar proliferations of exuberant tissue arise from the marginal and attached gingiva. The well-demarcated swellings are soft, red, irregular, and sometimes hemorrhagic. The surface of the hyperplastic tissue is bulbous or papulonodular. The base of the tissue may be sessile or stalklike. The condition is often accompanied by dry mouth, breath odor changes, and alveolar bone loss because of periodontitis. The gingivitis is difficult to manage when blood glucose levels remain elevated as the inflammatory response in the periodontal tissues is altered. Successful treatment requires meticulous home care and control of the blood glucose level with diet, hypoglycemic agents, or insulin. Oral surgical procedures should be limited to when the blood glucose level is below 200 mg/dL and the patient's condition is considered stable.

Gingival Edema of Hypothyroidism (Figs. 35.7 and 35.8) Hypothyroidism is a relatively common disorder in which clinical manifestations depend on the age at onset, duration, and severity of the thyroid insufficiency. When the patient is deficient in thyroid hormone (triiodothyronine [T_3] or thyroxine [T_4]) at an early age, cretinism results. This disease is characterized by short stature, mental retardation, disproportionate head-to-body size, delayed tooth eruption, mandibular micrognathism, and swollen lips and tongue. Regardless of the age of onset, hypothyroid patients have coarse, dry, yellowish skin; coarse hair; intolerance to cold; and lethargy. Adult-onset hypothyroidism is also characterized by dull expression, loss of eyebrow hair, slow physical and mental activity, and elevated cholesterol. Soft tissue swelling is the classic feature and is most prominent in the face, particularly around the eyes. It is caused by accumulation of subcutaneous fluid.

In affected patients, the palpated thyroid gland is most often normal in size, but can be enlarged. Enlarged thyroid glands that are deficient in thyroid hormone production are often caused by an autoimmune lymphocytic infiltration (**Hashimoto's thyroiditis**). In this disease, the thyroid glandular cells are eventually replaced by lymphocytes.

Hypothyroidism can produce oral manifestations. Within the mouth, macroglossia and macrocheilia are common and may cause an altered speech pattern. The gingiva appears uniformly enlarged, pale pink, and compressible. Swelling occurs in all directions on both the facial and lingual sides of the dental arches. When secondary inflammation is present, the tissues become red and boggy and have a tendency to bleed easily. Treatment for the gingival condition depends on the degree of thyroid deficiency. Patients with marginal deficiency require only strict oral hygiene measures, whereas frank cases require supplemental replacement thyroid therapy (thyroxin or levothyroxin) to achieve resolution of the systemic and oral condition.

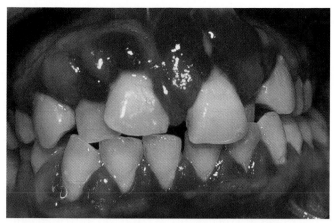

Fig. 35.1. **Hormonal gingivitis:** during pregnancy.

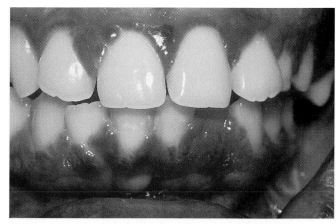

Fig. 35.2. **Hormonal gingivitis:** 3 weeks postpartum.

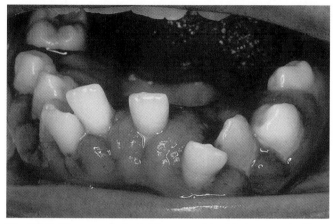

Fig. 35.3. **Hormonal gingivitis:** caused by birth control pills.

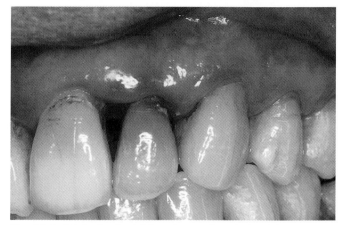

Fig. 35.4. **Diabetic gingivitis:** advanced periodontitis.

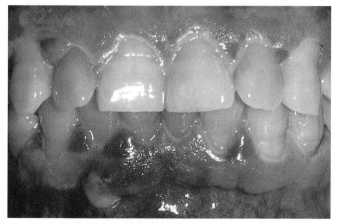

Fig. 35.5. **Diabetic gingivitis:** with periodontal abscess.

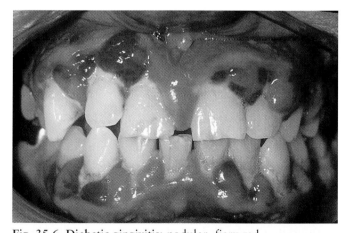

Fig. 35.6. **Diabetic gingivitis:** nodular, fiery red.

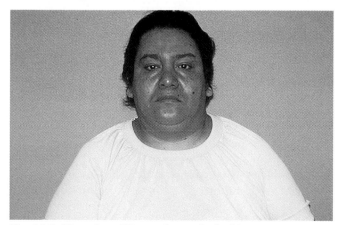

Fig. 35.7. **Hypothyroidism:** edema, thick skin.*

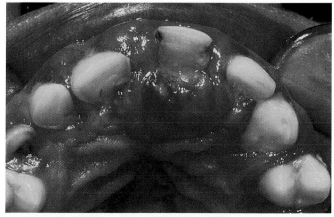

Fig. 35.8. **Hypothyroidism:** gingival edema.*

Spontaneous Gingival Bleeding

Leukemic Gingivitis (Figs. 36.1 and 36.2)

Leukemia, a malignant condition characterized by overproduction of leukocytes, is classified according to cell morphology (monocytic, myelogenous, or lymphoblastic) and the clinical course of the disease (acute or chronic). Oral manifestations are more frequently encountered in acute leukemia of the monocytic and myelogenous subtypes. Oral features occur early in the course of the disease because of neoplastic proliferation of one blood cell type that deposits in oral tissue. Systemic symptoms develop as the neoplastic cell type overwhelms the normal production of the other hematopoietic cells.

Consistent signs of acute leukemia are cervical lymphadenopathy, malaise, anemic pallor, leukopenia-induced ulcerations, and gingival changes. Leukemic gingival tissues are usually red, tender, and spongy and tend to peel away from the teeth. With progression of the disease, the swollen gingiva becomes purple and shiny. Stippling of the tissue is lost, and spontaneous bleeding from the gingival sulcus eventually occurs. The edematous tissue is most prominent interdentally and results from leukemic infiltration of leukocytes. In certain patients the neoplastic cells may invade pulpal and osseous tissue, inducing vague symptoms of pain without corresponding radiographic evidence of pathosis. Purpuric features, such as petechial lesions and ecchymoses on pale mucosal membranes, together with gingival hemorrhage, occur frequently. Systemic control of leukemia often involves intensive radiotherapy, chemotherapy, blood transfusions, and bone marrow transplantation. Difficulty may be encountered in maintaining optimal oral health because of the chemotherapy-induced oral ulcerations. Meticulous oral hygiene combined with antimicrobial rinses is recommended to reduce the inflammatory and ulcerative sequelae of chemotherapy.

Agranulocytosis (Neutropenia)

Agranulocytosis (also known as neutropenia) is a disease characterized by a decrease in the number of circulating polymorphonuclear neutrophils. In most instances, the condition is recognized by its clinical symptoms, which consist of chronic infections and an almost complete absence of neutrophils in laboratory blood tests. Antimetabolic, antibiotic, and cytotoxic drugs are the etiologic agents involved in more than half of all cases. In rare instances the condition may be congenital. An uncontrollable infection in the neutropenic patient can result in bacterial pneumonia, sepsis, and death.

Cyclic Neutropenia (Figs. 36.3 and 36.4)

A distinct form of agranulocytosis is cyclic neutropenia, which is characterized by a periodic diminution of circulating polymorphonuclear neutrophils that occurs about every 3 weeks and lasts for about 5 days. The condition is idiopathic and usually begins in childhood. It is sometimes accompanied by arthritis, pharyngitis, fever, headache, and lymphadenopathy. A history of repeated infections of the ear and upper respiratory tract is common. Oral manifestations include inflammatory gingival changes and mucosal ulcerations. The ulcerations are usually large, oval, and persistent. They vary in size and location; they are sometimes found on the attached gingiva and other times on the tongue and buccal mucosa. The gingivitis is periodic and ulcerative. At stages that correspond to elevated levels of polymorphonuclear neutrophils, minimal inflammation is evident. In contrast, when the polymorphonuclear neutrophil count decreases precipitously, generalized inflammatory hyperplasia and erythema occur. If left untreated, the condition is exacerbated by the presence of local factors such as plaque and calculus, which result in alveolar bone loss, tooth mobility, and early exfoliation of teeth.

The periodic appearance and spontaneous regression of signs and symptoms should cause the clinician to suspect cyclic neutropenia. Daily measurement of the leukocyte count is required to diagnose this condition. Curative treatment is unavailable. Management is therefore palliative and consists of antibiotic and antimicrobial therapy and repeated oral prophylaxis.

Thrombocytopathic and Thrombocytopenic Purpura (Figs. 36.5–36.8)

Platelets play an integral role in maintaining hemostasis by providing the primary hemostatic plug and by activating the intrinsic system of coagulation. A decrease in the number of circulating platelets (thrombocytopenia) may be idiopathic or may be the result of decreased platelet production in the bone marrow, increased peripheral destruction, or increased splenic sequestration. Decreased function of circulating platelets (thrombocytopathia) is often related to hereditary syndromes or acquired states such as drug-induced bone marrow suppression, liver disease, or dysproteinemic states like uremia. Mild thrombocytopathia is caused by daily use of aspirin.

The normal platelet count is 150,000 to 400,000 cells/mm^3. Vascular-related clinical manifestations of platelet disorders usually do not develop until the count decreases to less than 75,000 cells/mm^3. These features include petechiae, ecchymoses, epistaxis, hematuria, hypermenorrhea, and gastrointestinal bleeding resulting in melena. Spontaneous gingival bleeding is a frequent, early, and dramatic occurrence. Blood profusely oozes from the gingival sulcus, either spontaneously or after minor trauma such as toothbrushing. The fluid then turns into purplish-black globs of clotted blood that adhere to the oral structures. Clotted blood is sometimes swallowed, which results in nausea. Mild traumas, particularly at the occlusal line of the buccal mucosa and tongue, are sites of extensive hemorrhage. Multifocal red petechial spots on the soft palate are another frequent clinical sign of bleeding disorders. Measurement of the platelet count, clot retraction time, tourniquet test, and template bleeding time should be done to diagnose a platelet disorder. Platelet transfusions may be necessary if local measures do not control oral bleeding.

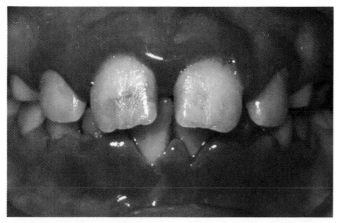

Fig. 36.1. Leukemic gingivitis: acute myelogenous leukemia.

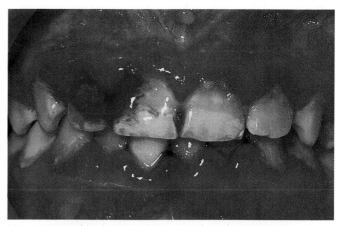

Fig. 36.2. Leukemic gingivitis: acute lymphocytic leukemia.

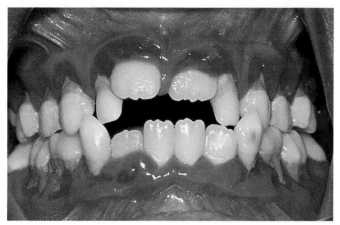

Fig. 36.3. Cyclic neutropenia: gingival erythema.*

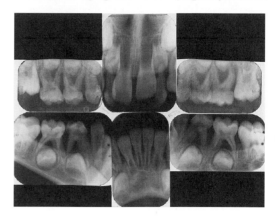

Fig. 36.4. Cyclic neutropenia: floating teeth.*

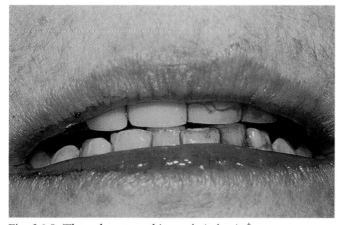

Fig. 36.5. Thrombocytopathia: and cirrhosis.‡

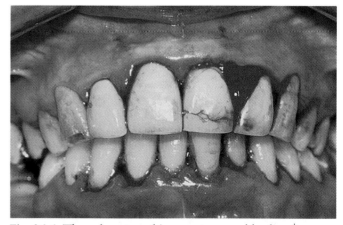

Fig. 36.6. Thrombocytopathia: spontaneous bleeding.‡

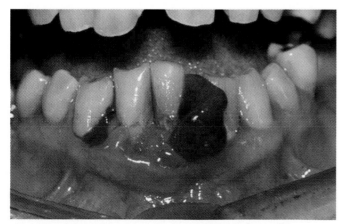

Fig. 36.7. Thrombocytopenia: 26,000 platelets/mm^3.]

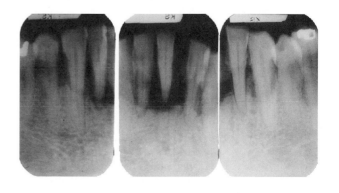

Fig. 36.8. Thrombocytopenia evidence of chronic irritants.]

Abnormalities by Location

Conditions Peculiar to the Tongue

Scalloped Tongue (Crenated Tongue) (Figs. 37.1 and 37.2)

A scalloped tongue is a common finding characterized by indentations on the lateral margins of the tongue. The condition is caused by abnormal pressure (e.g., suction) within the mouth of persons who clench or brux their teeth. It is usually bilateral but may be unilateral or isolated to a region where the tongue is held in close contact with the teeth. The abnormal pressure on the tongue imprints a distinctive pattern that appears as depressed ovals that are sometimes circumscribed by a raised white scalloped border. Causes of scalloped tongue include situations that produce abnormal tongue pressure, such as frictional movement of the tongue against teeth and diastemata, tongue thrusting, tongue sucking, clenching, bruxing, or an enlarged tongue. A prominent linea alba on the buccal mucosa is a frequent coexisting finding caused by the negative intraoral pressure associated with tongue sucking in persons who clench or brux their teeth. A crenated tongue may be seen in association with temporomandibular joint disorders, systemic conditions such as acromegaly and amyloidosis, and genetic disorders such as Down's syndrome, as well as in normal patients. The condition is harmless and asymptomatic. Treatment is aimed at habit elimination.

Macroglossia (Figs. 37.3 and 37.4)

Macroglossia involves an abnormally enlarged tongue. For assessment of tongue size, the tongue should be completely relaxed. The normal height of the dorsum of the tongue should be even with the occlusal plane of the mandibular teeth; the lateral borders of the tongue should be in contact with, but not overlapping, the lingual cusps of the mandibular teeth. A tongue that extends beyond these dimensions is said to be enlarged.

Macroglossia is either congenital or acquired. Congenital macroglossia can be caused by idiopathic muscular hypertrophy, muscular hemihypertrophy, benign tumors, hamartomas, or cysts. Idiopathic muscular hypertrophy is often associated with a mental deficiency or may be a component of a syndrome such as Beckwith-Wiedemann's syndrome. Acquired macroglossia may be the result of passive enlargement of the tongue when mandibular teeth are lost. In this case, the enlargement may be localized or diffuse, depending on the size of the edentulous area. Systemic disease, such as acromegaly, cretinism, and amyloidosis, or malignant neoplasms, which can occlude lymphatic drainage and produce a swollen tongue, can cause macroglossia. Indicators of an enlarged tongue are speech difficulties, displaced teeth, malocclusion, or a scalloped tongue. The affected region of the tongue often demonstrates enlarged fungiform papillae. If the enlarged tongue is hindering function, elimination of the primary cause or surgical correction may be necessary. An enlarged tongue can cause patients to have difficulty accommodating a removable prosthesis.

Hairy Tongue (Lingua Villosa, Coated Tongue) (Figs. 37.5 and 37.6)

Hairy tongue is an abnormal elongation of the filiform papillae that gives the dorsum of the tongue a hairlike appearance. The cause of the hypertrophic response of the filiform papillae is poorly understood but seems to be related to either increased keratin deposition or delayed shedding of the cornified layer. Patients who do not cleanse their tongues are most commonly affected. Cancer therapy, infection with *Candida albicans*, irradiation, poor oral hygiene, change in oral pH, smoking, and the use of antibiotics have also been associated with this condition.

Hairy tongue may be white, yellow, green, brown, or black, hence the names white-coated tongue and yellow, brown, or black hairy tongue. The color of the lesion is a result of intrinsic factors (chromogenic organisms) combined with extrinsic factors (food and tobacco stains). Hairy tongue occurs more frequently in men, primarily in persons older than age 30 years, and the prevalence seems to increase with age. The condition begins near the foramen cecum on the dorsal surface of the tongue and spreads laterally and anteriorly. The affected filiform papillae discolor, progressively elongate, and may reach a length of several millimeters. Generally, hairy tongue is only of cosmetic concern and the tongue remains asymptomatic. Vigorous brushing with abrasive pastes and topical antifungal agents leads to resolution. In refractory cases, an underlying endocrinopathy such as diabetes mellitus should be sought.

Hairy Leukoplakia (Figs. 37.7 and 37.8)

Hairy leukoplakia is a significant leukoplakic-like finding that indicates immunosuppression. The lesion is seen almost exclusively in patients infected with HIV or persons with immunosuppression resulting from drugs taken for organ transplantation or systemic disease. The white lesion is primarily located on the lateral borders of the tongue but may extend to cover the dorsal and ventral surfaces. Replication of Epstein-Barr virus within the affected epithelial cells appears to be causative. Hairy leukoplakia is so named because hairlike peeling of the parakeratotic surface layer is evident histologically. *C. albicans* is frequently associated with this lesion.

Hairy leukoplakia produces white vertical raised folds on the lateral border of the tongue. The lesion initially has alternating faint white folds and adjacent normal pink troughs that produce a characteristic vertical white-banded washboard appearance. The bands eventually coalesce to form discrete white plaques or extensive thick white corrugated patches. Large lesions are usually asymptomatic, have poorly demarcated borders, and do not rub off. Bilateral occurrence is common, but unilateral lesions are possible. Hairy leukoplakia has been documented on the palate and buccal mucosa. Antiviral agents that block or limit replication of Epstein-Barr virus are useful in reducing the size of, or eliminating, the lesions. Discontinuation of drug therapy can result in return of the lesions.

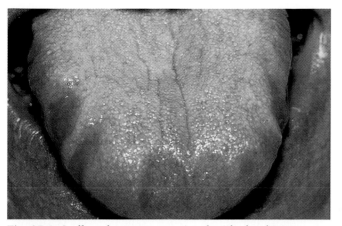

Fig. 37.1. **Scalloped tongue:** associated with clenching.

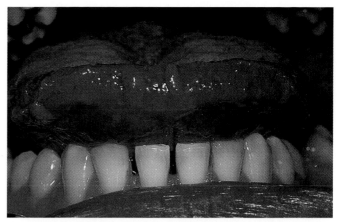

Fig. 37.2. **Scalloped tongue:** caused by tongue sucking.

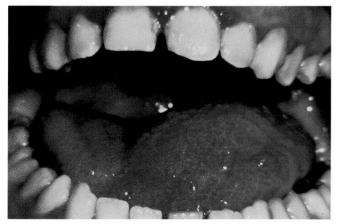

Fig. 37.3. **Macroglossia:** congenital hemihypertrophy.

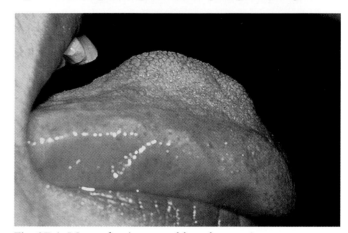

Fig. 37.4. **Macroglossia:** caused by a hemangioma.

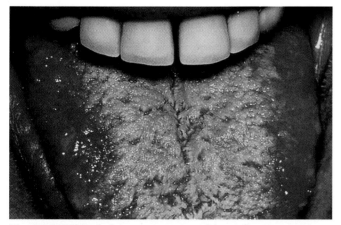

Fig. 37.5. **White hairy tongue:** stomatitis medicamentosa.

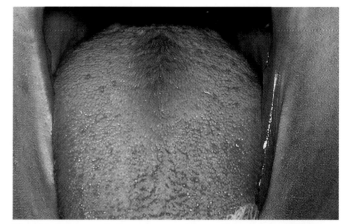

Fig. 37.6. **Brown hairy tongue:** after antibiotics.

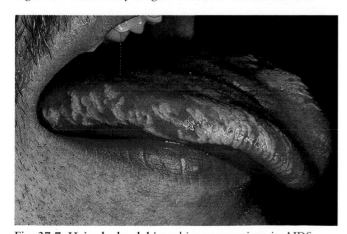

Fig. 37.7. **Hairy leukoplakia:** white corrugations in AIDS.

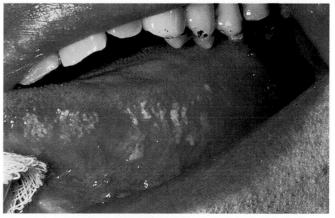

Fig. 37.8. **Hairy leukoplakia:** seen during dental treatment.

Conditions Peculiar to the Tongue

Geographic Tongue (Benign Migratory Glossitis, Erythema Migrans) (Figs. 38.1–38.4)

Geographic tongue is a benign inflammatory condition associated with desquamation of superficial keratin and filiform papillae. The cause is unknown, but emotional stress, nutritional deficiencies, and hereditary factors are suggested. Histologically, the lesion resembles psoriasis, but it is generally accepted that these conditions are distinct. The condition is restricted to the dorsal and lateral borders of the anterior two thirds of the tongue, affecting only the filiform and leaving the fungiform papillae intact.

Geographic tongue manifests in three patterns: 1) patchy areas of desquamated filiform papillae; 2) patchy desquamated areas delineated by raised, white, circinate lines; and 3) patchy areas of desquamated filiform papillae, with or without white circinate lines, bordered by an erythematous band of inflammation. Mixtures of these patterns may be present, and continuously changing patterns and migration from site to site are usual. Symptoms are uncommon in the first two patterns, but presence of the red inflammatory band is often associated with irritation by spicy foods and reports of pain.

Geographic tongue is common, affecting approximately 1% of the population. Women and young adults are most frequently affected. The condition may appear suddenly and persist for months or years. Spontaneous remissions and recurrences are typical.

Geographic Stomatitis (Figs. 38.5 and 38.6)

Geographic tongue is occasionally seen in association with a mucosal counterpart, **geographic stomatitis** (areata erythema migrans, ectopic geographic tongue), and fissured tongue. It produces red annular patches of the labial and buccal mucosa, soft palate, and occasionally floor of mouth. The patches are mild erosions of the mucosa. When asymptomatic, geographic tongue or stomatitis requires no treatment. However, mild burning is common and generally responds to topical anesthetics or topical steroids, in combination with stress reduction.

Anemia (Fig. 38.7)

Anemia is a condition of impaired oxygen delivery to bodily tissues that results from a deficiency in erythrocytes, hemoglobin, or total blood volume. Underlying causes of anemia include increased destruction of erythrocytes caused by hemolysis, increased blood loss caused by hemorrhage, or a decreased production of erythrocytes caused by a nutritional deficiency state or bone marrow suppression. Anemia is a sign of an underlying disease; thus, the cause of anemia must always be sought. Iron deficiency is the most common type of anemia, frequently affecting middle-aged women and young teenagers. It produces a microcytic (small red blood cells) anemia. Deficiencies in vitamin B_{12} and folic acid cause anemia, known as macrocytic anemia (large red blood cells).

Anemia produces changes in the oral mucosal membranes. These alterations, although characteristic, are not helpful in distinguishing the type of anemia causing the features seen. Analysis of erythrocyte indices is required for an accurate diagnosis.

Intraoral manifestations of anemia are most prominent on the tongue. The dorsum of the tongue initially appears pale, with flattening of the filiform papillae. Continued atrophy of the papillae results in a surface that is devoid of papillae and appears smooth, dry, and glazed. This condition is commonly called bald tongue. In the final stage, a beefy or fiery red tongue is seen, sometimes with concurrent oral aphthae.

Anemia may produce a sore, painful (glossodynia) or burning tongue (glossopyrosis). The lips may be thinned and taut, and the width of the mouth may develop a narrowed appearance. Other clinical signs associated with anemia include angular cheilitis, aphthous, dysphagia, mucosal erythema and erosions, pallor, shortness of breath, fatigue, dizziness, and a bounding pulse. Patients with a vitamin B_{12} deficiency may report weight loss, weakness, neurologic disturbances such as numbness and tingling of the extremities, and difficulty in walking. Therapy should be directed toward correcting the underlying cause. Improvement after therapy is reflected by changes in the oral appearance.

Xerostomia (Fig. 38.8)

Saliva keeps the oral cavity moist and aids in mastication, deglutition, digestion, speech, and immunologic neutralization. When impaired salivary function causes a dry mouth, the condition is called **xerostomia**. Manifestations of decreased salivary flow can be subtle with no symptoms or severe with myriad symptoms. Hyposalivation may result from advancing age, anemia, avitaminosis, dehydration, diabetes, emotional stress, mechanical blockage, surgery, collagen vascular disease, ectodermal dysplasia, mumps, Mikulicz's disease, multiple sclerosis, Sjögren's syndrome, AIDS, and head and neck irradiation. Many therapeutic drugs, primarily antidepressant agents, antihistamines, antihypertensive and cardiac agents, decongestants, ganglionic blocking agents, and tranquilizers, also produce xerostomia.

Mild cases of xerostomia are relatively free of symptoms, and the mucosa appears normal. In moderate cases the tongue is dry, pale, red, and atrophic. In severe cases the tongue may be devoid of papillae, fissured, and inflamed. The mucosa appears dry, shiny, and sticky, and the lips appear cracked and fissured. Ropelike accumulations of saliva on the tongue along with burning tongue (glossopyrosis) and alterations in taste are usually present. Progression of xerostomia can result in halitosis, candidiasis, multiple carious lesions evident at the cervical margin, and difficulty with speech, mastication, and retention of prosthodontic appliances. Chronic xerostomia requires long-term multiphasic support, including alternative drug therapy, as well as use of emollients, artificial saliva, sialogogues (pilocarpine, bethanechol, cevimiline), fluoride treatment, oral hygiene instructions, antifungal agents, and nutritional counseling.

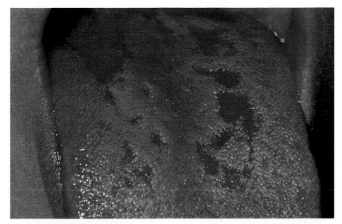

Fig. 38.1. **Geographic tongue:** asymptomatic denuded areas.

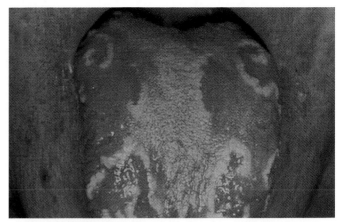

Fig. 38.2. **Geographic tongue:** asymptomatic white regions.

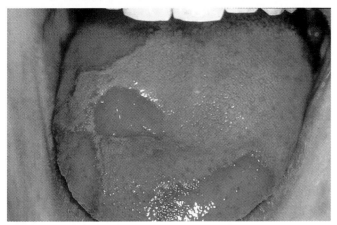

Fig. 38.3. **Geographic tongue:** red and painful.

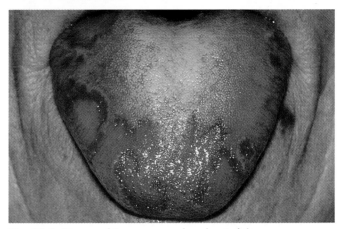

Fig. 38.4. **Geographic tongue:** red and painful.

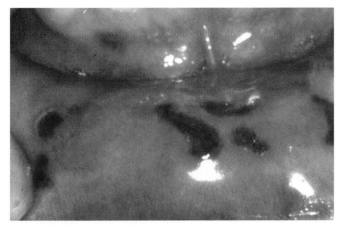

Fig. 38.5. **Geographic stomatitis:** symptomatic labial mucosa.

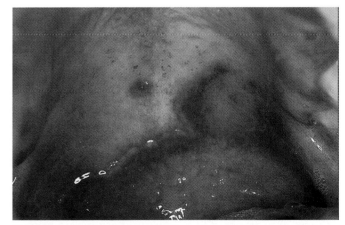

Fig. 38.6. **Geographic stomatitis:** annular pattern on palate.

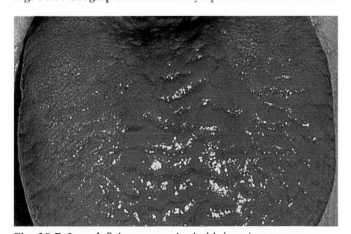

Fig. 38.7. **Iron deficiency anemia:** bald, burning tongue.

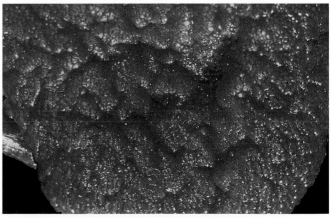

Fig. 38.8. **Xerostomia:** dry, fissured atrophic tongue.

Conditions Peculiar to the Tongue

Cyst of Blandin-Nuhn (Lingual Mucus-Retention Phenomenon) (Fig. 39.1) The glands of Blandin-Nuhn are accessory salivary glands on the ventral surface of the tongue composed of mixed serous and mucous elements. The cyst develops when trauma to the ventral tongue induces extravasation of saliva into the surrounding tissues. It appears as a small painless pink-red swelling with raised and well-demarcated borders. The lesion is soft and fluctuant. When superficial, the cyst has balloonlike features and a pedunculated base; deeper lesions have sessile bases. Although usually induced by trauma, the cyst of Blandin-Nuhn may be congenital. The congenital variant may represent a true epithelial-lined salivary duct cyst. These cysts rarely exceed 1 cm in diameter. Treatment is excisional biopsy.

Median Rhomboid Glossitis (Central Papillary Atrophy of the Tongue) (Figs. 39.2–39.4) Median rhomboid glossitis was once thought to be a developmental defect of incomplete descent of the tuberculum impar. This theory is no longer valid. It is now accepted that median rhomboid glossitis is a permanent result of a *C. albicans* infection in conjunction with other factors (possibly smoking or a change in oral pH). Median rhomboid glossitis frequently affects middle-aged men and rarely affects children. There is no racial predilection. The prevalence is often higher in patients who have diabetes, are immunosuppressed, or have completed a course of broad-spectrum antibiotics.

Median rhomboid glossitis is a smooth, denuded, beefy red patch devoid of filiform papillae. With time the lesion becomes granular and lobular. The most common location is the midline of the dorsum of the tongue, just anterior to the circumvallate papillae. The size and shape of the lesion varies, but the lesion frequently appears as a well-demarcated 1- to 2.5-cm oval or rhomboid with irregular but rounded borders. The condition is generally asymptomatic. An erythematous palatal candidal lesion is sometimes observed directly over the lesion of the tongue. In this case, the condition is termed **chronic multifocal candidiasis** (Figs. 39.3 and 39.4).

Median rhomboid glossitis is easily recognized by its clinical appearance, characteristic location, and asymptomatic nature. Early recognition and treatment with antimonilial agents usually leads to resolution. End-stage median rhomboid glossitis is usually asymptomatic but refractory to antifungal treatment as the lesion becomes fibrotic and hypovascular.

Granular Cell Tumor (Figs. 39.5 and 39.6) The granular cell tumor is a rare benign soft tissue tumor composed of oval cells that have an extremely granular cytoplasm. This tumor may occur in cutaneous, mucosal, and visceral sites, but about 50% of cases occur in the dorsal-lateral surface of the tongue. Its histogenesis is controversial. Most investigators believe that the tumor is a benign proliferation of neurogenic cells.

The granular cell tumor can occur at any age and in any race, but it has a slight predilection for women.

Usually the lesion consists of an asymptomatic, solitary, dome-shaped submucosal nodule covered clinically by normal, yellow, or white tissue. The surface may be ulcerated when it has been traumatized. The granular cell tumor is often sessile, well circumscribed, and firm to compression. Growth is very slow and painless; some tumors grow to several centimeters in size. Larger lesions may demonstrate a slightly depressed central area. In rare cases, these lesions are found on the ventral surface of the tongue or buccal mucosa. Approximately 10% of affected patients experience multiple lesions.

The granular cell tumor is characterized by pseudoepitheliomatous hyperplasia and granular cells that may histologically resemble epidermoid carcinoma or the congenital epulis of the newborn. Conservative local excision is the preferred treatment. These lesions do not tend to recur.

Lingual Thyroid (Fig. 39.7) Lingual thyroid is an uncommon nodule of thyroid tissue found just posterior to the foramen cecum on the posterior third of the tongue. It occurs when embryonic tissue from the thyroid gland fails to migrate to the anterolateral surface of the trachea. Persistent thyroid tissue occurs much more frequently in women than in men (the ratio is 4:1) and may appear at any age. If the remnant tissue becomes cystic the condition becomes a **thyroglossal duct cyst**.

The lingual thyroid is a raised asymptomatic mass that is usually about 2 cm in diameter. Increased surface vascularity is a prominent feature. Hemorrhage, dysphagia, dysphonia, symptoms of hypothyroidism, and (rarely) pain can be associated with the condition. Clinicians can differentiate the lesion from similar lesions by confirming its distinctive location posterior to the circumvallate papillae and by using uptake studies of radioactive iodine. Biopsy should be deferred until it is ascertained that the rest of the thyroid gland is present and functioning. In more than 50% of patients with ectopic thyroid, the lingual thyroid is the only active thyroid tissue present.

Body Piercing (Tongue Barbell) (Fig. 39.8) Body piercing is the placement of a foreign object through tissue of the body. The object(s) is placed for cosmetic and social reasons, with some cultures initiating piercing in the very young, whereas others elect to be pierced during adolescence or throughout life. In the United States, body piercing is usually performed in tattoo parlors without anesthesia and minor regard for infection control. Common extraoral locations include the ears, eyebrows, ala of the nose, belly button, and breast nipple. Intraorally, the mucobuccal fold of the lower lip and the tongue are common sites. A popular object placed in the pierced tongue is the metallic barbell. Common adverse events associated with piercing include infection, swelling and bleeding, allergic reactions, and tooth fractures. They need to be removed before taking radiographs, and patients should be advised of the potential adversities associated with these objects.

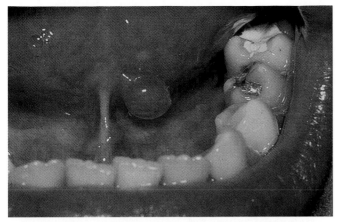

Fig. 39.1. Cyst of Blandin-Nuhn: variant of a mucocele.

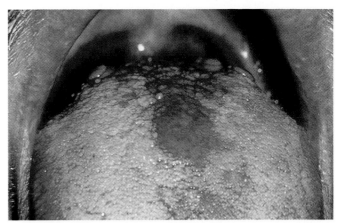

Fig. 39.2. Median rhomboid glossitis: typical presentation.

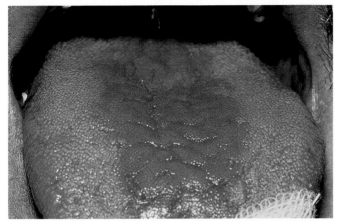

Fig. 39.3. Median rhomboid glossitis: smooth denuded patch.*

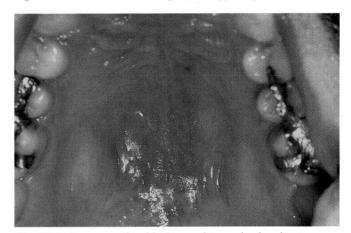

Fig. 39.4. Contact palatal lesion: red irregular border.*

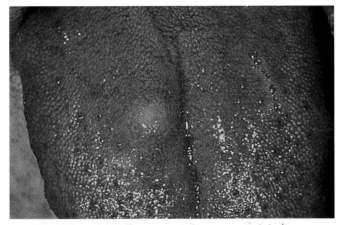

Fig. 39.5. Granular cell tumor: pink tongue nodule.‡

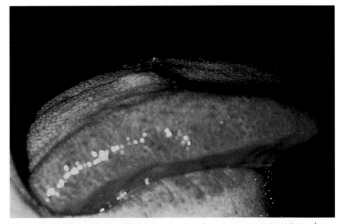

Fig. 39.6. Granular cell tumor: raised appearance evident.‡

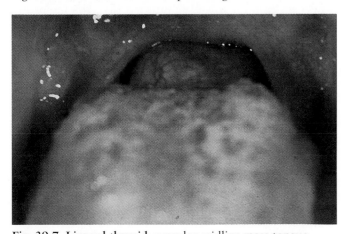

Fig. 39.7. Lingual thyroid: vascular midline mass tongue.

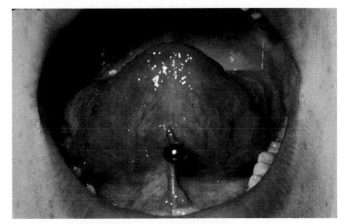

Fig. 39.8. Body piercing: tongue barbell.

Conditions Peculiar to the Lip

Actinic Cheilosis (Actinic Cheilitis) (Figs. 40.1 and 40.2) Actinic cheilosis is a clinical lesion of the lower lip caused by excessive solar radiation damage. Older, fair-skinned men with outdoor occupations are typically affected. In early stages, the lower lip is mildly keratotic with a subtle blending of the vermilion border with the adjacent skin. With increased exposure to the sun, focal white zones that have distinct or diffuse borders become apparent. The lip slowly becomes firm, scaly, slightly swollen, fissured, and everted. Ulceration with encrustation is typical of the chronic condition. The ulcers may be caused by loss of elasticity, or they may be an early sign of dysplastic or carcinomatous transformation. Histologic features include atrophic thinning of the epithelium, subepithelial basophilic degeneration of collagen, and increased elastin fibers. Biopsy is recommended to rule out similar sun-related diseases such as epithelial dysplasia, carcinoma in situ, basal cell carcinoma, squamous cell carcinoma, malignant melanoma, keratoacanthoma, cheilitis glandularis, and herpes labialis.

Actinic cheilosis is considered a precancerous condition. Clinicians should warn the patient of the likelihood of disease progression without the use of sunscreen protective agents. Dysplastic changes should be treated surgically or by topical application of 5-fluorouracil.

Candidal Cheilitis (Figs. 40.3 and 40.4) Candidal cheilitis is an inflammatory condition of the lips associated with *C. albicans* and a lip-licking habit. It is believed that the candidal organisms obtain access to the surface layers of the labial epithelium after mucosal breakdown, which is caused by repeated wetting and drying of the labial tissues. Desquamation and fissuring of surface epithelium results, and a fine whitish scale consisting of dried salivary mucous may be seen. In children, the affected perilabial skin appears red, atrophic, and fissured. Chapped, dry, itchy, burning lips and the inability to eat hot spicy foods are frequent symptoms. Chronic infection is characterized by painful vertical fissures that ulcerate and are slow to heal. A hypersensitivity reaction to ingredients contained in lip balms or lipsticks may mimic the condition. In candidal cheilitis the lip-licking habit perpetuates the condition. Although nystatin ointment is helpful, ultimate resolution requires elimination of the habit. In persistent cases, an underlying systemic problem such as diabetes mellitus or human immunodeficiency virus infection should be ruled out.

Angular Cheilitis (Perleche) (Figs. 40.5 and 40.6) Angular cheilitis is a painful condition consisting of radiating erythematous fissures at the corners of the mouth. The condition is most commonly seen after the age of 50 years and is usually encountered in women and denture wearers. The cause is believed to be associated with a mixed infection of *C. albicans* and *Staphylococcus aureus*.

Angular cheilitis results from repeated pooling of saliva and carriage of pathogens from the mouth to the region. Licking the corners of the mouth (perleche: to lick in French) contributes to the perpetuation of this disease. Patients often perform this unconscious habit in an effort to provide relief to the area.

Angular cheilitis initially produces soft, red, and ulcerated mucocutaneous tissue at the corners of the mouth. With time the erythematous fissures become deep and extend several centimeters from the commissure onto the perilabial skin or ulcerate and involve the labial and buccal mucosa. The ulcers frequently develop crusts that split and reulcerate during normal oral function. Small yellow-brown granulomatous nodules may eventually appear. Bleeding is infrequent.

Angular cheilitis is chronic and usually bilateral and is often associated with denture stomatitis or glossitis. Predisposing conditions include anemia, poor oral hygiene, frequent use of broad-spectrum antibiotics, decreased vertical dimension, high sucrose intake, dry mouth, flaccid perioral folds, and vitamin B deficiency. Treatment should include preventive measures (such as elimination of traumatic factors, meticulous oral hygiene, reestablishment of the correct vertical dimension and salivary flow) combined with topical antifungal and antibiotic therapy. Vitamin supplementation may also prove beneficial. Elimination of any lip-licking habit is also part of the management protocol.

Exfoliative Cheilitis (Figs. 40.7 and 40.8) Exfoliative cheilitis is a persistent condition affecting the lips that is characterized by fissuring, desquamation, and the formation of hemorrhagic crusts. *C. albicans*, oral sepsis, stress, and habitual lip-licking and biting are etiologic agents. An association with psychological and thyroid disorders has been reported. This condition usually begins as a single fissure near the midline of the lower lip and spreads to produce multiple fissures. The fissures may ultimately develop a yellow-white scale or ulcerate and form hemorrhagic crusts over the entire lip. The condition is often bothersome and unsightly; the lower lip is more adversely affected than the upper lip. When the condition is symptomatic, burning is the usual chief symptom. Exfoliative cheilitis has a predisposition for teenage girls and young women, and stress has been reported to cause acute exacerbations. Because the cause of the condition appears to be multifactorial, exfoliative cheilitis is difficult to manage and may persist for many years. Treatment is best rendered through the elimination of predisposing systemic or psychological factors together with topical application of antifungal ointments.

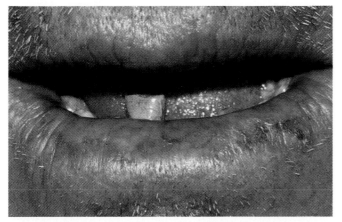

Fig. 40.1. **Actinic cheilosis:** vermilion border lost and scaly.

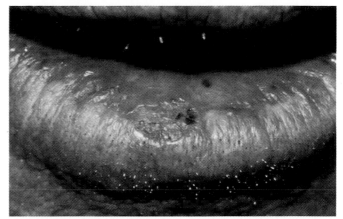

Fig. 40.2. **Actinic cheilosis:** everted, thickened with crusts.

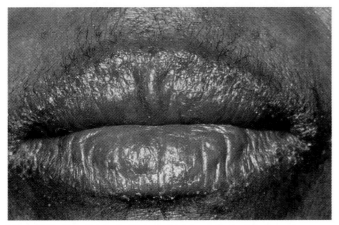

Fig. 40.3. **Candidal cheilitis:** whitish scale is dried mucin.

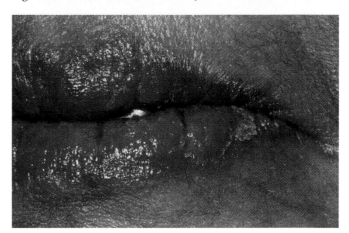

Fig. 40.4. **Candidal cheilitis:** in an uncontrolled diabetic.

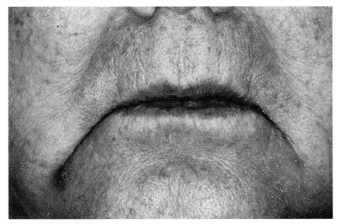

Fig. 40.5. **Angular cheilitis:** flaccid perioral folds.*

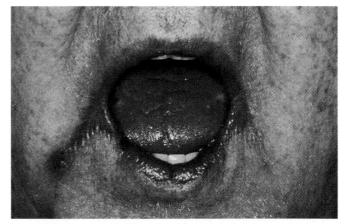

Fig. 40.6. **Angular cheilitis:** in older adult.*

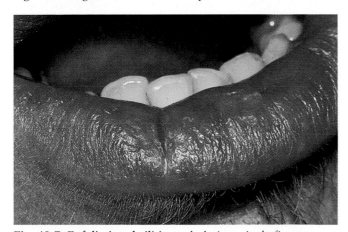

Fig. 40.7. **Exfoliative cheilitis:** early lesion; single fissure.

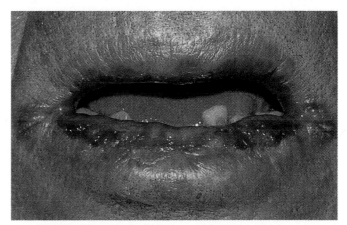

Fig. 40.8. **Exfoliative cheilitis:** hemorrhagic crusts.

Nodules of the Lip

Mucocele (Mucus Extravasation Phenomenon) (Figs. 41.1 and 41.2)

The mucocele results from retention of mucous secretions in subepithelial tissue when a salivary gland duct is severed. Most mucoceles are associated with traumatized accessory salivary gland ducts of the mandibular labial mucosa. They lack an epithelial lining and are usually surrounded by granulomatous tissue. The **ranula** is a variant mucocele of the floor of the mouth caused by trauma to a sublingual gland duct (Bartholin's duct) and rarely Wharton's duct of the submandibular gland. Mucoceles are distinguished from the rare salivary duct cyst (mucous retention cyst), which is a true cyst with an epithelial lining (Fig. 39.1).

The mucocele constitutes the most common nodular swelling of the lower lip. These swellings are asymptomatic, soft, fluctuant, bluish-gray, and usually less than 1 cm in diameter. Enlargement coincident with meals may be an occasional finding. The most common location is the lower lip midway between the midline and commissure, but other locations include the buccal mucosa, palate, floor of the mouth, and ventral tongue. Children and young adults are most frequently affected. Trauma is the etiologic agent.

Superficial mucoceles often regress spontaneously, whereas deep-seated mucoceles tend to persist and exacerbate with repeated trauma. Persistent mucoceles are treated by surgical excision. Recurrence is possible if the involved accessory salivary glands are not removed or if other ducts are severed during the procedure.

Accessory Salivary Gland Tumor (Figs. 41.3 and 41.4)

Nodular swellings of the upper lip are infrequent and are usually caused by benign neoplasia of the minor salivary glands, such as the canalicular adenoma and pleomorphic adenoma. Benign accessory salivary gland tumors constitute approximately 10% of all salivary gland tumors and are characterized by encapsulation, slow growth, and long duration (several months). Persons older than age 30 years are more commonly affected. Clinical examination shows the pleomorphic adenoma to be a pink to purple dome-shaped or multinodular lesion that protrudes from the inner aspect of the lip or vestibule. It is usually semisolid, freely movable, painless, and especially firm on palpation. The border is well circumscribed. Although it has unlimited potential for growth, the tumor generally remains less than 2 cm in diameter. Fluctuance and surface ulceration are not usual clinical features.

Malignant salivary gland tumors, such as mucoepidermoid carcinoma and adenocarcinoma, are rare in the upper lip and may be distinguished from benign neoplasia by their rapid and aggressive growth, short duration, and tendency to ulcerate and cause neurologic symptoms. Treatment of salivary gland neoplasia consists of surgical excision. If the excision is incomplete, recurrences are possible.

Nasolabial Cyst (Nasoalveolar Cyst) (Figs. 41.5 and 41.6)

The nasolabial cyst is a developmental cyst of soft tissue located in the cuspid–lateral incisor region of the upper lip. The cause is uncertain, and two theories have been suggested. The most accepted theory is that epithelial remnants become entrapped during the embryologic fusion of the lateral nasal, globular, and maxillary processes. A more recent theory suggests that the tissue originates from the nasolacrimal duct. Proliferation and cystic degeneration of the entrapped tissue usually do not become clinically evident until after age 30 years, even though the tissue has been entrapped since birth. The condition has a slight female predilection.

The nasolabial cyst is a palpable soft tissue mass under the upper lip that may cause elevation of the ala of the nose, as well as dilatation of the nostril and alteration of the nasolabial fold. The intraoral cyst may be tense or fluctuant, depending on size, and can affect the fit of a maxillary denture. Aspiration yields a yellowish or straw-colored fluid. The cyst is most often unilateral and is generally not in contact with the adjacent bone; thus, the maxillary teeth remain vital. Infrequently, if the nasolabial cyst applies pressure to the adjacent bone, local resorption of osseous structures can result. Treatment is simple excision.

Implantation Cyst (Epithelial Inclusion Cyst) (Fig. 41.7)

An implantation cyst is an unusual cyst arising from a foreign-body reaction to surface epithelium that is implanted within epidermal structures after traumatic laceration. The cyst can occur intraorally or extraorally, at any age, and in any race or sex. Within the mouth, the lesion appears as a firm, dome-shaped, freely movable nodule located at the site of impetus, which is often the lip. Implantation cysts are usually small, solitary, and asymptomatic. Growth appears to remain constant, and the overlying mucosa appears smooth and pink. There is no swelling at mealtimes nor is there spontaneous drainage of mucin as seen in mucocele. A history of trauma should also lead the clinician to suspect this lesion. Surgical excision and histopathologic examination are recommended.

Mesenchymal Nodules and Tumors (Fig. 41.8)

A variety of mesenchymal tumors, such as fibroma, lipofibroma, and neuroma, can cause nodular swellings of the lip. The example shown here is a neurofibroma. Neurofibromas may be solitary or found in conjunction with **von Recklinghausen's disease** (Figs. 62.7 and 62.8). When solitary, the neurofibroma is usually an asymptomatic, sessile, smooth-surfaced nodule of the buccal mucosa, gingiva, palate, or lips. Histologic examination of the tumor shows connective tissue and nerve fibrils. The discovery of a solitary neurofibroma requires close examination for multiple neurofibromatosis because the latter condition is associated with a marked tendency toward malignant transformation.

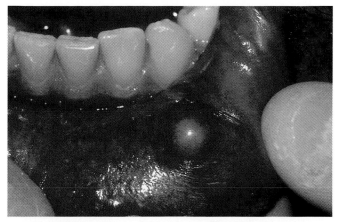

Fig. 41.1. Mucocele: small bluish superficial swelling.

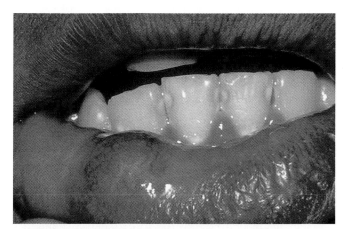

Fig. 41.2. Mucocele: bluish larger and deeper lesion.

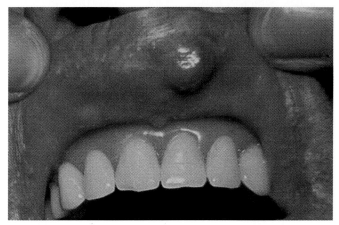

Fig. 41.3. Pleomorphic adenoma: a firm bluish nodule.

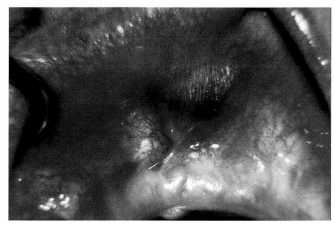

Fig. 41.4. Canalicular adenoma: purplish labial nodule.

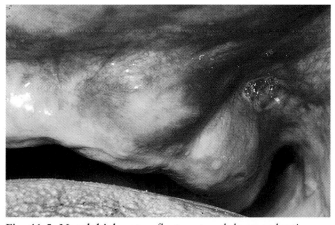

Fig. 41.5. Nasolabial cyst: a fluctuant nodule on palpation.

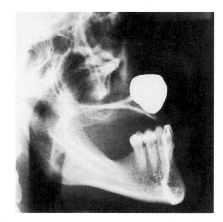

Fig. 41.6. Nasolabial cyst: injected with contrast medium.

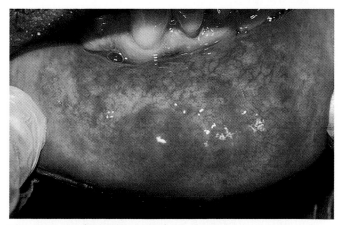

Fig. 41.7. Implantation cyst: from trauma.

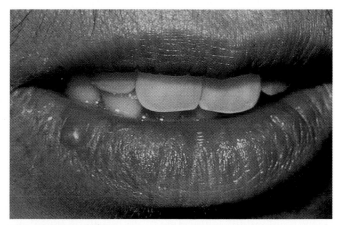

Fig. 41.8. Neurofibroma: sessile base, normal color.

Swellings of the Lip

Angioedema (Angioneurotic Edema) (Figs. 42.1 and 42.2)
Angioedema is a hypersensitivity reaction characterized by the accumulation of fluid within the facial tissues that results in soft, swollen areas under the skin. It occurs in hereditary and acquired forms and may be generalized or localized. Most cases of angioedema are acquired and result from IgE-mediated mast cell degranulation and release of histamine because of antigenic stimuli introduced systematically (such as through food consumption) or by contact, infection, or stress. Histamine mediates capillary permeability and the leakage of plasma into the soft tissues. Swelling develops within minutes or gradually over a few hours and is of transient duration. When swelling affects the lips it is usually uniform and diffuse but may be asymmetrical. The vermilion border appears stretched, everted, pliable, and less distinct; the surface epithelium remains normal in color or is slightly red. Swellings of the tongue, floor of the mouth, eyelids, face, and extremities may accompany the condition. Acquired angioedema is usually recurrent and self-limiting and poses little threat to the patient. Symptoms are limited to burning or itching. Management involves prescription of antihistamines, identification and withdrawal of allergenic stimuli, and stress reduction.

Angiotensin-converting enzyme drugs that are used for treating hypertension can cause angioedema in association with increased bradykinin levels. Infections and autoimmune disease can also induce angioedema by triggering capillary permeability via the formation of antigen-antibody complexes or by elevating numbers of eosinophils.

There are two types of the rare hereditary form of angioedema (type I and type II). Both are autosomal dominant. They occur in association with activation of the complement pathway. Pharyngeal and laryngeal involvement are usual and may be life-threatening. Hereditary angioedema responds poorly to epinephrine, corticosteroids, and antihistamines. Management involves avoidance of violent physical activity; androgenic drugs, such as danocrine (Danazol), help to prevent attacks.

Cheilitis Glandularis (Fig. 42.3)
Cheilitis glandularis is a chronic inflammatory disorder of the accessory labial salivary glands that most frequently affects older men. The lower lip is particularly susceptible and is characterized by diffuse enlargement and eversion of the lip. Although the cause remains poorly understood, the condition is associated with chronic exposure to the sun and wind and, less frequently, with smoking, poor oral hygiene, bacterial infection, and congenital predisposition.

Clinical manifestations of cheilitis glandularis include a symmetrically enlarged, everted, and firm lower lip. With time, the inflamed labial accessory salivary glands become dilated and appear as multiple small red spots. From these ductal openings a viscous, yellowish, mucopurulent exudate is secreted that makes the lip sticky. Progression of the condition causes the lip to appear atrophic, dry, fissured, and scaly and to become painful. Distinction of the vermilion border is eventually lost, and secondary infection of a deep labial fissure often results in fistulation and scarring. Emollients and sunscreens afford protection; severe cases require vermilionectomy, which produces an excellent esthetic result. These patients are at an increased risk for malignant transformation to squamous cell carcinoma.

Orofacial Granulomatosis (Cheilitis Granulomatosa) (Figs. 42.4–42.6)
Orofacial granulomatosis is a noncaseating granulomatous condition resulting in nonpainful symmetric enlargement of orofacial tissues. The condition has two clinical variants: cheilitis granulomatosa, which usually involves only the lips, and **Melkersson-Rosenthal syndrome**, which has the features of unilateral facial paralysis, fissured pebbly tongue, and persistent labiofacial swelling. The cause of orofacial granulomatosis is unknown, and there is no gender predilection. The labial swelling develops slowly at a young age. Both lips may be firm and swollen, but symmetric enlargement of the lower lip is more common. The diffuse enlargement is asymptomatic and does not affect the color of the lip, but discrete nodules can often be palpated. The tongue, buccal mucosa, gingiva, palatal mucosa, and face have also been associated with this condition. Steroids and surgery have been used with limited success. Select patients have responded to elimination of odontogenic infection and management of systemic disorders. Spontaneous regression is possible.

Trauma (Fig. 42.7)
Trauma to the lips often results in edema that is fluctuant, irregular, and exquisitely painful. The trauma may originate from an external source or may be self-induced. External trauma may damage the soft tissue of the lip, resulting in laceration or hemorrhage. Tooth fracture may accompany the condition.

Traumatic enlargement of the lip is often a problem of children and mentally handicapped patients who inadvertently chew their lip while under local anesthesia. The best management for this type of lip injury is to limit the traumatic influence, apply ice compresses, and treat any lacerations or hemorrhage as soon as possible.

Cellulitis (Fig. 42.8)
Cellulitis means inflammation of cellular tissue. This degenerative process is caused by a bacterial infection in which localization of purulent material has yet to occur. When of dental origin, cellulitis typically produces grossly edematous facial tissue that is warm and painful to touch and is extremely hard to palpation. A firm, diffusely swollen lip may be the first sign of cellulitis of odontogenic origin in the anterior region. A nonvital tooth is usually the root of the problem. Failure of host defense mechanisms to control the infection can result in an abscess or spread of infection. Treatment involves extirpation of necrotic pulpal tissue, drainage, culture, antibiotic sensitivity testing, and antibiotic therapy. Injection of local anesthetic into the inflammatory region should be avoided to minimize spread of the infection.

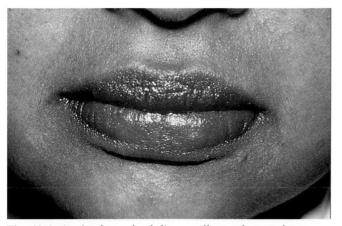

Fig. 42.1. **Angioedema:** both lips swollen and everted.

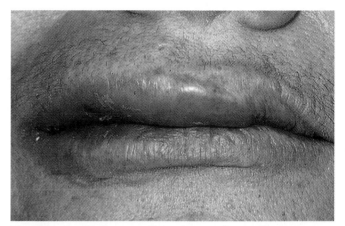

Fig. 42.2. **Angioedema:** unilateral upper lip swelling.

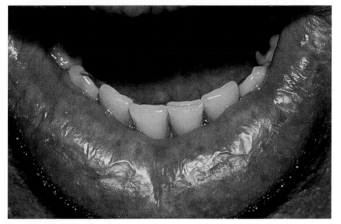

Fig. 42.3. **Cheilitis glandularis:** everted lip; red spots.

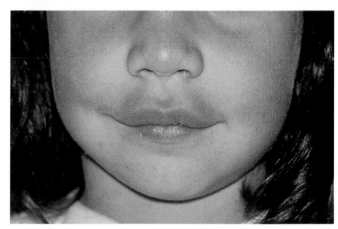

Fig. 42.4. **Melkersson-Rosenthal syndrome:** facial paralysis.*

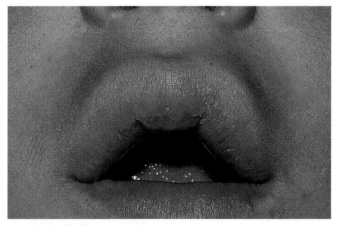

Fig. 42.5. **Cheilitis granulomatosa.***

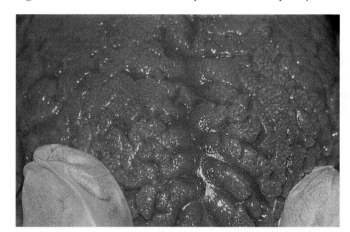

Fig. 42.6. **Melkersson-Rosenthal syndrome:** fissured tongue.*

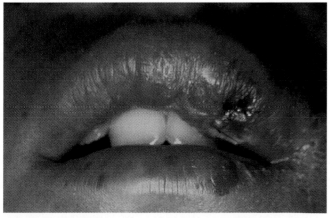

Fig. 42.7. **Trauma:** swollen, ulcerated upper lip.

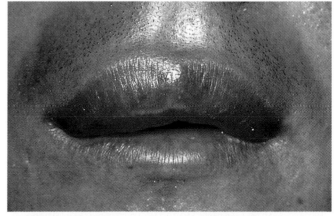

Fig. 42.8. **Cellulitis:** lip swelling; abscessed incisor.

Swellings of the Floor of the Mouth

Dermoid Cyst (Figs. 43.1 and 43.2) The dermoid cyst is a developmental cyst classified as a cystic form of teratoma. The cyst may occur anywhere on the skin but has a propensity for the floor of the mouth. Although a few appear very early in life, most occur in adults younger than 35 years of age. There is no sex predilection.

When the dermoid cyst arises above the mylohyoid muscle, it appears as a painless midline, dome-shaped mass arising in the floor of the mouth. The overlying mucosa is a natural pink, the tongue is slightly elevated, and palpation yields a doughlike consistency. Patients may report difficulties in eating and speaking. The cyst grows slowly, but diameters in excess of 5 cm may be seen. Dermoid cysts may appear below the floor of the mouth if the original site of development is inferior to the mylohyoid muscle. In this instance a submental swelling is noted. The lesion is histologically distinguished from an epidermoid cyst by the presence of adnexal structures such as sebaceous glands, sweat glands, and hair follicles in the fibrous wall. The lumen contains semisolid keratin and sebum that accounts for the doughy consistency and makes aspiration difficult. Surgical enucleation is the preferred treatment.

Ranula (Mucocele of the Sublingual Gland) (Figs. 43.3 and 43.4) Ranula refers to large mucoceles of the floor of the mouth. Like other mucoceles, a ranula is caused by pooling of saliva within submucosal tissue, and arises after trauma to a salivary gland duct. A ranula is usually much larger than a mucocele. Most involve the major excretory duct of the sublingual gland (ducts of Bartholin) or submandibular gland (Wharton's duct). Less commonly they arise from severed ducts of accessory salivary glands in the floor of mouth. No sex predilection is apparent, and persons younger than 40 years of age are most commonly affected.

There are two types of ranulae: the more common superficial ranula that appears as a soft compressible swelling rising up from the floor of mouth, and the dissecting or plunging ranula that penetrates below the mylohyoid muscle to produce a submental swelling. The superficial ranula is characteristically translucent or bluish; it is unilateral, dome-shaped, and fluctuant. As the asymptomatic lesion enlarges, the mucosa becomes stretched, thinned, and tense. Unlike with a dermoid cyst, digital pressure does not cause the lesion to pit. However, it can rupture causing mucous fluid to escape. The entire floor of the mouth may be filled by the swelling, which elevates the tongue and hinders movement. This impairs mastication, deglutition, and speech.

A ranula should be differentiated from other floor-of-the-mouth swellings such as dermoid cysts and salivary gland tumors (i.e., mucoepidermoid carcinoma of the submandibular gland). Sialography and biopsy aid in the diagnosis. Treatment is excision or marsupialization (Partsch operation), which consists of excising the overlying mucosa and suturing the remaining cystic lining to the floor of the mouth along the margins of the incision.

Incision and drainage are not the treatment of choice as they may reaccumulate fluid. Recurrences are common in ill-managed cases involving a plunging ranula or superficial ranula. Removal of the affected major salivary gland is required for recurrent and plunging ranulae.

Salivary Duct Cyst (Fig. 43.5) The salivary duct cyst is an epithelium-lined recess that arises within salivary gland ductal tissue, either the major or minor glands. They are slow-growing and asymptomatic fluctuant swellings that frequently develop in the lip, buccal mucosa, floor of the mouth, or parotid gland. When superficial they are blue or amber in color; deep lesions do not alter the color of the mucosa. Treatment is excision.

Salivary Calculi (Sialoliths) (Fig. 43.6) Sialoliths or salivary stones are accretions of calcium complexes within a salivary gland or duct that may obstruct salivary flow and cause floor-of-the-mouth swelling. They are usually round or oval and smooth or rough surfaced. Concentric laminations of different densities are often seen. Stones occur most frequently after age 25 years, twice as often in men as in women, and usually in the submandibular gland. The ascending course of the excretory duct, along with high mucous content and alkaline pH of the saliva, are significant factors in stone formation.

Obstruction of salivary flow by a calculus in Wharton's duct results in a floor-of-the-mouth swelling that is firm, tender, and painful. Acute symptoms often recur at meal time. Swelling may extend along the course of the excretory duct and last for hours or days, depending on the blockage. The overlying mucosa usually remains pink, unless secondarily infected. In this case, the mucosa may turn red and pus may emanate from the ductal opening. Another sequela is the development of salivary duct cyst that represents ductal dilatation caused by increased intraductal pressure. Management of calculi involves appropriate occlusal radiographs, sialography (if no infection is present), and surgical removal of the sialolith. Localized cellulitis and fever require the use of antibiotics before invasive procedures.

Mucocele (Mucus-Retention Phenomenon) (Figs. 43.7 and 43.8) The mucocele is a soft fluctuant lesion involving the retention of mucus in subepithelial tissue, usually as a result of trauma (possibly iatrogenic) to a salivary gland duct. These clear or bluish swellings may occur on the lip, floor of the mouth, ventral tongue, palate, or buccal mucosa. They are usually asymptomatic and less than 1 cm in diameter. The base of the mucus-retention phenomenon is commonly sessile, although pedunculated bases are possible. Children and young adults are most frequently affected. Superficial lesions may heal spontaneously, whereas persistent lesions should be excised and examined microscopically. If the condition is managed properly, recurrences are rare.

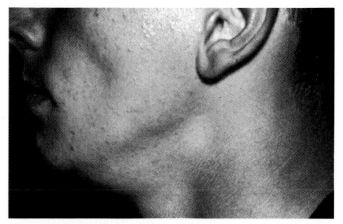

Fig. 43.1. **Dermoid cyst:** below mylohyoid muscle.

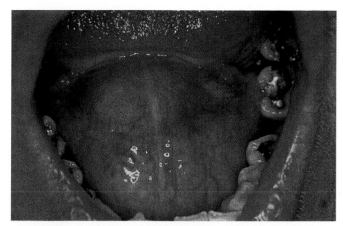

Fig. 43.2. **Dermoid cyst:** above mylohyoid muscle.

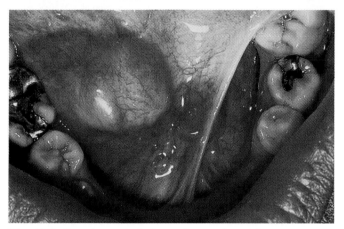

Fig. 43.3. **Ranula:** typical size, color, and translucency.

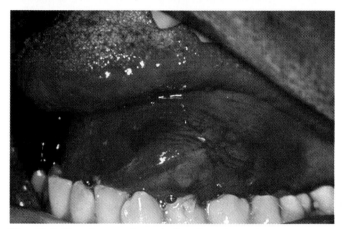

Fig. 43.4. **Ranula:** rare large lesion; impairs eating.

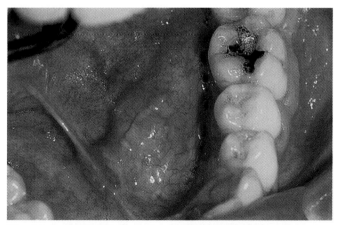

Fig. 43.5. **Salivary duct cyst:** caused by sialolith.

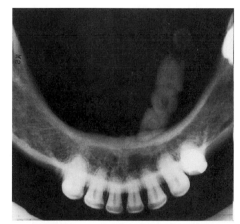

Fig. 43.6. **Sialoliths:** concentric laminations of several calculi.

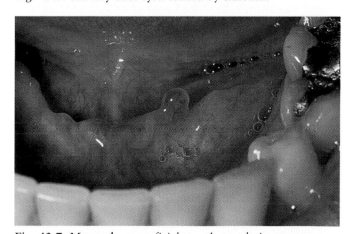

Fig. 43.7. **Mucocele:** superficial translucent lesion.

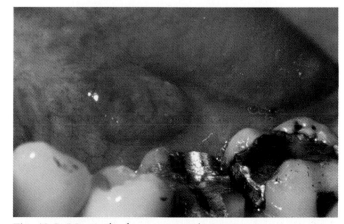

Fig. 43.8. **Mucocele:** from trauma during crown preparation.

Swellings of the Palate

Palatal Torus (Torus Palatinus) (Fig. 44.1) A palatal torus is a bony exostosis located in the midline of the hard palate adjacent to bicuspid or molar teeth. It affects approximately 20% of adults. They are frequently inherited. The incidence is higher in women than men. After puberty there is a tendency for slow growth.

Tori vary greatly in size and shape. The flat torus sits on a broad base; the surface is smooth and minimally convex. The spindle torus is an enlarged, narrow, bony ridge along the midline of the palate. The lobular torus sits on a single base and is divided into lobules by one or several grooves. The covering mucosa is pale pink, thin, and delicate; the boundary of the lesion is distinct.

The palatal torus is frequently asymptomatic unless traumatized, with some patients unaware of the torus until after the traumatic episode. Palatal tori should be removed if they interfere with mastication, phonetics, playing a musical instrument, or a prosthetic appliance.

Lipoma (Fig. 44.2) The lipoma is a common benign mesenchymal tumor, but an uncommon intraoral finding. It is composed of adipocytes and appears as a well-circumscribed, dome-shaped yellowish submucosal mass. The buccal mucosa, tongue, floor of the mouth, and alveolar fold are common sites. The palate is a rare site of involvement. Treatment is excision. (See Fig. 62.3 for complete description.)

Nasopalatine Duct Cyst (Incisive Canal Cyst) (Figs. 44.3 and 44.4) The nasopalatine duct cyst is a developmental cyst that arises from entrapped squamous or respiratory epithelial remnants of the nasopalatine duct within the incisive canal. It is the most common nonodontogenic cyst in the oral cavity. It may occur at any age and anywhere along the course of the incisive canal. However, the cyst is generally confined to palatal bone between the maxillary central incisors at the height of the incisive canal.

The nasopalatine duct cyst is usually asymptomatic and discovered as an incidental finding during routine examination. Symptomatic cysts are usually bacterially infected. Infrequently, the cyst arises entirely in soft tissue of the incisive papilla, where it appears as a small, superficial, fluctuant swelling. A well-developed incisive canal cyst may swell the entire anterior third of the palate.

Radiographically, the cyst appears as a well-delineated, midline, symmetrically oval or heart-shaped radiolucency located between the roots of vital maxillary central incisors. The margin is sclerotic and contiguous with the incisive canal. Root divergence and root resorption of the central incisors are occasional findings associated with large lesions. A similar cyst that is located more posteriorly in the palate has been called the **median palatal cyst.** Current beliefs are that both cysts represent the same entity found in slightly different locations. Both conditions are treated by surgical enucleation.

Periapical Abscess (Figs. 44.5 and 44.6) A periapical abscess is a fluctuant soft-tissue swelling consisting of purulent and necrotic material resulting from bacterial infection of the pulp. It appears at the periapex of a diseased tooth that is often tender to percussion, mobile, and slightly high in occlusion. Regional lymphadenopathy, fever, malaise, and trismus are common accompanying features. Examination of the teeth and supporting tissues along with diagnostic testing reveals the offending nonvital tooth. Radiography often shows an oval periapical radiolucency.

Any abscessed maxillary tooth may produce a swelling of the palate. Generally, the swelling is red-purple, soft, tender, and lateral to the midline if a maxillary posterior tooth is involved. In contrast, an abscessed maxillary incisor may cause a midline swelling in the anterior third of the palate. Aspiration or incision produces a creamy yellow or yellow-green purulent discharge. Immediate drainage, root canal therapy, or extraction is indicated to prevent spread of the infection. Antibiotics, analgesics, and antipyretic agents may also be needed.

Periodontal Abscess The differential diagnosis for a unilateral palatal swelling should include periodontal abscess. This entity is discussed under Periodontitis (Figs. 30.7 and 30.8).

Lymphoid Hyperplasia (Benign Lymphoid Hyperplasia) (Fig. 44.7) Lymphoid hyperplasia is a rare, benign, reactive process that involves proliferation of normal lymphoid tissue of the oropharynx (enlarged tonsils), tongue, floor of mouth, or soft palate in response to some antigenic (often unknown) stimulus that usually was inhaled or ingested. Persons older than 30 years are most often affected. Clinical examination reveals a soft to firm swelling arising at the posterior extent of the hard palate that grows slowly (up to 3 cm), either unilaterally or bilaterally. The surface of the mature lesion is pink to purple, nonulcerated, and dome-shaped or lumpy. Patients rarely report pain. Biopsy is recommended; however, the condition resolves spontaneously.

Primary Lymphoma of the Palate (Fig. 44.8) Primary lymphoma of the palate is a malignant neoplastic growth of lymphocytes or histiocytes. They are classified into Hodgkin's or non-Hodgkin's lymphoma and subdivided into nodal and extranodal disease. Non-Hodgkin's lymphoma may develop at any lymphoid site, including cervical lymph nodes, mandible, palate, and rarely the gingiva. Primary lymphomas of the palate occur most commonly in patients older than 60 years but may be seen in younger patients, especially those with AIDS. The tumor arises at the junction of the hard and soft palates as an asymptomatic, soft, spongy, nonulcerated swelling; rarely does it affect the underlying palatal bone. The surface is often lumpy and purplish. Early recognition and biopsy are important so that treatment may be initiated when the lesion is confined entirely to the palate. Irradiation is used to treat palatal lymphomas, whereas chemotherapy is used for disseminated disease.

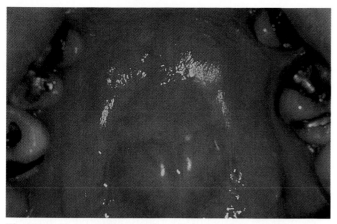

Fig. 44.1. **Torus palatinus:** flat, slight lobulation.

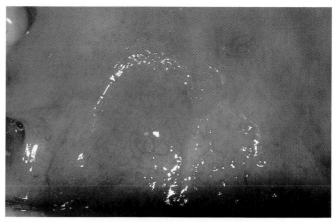

Fig. 44.2. **Lipoma:** palatal nodule; hypervascular surface.

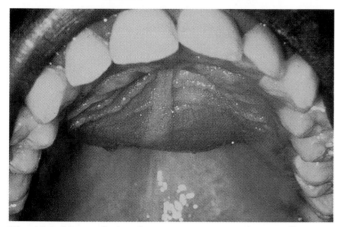

Fig. 44.3. **Nasopalatine duct cyst:** anterior palate swelling.

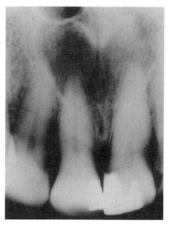

Fig. 44.4. **Nasopalatine duct cyst:** classic heart shape.

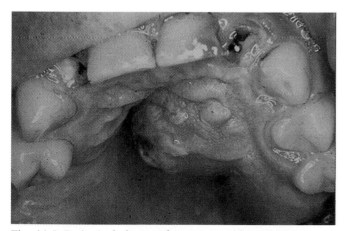

Fig. 44.5. **Periapical abscess:** from nonvital lateral incisor.

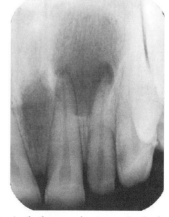

Fig. 44.6. **Periapical abscess:** large periapical radiolucency.

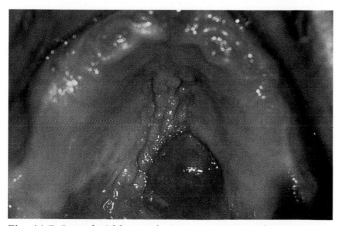

Fig. 44.7. **Lymphoid hyperplasia:** at posterior palate.

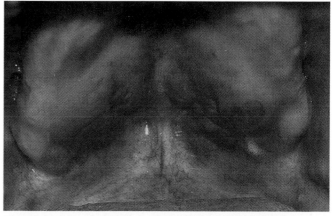

Fig. 44.8. **Primary lymphoma of palate:** with telangiectasia.

Swellings of the Palate: Salivary Gland Lesions

Subacute Sialadenitis (Figs. 45.1) Sialadenitis is inflammation of a salivary gland. It is often caused by bacterial infection (**bacterial sialadenitis**) that arises when salivary flow is low because of dehydration or debilitation. This state allows pathogens (*Staphylococcus aureus*, *Streptococcus viridans*, and *Streptococcus pneumoniae*) to travel up the duct system and replicate. Viruses (mumps, coxsackie, echo) also can be causative. A distinct type of sialadenitis, **subacute sialadenitis**, affects the minor salivary glands of the palate of young men. It appears as a painful, reddish nodular swelling (up to 1 cm) that has an intact, nonulcerated surface. The cause is unknown, and biopsy is recommended.

Necrotizing Sialometaplasia (Figs. 45.2 and 45.3) Necrotizing sialometaplasia is a benign reactive lesion, chiefly of accessory palatal salivary glands, that has histologic features that resemble malignancy. The inflammatory lesion begins after trauma as a rapidly growing nodular swelling on the lateral aspect of the hard palate, particularly in men older than 40 years. Tissue infarction as a result of vasoconstriction and ischemia caused by trauma or dental injection appears causative. Rarely, the soft palate or buccal mucosa is involved; bilateral cases have been reported.

Necrotizing sialometaplasia appears as a small painless nodule that eventually enlarges and causes pain. Within a few weeks it ulcerates and the pain diminishes. The size of the swelling varies, and growth to a diameter of 2 cm is possible. A deep central ulcer with a grayish pseudomembrane is characteristic. The ulcer is irregular and pebbly; the border is often rolled. Healing occurs spontaneously over 4 to 8 weeks or after a biopsy. Biopsy is recommended to rule out similar-appearing lesions such as salivary gland tumors and malignant lymphoma. Histologically, it demonstrates squamous metaplasia of ductal epithelium, which may be misdiagnosed as mucoepidermoid carcinoma.

Benign Accessory Salivary Gland Neoplasm (Figs. 45.4 and 45.5) There are at least 10 different types of benign salivary gland tumors. Up to 80% occur within the parotid gland, 10% in the submandibular gland, and about 10 to 20% in minor salivary glands. Most are pleomorphic adenoma, Warthin's tumor, oncocytoma, or basal cell adenoma. Two of the more common types are discussed.

The basal cell (monomorphic) adenoma is a benign salivary gland tumor that can develop in the palate, most commonly in older women. It appears as a slow-growing dome-shaped mass. The tumor is encapsulated and consists of a regular glandular pattern, usually only one cell type, and lacks a mesenchymal component as seen in pleomorphic adenoma. Treatment is surgical excision.

The pleomorphic adenoma, or benign mixed tumor, is the most common benign neoplasm of accessory salivary glands. It occurs in major or minor salivary glands, the palate being the most common location when accessory salivary glands are affected. Occurrences are most frequent in women between the ages of 30 and 60 years. These neoplasms tend to occur lateral to the midline and distal to the anterior third of the hard palate.

The clinical presentation of the pleomorphic adenoma is a firm, painless, slow-growing, nonulcerated, dome-shaped swelling. Palpation reveals isolated softer areas and a smooth or lobulated surface. Slow persistent enlargement over a period of years is typical, and lesions may achieve sizes greater than 1.5 cm in diameter. Histologically, it shows epithelial cells in a nestlike arrangement, with pools of myxoid, chondroid, and mucoid material. A distinct fibrous connective tissue capsule containing tumor cells surrounds and usually limits the extension of the tumor. Thorough excisional biopsy is recommended because the condition frequently recurs after simple enucleation or incomplete excision. Tumorous involvement of the capsule may play a role in recurrence.

Malignant Accessory Salivary Gland Neoplasm (Figs. 45.6–45.8) There are more than 15 different types of malignant salivary gland tumors. Adenoid cystic carcinoma (cylindroma) and mucoepidermoid carcinoma are the two most common intraoral malignant neoplasms of the accessory salivary glands. Persons between the ages of 20 and 50 years are most frequently affected by mucoepidermoid carcinoma; the adenoid cystic carcinoma usually occurs after age 50 years. The adenoid cystic carcinoma occurs also in respiratory, gastrointestinal, and reproductive tissues, whereas mucoepidermoid carcinoma may occur in the skin, respiratory tract, or centrally within bone, particularly the mandible.

Malignant accessory salivary gland neoplasms occur frequently in the posterior palate. These neoplasms are usually asymptomatic, firm, dome-shaped swellings that occur lateral to the midline. The overlying tissue appears normal in the early stages, but the mucosa later becomes erythematous, with several small telangiectactic surface vessels. These neoplasms grow more quickly and are more painful than benign salivary gland tumors. Induration and eventual spontaneous ulceration are common. A bluish appearance or a mucus exudate emanating from the ulcerated tumor surface are distinctive features of mucoepidermoid carcinoma.

Treatment is radical excision. The prognosis varies depending on the degree of histologic differentiation, the extent of the lesion, and the presence of metastasis. Adenoid cystic carcinoma rarely metastasizes but is an infiltrating malignant condition with a propensity for distant spread by perineural invasion; thus, lifetime follow-up is necessary. In contrast, the mucoepidermoid tumor infrequently metastasizes and is more easily cured by surgical means. Other malignant accessory salivary gland neoplasms include the acinic cell adenocarcinoma, polymorphous low-grade adenocarcinoma, carcinoma ex pleomorphic adenoma, carcinosarcoma, and malignant mixed tumor.

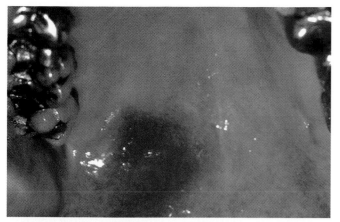

Fig. 45.1. **Subacute sialadenitis:** in young man.

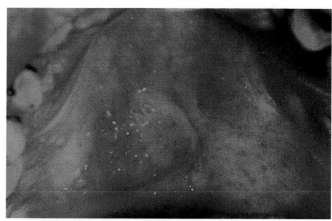

Fig. 45.2. **Necrotizing sialometaplasia:** painful swelling.

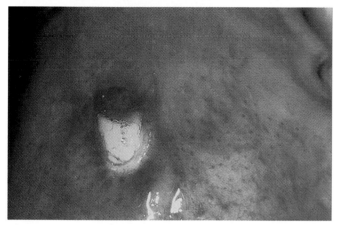

Fig. 45.3. **Necrotizing sialometaplasia:** ulcerative phase.

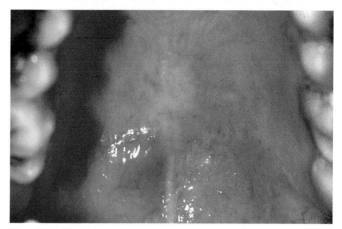

Fig. 45.4. **Basal cell adenoma:** painless nodule.

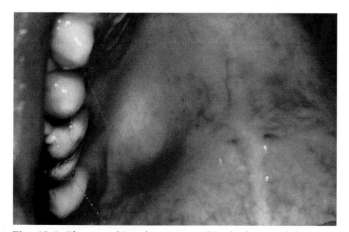

Fig. 45.5. **Pleomorphic adenoma:** strikingly firm nodule.

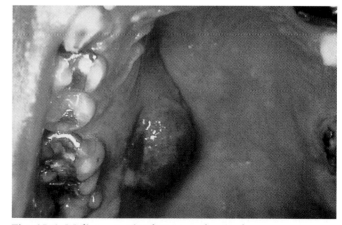

Fig. 45.6. **Malignant mixed tumor:** ulcerated.

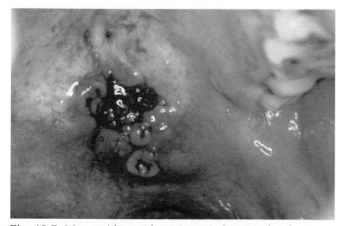

Fig. 45.7. **Mucoepidermoid carcinoma:** draining fistulas.

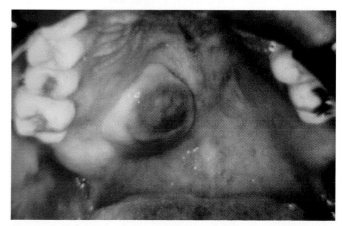

Fig. 45.8. **Adenoid cystic carcinoma:** surface ulceration.

105

Swellings of the Face

Odontogenic Infection (Figs. 46.1–46.8)
Orofacial infections arise when microbes invade tissue, replicate, and overwhelm the local immune response. Infections are promoted by poor health and systemic disease, poor oral hygiene, and traumatic surgery. Oral infections are called odontogenic when they are tooth-related. Most odontogenic infections arise as a consequence of pulpal necrosis, sulcular and apical periodontitis, and pericoronitis. Almost all odontogenic infections are polymicrobial, consisting of anaerobic (65%) and aerobic (35%) bacteria. Obligate Gram-negative anaerobes (such as *Bacteroides*, *Fusobacterium* species), anaerobic Gram-positive organisms (such as *Peptostreptococcus* species), and facultative anaerobic Gram-positive streptococci (such as *Streptococcus milleri*) are the organisms most frequently identified in odontogenic infections. Other contributors are *Lactobacillus*, *Diphtheroids*, *Actinomyces*, and *Eikenella* species. It is common for these organisms to be resistant to one or more frequently used antibiotics.

Odontogenic infections produce four classic features: calor (heat), dolor (pain), rubor (redness), and tumor (swelling). They begin as a swelling that slowly enlarges. Patients complain of dull pain and a bad taste. It may remain localized for a long time or progress to an abscess, parulis, cellulitis, or space infection. An **abscess** is an acute swelling that contains pus and necrotic debris. It appears as a well-localized swelling that is soft and occasionally pointed. It is visible in or outside the mouth and drains spontaneously or when incised. The **parulis** is similar to the abscess, but the bacterial infection drains through a sinus tract onto the mucosal surface as a yellow-red papule. In most cases the parulis represents chronic infection and is asymptomatic. **Cellulitis** is an early feature of a spreading odontogenic infection; it represents a diffuse inflammatory response that has not yet localized. Cellulitis produces a diffuse, red, warm, hard swelling (generally over the cheek or mandible) that is firm and tender to palpation. It may mature into an abscess and drain or become aggressive and spread. Spread of the infection beyond anatomic boundaries through fascial (spaces) planes is called a **space infection**.

Buccal Space Infection (Figs. 46.1 and 46.2)
A buccal space infection is most often caused by an odontogenic infection that has spread externally to the cortical plate, laterally to the buccinator muscle, and anteriorly to the masseter muscle. It frequently arises from lateral migration of pathogenic bacteria that infect the periapex of a maxillary or mandibular molar. Entry into the space is usually gained at the posterior insertion of the buccinator muscle. Pain, swelling, fever and chronic inflammation of a mandibular molar are the most prominent features.

Masseteric (Submasseteric) Space Infection (Figs. 46.3 and 46.4)
A masseteric space infection is generally the result of an odontogenic infection that has spread posteriorly from an infected mandibular molar or buccal space to a region between the masseter muscle and the lateral aspect of the ramus. The swelling is firm and nonfluctuant and overlies the angle of the mandible. Masseteric muscle involvement produces marked trismus (difficulty in opening). Computed tomography and magnetic resonance imaging are useful in defining this condition.

Infraorbital Space Infection (Figs. 46.5 and 46.6)
This space infection involves the region lateral to the nasal ala and below the eye as a result of an infected maxillary tooth (usually a tooth anterior to the first molar) that has spread superiorly. Grave concern is raised when the infection encroaches on the eyelid or affects vision, because the ophthalmic (angular) veins lack valves and spread of infection to the brain is possible. **Cavernous sinus thrombosis** is a severe infection resulting from spread of infection via the angular veins to the brain.

Treatment of odontogenic infection involves four steps: 1) removal of the source of the infection, 2) establishment of drainage, 3) provision of antibiotics when needed, and 4) provision of supportive care. The infection is often controlled by instituting root canal therapy or extraction of the offending tooth when the source of infection is localized (for example, parulis, apical periodontitis). These treatments provide a pathway for exudate drainage and reduce or remove the microbial load. Alternatively, incision and drainage can be performed to drain an abscess. If the condition is diffuse, as in cellulitis or pericoronitis, incision and drainage are generally unsuccessful and not recommended. Root canal therapy or extraction are used to treat cellulitis caused by a nonvital tooth, whereas pericoronitis is generally first managed with irrigation and antibiotics. When the pain of pericoronitis remits, extraction is performed. Guidelines for prescribing antibiotics for odontogenic infection include the presence of a spreading infection (regional lymphadenopathy, fever, swelling beyond anatomic boundaries) in combination with inability to establish drainage. Penicillin VK is the drug of choice, generally prescribed as 500 mg orally four times daily for 7 days.

Ludwig's Angina (Figs. 46.7 and 46.8)
Ludwig's angina is a severe and spreading infection that involves the submandibular, submental, and sublingual spaces bilaterally. These spaces are located between the tongue, hyoid bone, and lingual cortical plates of the mandible. It generally arises from an infected mandibular molar or a fractured (and infected) mandible. Spreading infection forces the tongue superiorly and posteriorly and forces submandibular tissues apically. This impinges on the airway and can result in airway obstruction. Aggressive use of antibiotics, culture, sensitivity, and multiple incision and drainage may be required to control the infection. In some patients, emergency procedures, such as a tracheostomy, are needed to sustain life.

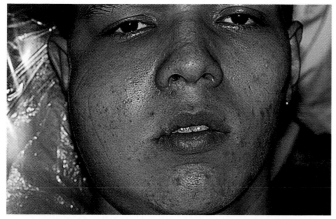

Fig. 46.1. **Buccal space infection:** infected mandibular molar.

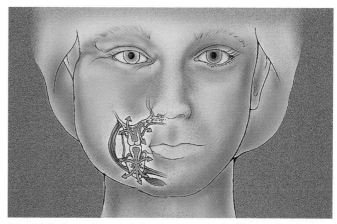

Fig. 46.2. **Buccal space infection:** anatomic illustration.

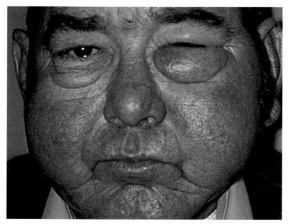

Fig. 46.3. **Masseteric space infection:** infected #19

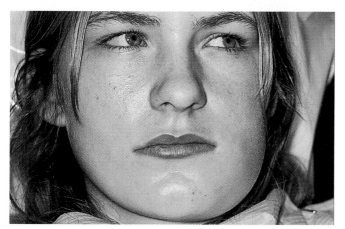

Fig. 46.4. **Masseteric space infection:** anatomic illustration.

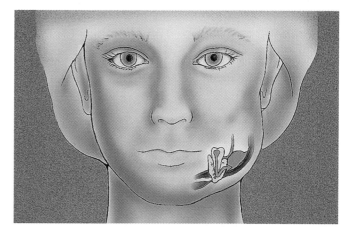

Fig. 46.5. **Infraorbital space infection:** impinging on the eye.

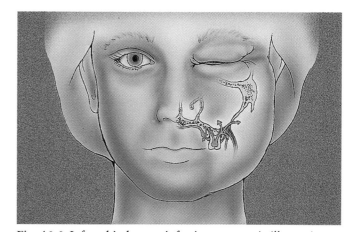

Fig. 46.6. **Infraorbital space infection:** anatomic illustration.

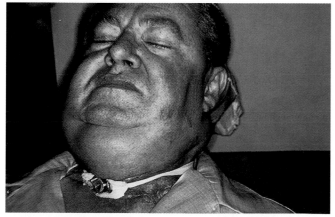

Fig. 46.7. **Ludwig's angina:** requiring tracheostomy.

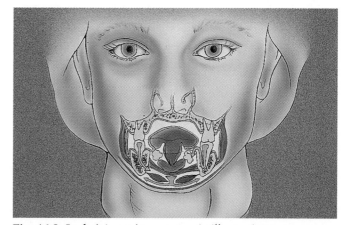

Fig. 46.8. **Ludwig's angina:** anatomic illustration.

Swellings of the Face

Sialadenosis (Fig. 47.1) Sialadenosis is an asymptomatic, noninflammatory enlargement of major salivary glands. The condition indicates an underlying systemic disorder, such as alcoholism, anorexia nervosa, bulimia, diabetes mellitus, drug reaction, malnutrition, or HIV infection. It arises when acinar cells swell, probably because of dysregulation of autonomic innervation of the gland. Most cases begin as slow-growing, painless swellings of the parotid gland. It is often bilateral but can be unilateral. Salivary flow may be reduced. Microscopy shows engorged and hypertrophied acinar cells or infiltration of fat. Treatment attempts to control the systemic disease and minimize gland growth.

Warthin's Tumor (Papillary Cystadenoma Lymphomatosum) (Fig. 47.2) Warthin's tumor is a benign salivary gland tumor that usually occurs after age 60 and almost exclusively in the parotid gland. It is thought to arise from glandular elements entrapped within a salivary gland lymph node. Smokers have more than five times the risk as nonsmokers. There is a slight predilection for men. The tumors arise mostly in the tail of the parotid gland as a slow-growing, doughy, nodular mass. About 6% of tumors occur in parotid glands bilaterally; the submandibular and minor salivary glands are rarely affected. The tumor is composed of bilayered, oncocytic ductal epithelium and a lymphoid stroma that forms numerous papillae and invaginating cystic spaces. Biopsy and surgical excision are recommended. Recurrence and malignant transformation are rare.

Sjögren's Syndrome (Inflammatory Exocrinopathy) (Fig. 47.3) Sjögren's syndrome is a chronic autoimmune disease characterized by progressive lymphocytic infiltration and dysfunction of exocrine glands. The disease is associated with polyclonal B-cell hyperactivity, certain histocompatibility antigens, and chronic viral infections (Epstein-Barr and retroviruses). It affects 1 in 2,000 persons, women in 90% of cases, and usually manifests between 35 and 50 years of age. The primary form, **sicca syndrome**, is limited to the salivary and lacrimal glands, producing dry eyes (xerophthalmia) and dry mouth (xerostomia). Oral and ocular disease accompanied by systemic disease (i.e., rheumatoid arthritis, systemic lupus erythematosus, and infiltrative disease of gastrointestinal and pulmonary exocrine glands) is known as **secondary Sjögren's syndrome.** The syndrome develops slowly and involves progressive enlargement of the major salivary glands, particularly the parotid glands bilaterally. The glands become firm but not painful. Involvement of the pancreas or gall bladder results in abdominal complaints. Biopsy specimens of minor labial salivary glands show multiple inflammatory aggregates adjacent to salivary acini. Serum markers, i.e., antinuclear antibodies (anti-SS-A and anti-SS-B) and rheumatoid factor, help confirm the diagnosis of secondary Sjögren's syndrome. Management of dryness is attempted with artificial tears and saliva. Pilocarpine, cevimeline, fluoride, and chlorhexidine are useful. Patients are at increased risk for caries and the development of lymphoma.

Cushing's Disease and Syndrome (Fig. 47.4) Cushing's disease is the persistent elevation of cortisol blood levels caused by cortisol hypersecretion by the adrenal gland. It is usually induced by a pituitary adenoma. Elevation of cortisol results in fluid retention, hypertension, and hyperglycemia. Clinical features include truncal obesity, a round (moon-shaped) face with plethora (red), facial and truncal acne, a buffalo hump at the back of the neck, and purple abdominal striae. These features are caused by collagen wasting, dermal weakening, capillary fragility, and fluid accumulation. Treatment is directed toward eradicating tumors and correcting daily cortisol levels.

Masseter Hypertrophy (Fig. 47.5) Masseter hypertrophy occurs as a result of chronic muscle activity induced by tooth clenching, gum chewing, or bruxism. The masseter muscles are firm and nontender. Enlargement is most prominent over the angle of the mandible.

Neurofibromatosis (von Recklinghausen's Disease) (Fig. 47.6) Neurofibromatosis is an autosomal dominant disease associated with loss of a tumor suppressor gene (NF1 or NF2) and multiple tumors (neurofibromas) of the skin, mouth, bone, and gastrointestinal tract and pigmentations of the skin (café au lait), iris (Lisch nodules), and axilla (axillary freckling or Crowe's sign). The tumors appear after puberty as papules, nodules, or pendulous growths. In the mandible they can expand the mandibular canal and cortical plates, producing facial swelling, or rarely undergoing malignant transformation.

Cystic (Lymphangioma) Hygroma (Fig. 47.7) Cystic hygroma is a hamartoma of lymphoid vessels (lymphangioma) that fail to communicate with the normal lymphatic system. As a result, lymph collects within the numerous dilated vessels. Most appear in the neck and axilla as soft, compressible swellings. Airway obstruction may be a concern. Excision is generally successful.

Ewing's Sarcoma (Fig. 47.8) Ewing's sarcoma is a malignant tumor derived from stem or primitive mesenchymal cells caused by a chromosomal translocation (i.e., chromosome 11 switches with chromosome 12 or 22). The tumor is related to the primitive neuroectodermal tumor. Persons younger than 30 years are most often affected. Most sarcomas arise in the femur and pelvic bones; fewer than 5% arise in jaws. They are sometimes found in soft tissue without bony involvement. In the jaws, the mandible is most often involved. Patients present with swelling, pain, paresthesia, loose teeth, fever, leukocytosis, and an elevated sedimentation rate. The mass is soft when the tumor has penetrated the bony cortical plate. Radiographs show displaced teeth and an osteolytic radiolucent mass with ill-defined tumor margins. Metastasis to lung, liver, and lymph nodes occurs frequently. Survival rates of 50 to 75% have been achieved with the combined use of radiation, surgery, and chemotherapy.

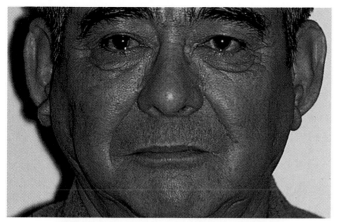

Fig. 47.1. **Sialadenosis:** of the parotid glands in a diabetic.

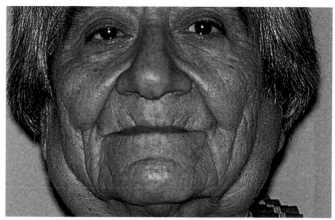

Fig. 47.2. **Warthin's tumor:** bilateral parotid enlargement.

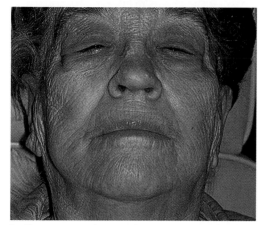

Fig. 47.3. **Sjögren's syndrome:** dry eyes, parotid enlargement.

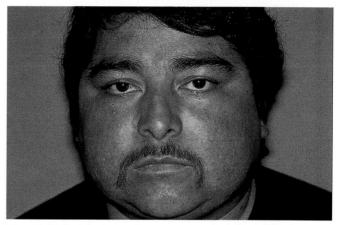

Fig. 47.4. **Cushing's syndrome:** acne and red swollen face.

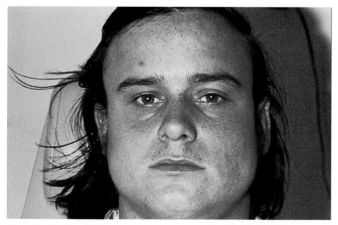

Fig. 47.5. **Masseter hypertrophy:** in a clench.

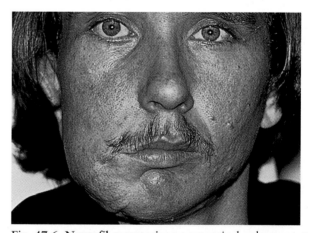

Fig. 47.6. **Neurofibromatosis:** asymmetrical enlargement.

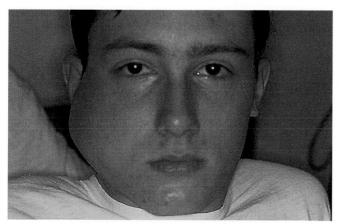

Fig. 47.7. **Cystic hygroma:** soft, present since birth.

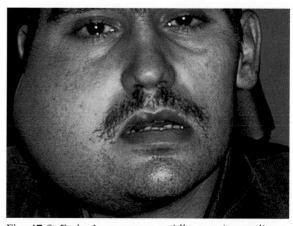

Fig. 47.8. **Ewing's sarcoma:** rapidly growing malignancy.

Conditions Peculiar to the Face

Angioedema (Fig. 48.1) Angioedema is a hypersensitivity reaction characterized by the accumulation of fluid within the facial tissues. The resulting tissues are soft, swollen, and itchy. It can be triggered by mechanical trauma, stress, infection, or an allergen. Most cases are acquired and result from IgE-mediated mast cell degranulation and release of histamine after exposure to antigenic stimuli (such as food) or physical contact. Histamine mediates capillary permeability and the leakage of plasma into soft tissues. Less commonly, infections and autoimmune disease trigger capillary permeability via the formation of antigen-antibody complexes or elevation in the number of circulating eosinophils.

Angioedema produces facial swelling that develops within minutes or over a few hours. The swellings are usually uniform, diffuse, and symmetric. The lips are commonly affected, producing overly full, stretched, pliable swellings. Generally the skin tone remains normal in color or is slightly red. The tongue, floor of the mouth, eyelids, face, and extremities may also be affected. Acquired angioedema is usually recurrent and self-limiting and poses little threat to the patient. Symptoms are limited to burning or itching. Management involves prescription of antihistamines, identification and withdrawal of allergenic stimuli, and stress reduction.

In the rare hereditary form, angioedema is inherited in an autosomal dominant pattern. It involves activation of the complement pathway caused by an enzyme deficiency (type I) or a dysfunctional enzyme (type II). Treatment involves avoidance of violent physical activity and trauma and prophylaxis with androgenic drugs, such as danocrine (Danazol). Angiotension-converting enzyme (ACE) drugs used for high blood pressure and nonsteroidal anti-inflammatory drugs have also been implicated in causing angioedema. The condition with ACE inhibitors appears to arise from increased bradykinin levels, not release of histamine. Management involves avoidance of these drugs or substitution with another type of antihypertensive agent.

Emphysema (Fig. 48.2) Emphysema is defined as the abnormal presence of air in tissue. In dentistry, emphysema is most commonly caused by a surgical procedure. The condition results when compressed air from a high-speed handpiece is forced under a mucoperiosteal flap, through an open pulp chamber, or intraalveolarly. The air becomes entrapped in subcutaneous tissue or a fascial plane. Under these circumstances, the soft tissues become distended adjacent to the surgical site within minutes of the procedure. The swelling is soft or mildly firm and yields a distinctive crackling sound on palpation. The entrapped air can migrate along fascial planes through the neck to the sternum, into the prevertebral fascia and mediastinum, toward the temporal and orbital regions, or into the vascular system. Emphysema is associated with risks for infection, air embolism, and death. Broad-spectrum antibiotics are recommended to prevent infection. Signs suggestive of embolic sequelae, such as sudden vision changes, dyspnea, altered heart rate, or loss of consciousness, warrant immediate transfer to an emergency care facility.

Postoperative Bleeding (Figs. 48.3–48.6) Bleeding is the result of trauma and surgery of the oral soft tissues. Facial swelling can result from orofacial bleeding when there is excess bleeding or blood that does not have an escape route through the epithelium. The end result is **purpura**, the accumulation of blood within the subcutaneous or submucosal tissues. Purpura is classified according to the size of the severed vessel and the size of the lesion produced. Rupture of capillaries produces punctate bleeds called **petechiae**. Subcutaneous bleeding that produces a nonraised lesion up to 1 cm in diameter is called an **ecchymosis** (bruise). A large area of subcutaneous bleeding (greater than 1 cm) that distends soft tissues is a **hematoma**.

In dentistry, hematomas are commonly caused by the inadvertent penetration of the needle into the posterior superior alveolar vein. Swelling occurs without pain within seconds or minutes of the trauma. The swelling grows uniformly and without color change in the posterior cheek region, over and in front of the mandibular ramus. The hematoma is slightly firm and compressible. It may cause tissue tenderness, nerve paresthesia, and muscle trismus. Pressure and ice should be applied to the hematoma during the first 24 hours. Thereafter, heat should be applied to dissipate the blood. Depending on its size, the lesion may take more than 1 week to resolve and may discolor the skin. During the healing phase, the skin color fades from purple to brown, then tan and yellow. Antibiotics should be considered if the hematoma is caused by severance of a vessel with a contaminated instrument.

Bell's Palsy (Figs. 48.7 and 48.8) Bell's palsy is unilateral paralysis of the seventh cranial (facial) nerve. The condition results in the inability to move the muscles of facial expression on the affected side. Trauma to the facial nerve caused by surgery, tooth extraction, infection, or exposure to cold is the most frequent cause. Some cases have been linked to the inflammatory response caused by reactivation of herpesvirus in the geniculate ganglion. All persons are susceptible, but the condition is seen most often in middle-aged adults (slightly more often in women). Patients develop abrupt onset of inability to raise the forehead skin, close the eye, and lift the corner of the mouth of the affected side. Eye watering (crocodile tears), mouth drooling, and loss of taste are common consequences. The palsy may be temporary or permanent. In 70% of cases of idiopathic Bell's palsy, normal function returns within 6 weeks. The few cases lasting longer than 1 year usually persist indefinitely. Palliative care is provided to protect the eye from corneal ulceration. Corticosteroids and surgical decompression of the facial nerve have lessened symptoms in some patients.

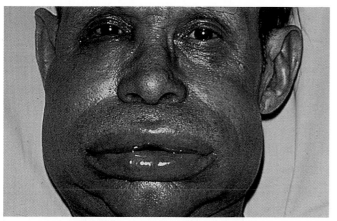

Fig. 48.1. **Angioedema:** caused by contact with latex rubber.

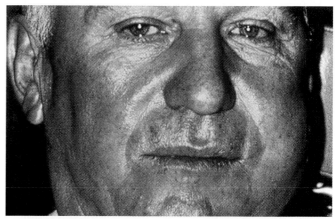

Fig. 48.2. **Air emphysema:** after flap surgery.

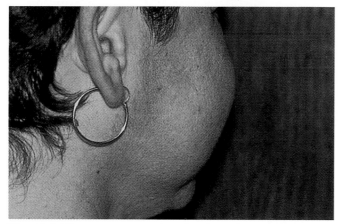

Fig. 48.3. **Hematoma:** posterior alveolar vein injured.*

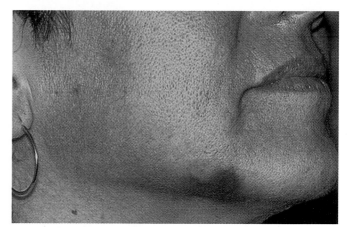

Fig. 48.4. **Hematoma:** 1 week later.*

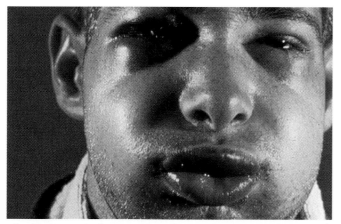

Fig. 48.5. **Surgical trauma:** swelling 2 days post oral surgery.‡

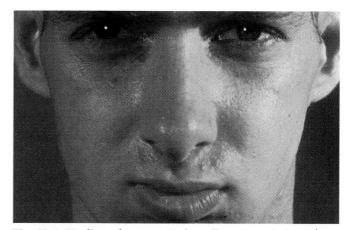

Fig. 48.6. **Healing of postsurgical swelling:** 2 weeks later.‡

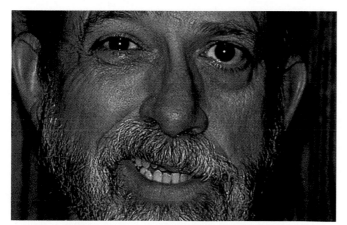

Fig. 48.7. **Bell's palsy:** inability to lift left side of face.

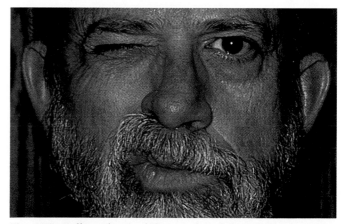

Fig. 48.8. **Bell's palsy:** inability to close left eyelids.

Intraoral Findings by Color Changes

White Lesions

Fordyce's Granules (Figs. 49.1 and 49.2)
Fordyce's granules are ectopic sebaceous glands found within the mouth that are considered a variation of normal oral mucosal anatomy. Technically speaking, these are sebaceous choristomas (i.e., normal tissue in an abnormal location). These asymptomatic granules consist of individual sebaceous glands that are 1 to 2 mm in diameter. Characteristically they appear as white, creamy white, or yellow slightly raised papules on the buccal mucosa and vermilion of the upper lip. They usually occur in multiples, forming clusters, plaques, or patches. Enlarged clusters may feel rough to palpation and to the patient's tongue. They are sometimes an isolated finding. Less common locations include the labial mucosa, retromolar pad, attached gingiva, tongue, and frenum.

Fordyce's granules arise from sebaceous glands embryologically entrapped during fusion of the maxillary and mandibular processes. They become more apparent after sexual maturity as the sebaceous system develops. Rarely, an intraoral hair may be seen in association with the condition.

Fordyce's granules occur in approximately 80% of adults, and no race or gender predilection has been reported. However, the density of granules per mucosal area is greater in men than women. Histologic examination shows rounded nests of clear cells, 10 to 30 per nest; darkly staining, small, centrally located nuclei are found encapsulated in the lamina propria and submucosa. The clinical appearance is adequate for diagnosis of Fordyce's granules; biopsy is not usually required.

Linea Alba Buccalis (Figs. 49.3 and 49.4)
The linea alba buccalis is a common intraoral finding that appears as a raised white wavy line of variable length and prominence located at the level of the occlusion on the buccal mucosa. Generally, this asymptomatic cornified entity is 1 to 2 mm wide and extends horizontally from the second molar to the canine region of the buccal mucosa. The lesion is most often found bilaterally and cannot be rubbed off. The thickened epithelial changes consist of hyperkeratotic tissue that is a response to frictional activity of the teeth. The condition is often associated with crenated tongue and may be a sign of bruxism, clenching, or negative oral pressure. The clinical appearance is diagnostic and requires no treatment.

Leukoedema (Figs. 49.5 and 49.6)
Leukoedema is an opalescent, milky-white, or gray surface change of the buccal mucosa. This common mucosal variant is associated with dark-pigmented persons but may be seen infrequently in lighter-pigmented persons. The incidence of leukoedema tends to increase with age, and 50% of African American children and 92% of African American adults are affected. The labial mucosa, soft palate, and floor of the mouth are less common locations of occurrence.

Leukoedema is usually faint and bilateral. Close examination of leukoedema reveals fine white lines and wrinkles. Exaggerated and long-standing cases have overlapping folds of tissue. Prominence of the lesion is related to the degree of underlying melanin pigmentation, level of oral hygiene, and amount of smoking. The borders of the lesion are irregular and diffuse; they fade into adjacent tissue, which makes it difficult to determine where the lesion begins and ends. The condition is diagnosed by stretching the mucosa, which causes the white appearance to significantly diminish or disappear in some cases. Wiping the lesion fails to remove it. The cause of leukoedema is unknown, although it is more severe in smokers and diminishes with smoking cessation. Histologic examination of biopsy specimens shows increased epithelial thickness with prominent intracellular edema of the spinous layer without evidence of inflammation. No serious complications are associated with this lesion, and no treatment is required.

Morsicatio Buccarum (Mucosal Chewing) (Figs. 49.7 and 49.8)
Morsicatio buccarum (cheek biting or chewing) is a common nervous habit that produces a progression of mucosal changes. Slightly raised irregular white plaques initially appear in a diffuse pattern that covers areas of trauma. Increased injury produces a hyperplastic response that increases the size of the plaque. A linear or striated pattern is sometimes observed, with thick and thin areas seen side by side. Persistent injury leads to an enlarging plaque with interadjacent traumatic erythema and ulceration.

Mucosal chewing is usually seen on anterior buccal mucosa and less frequently on the labial mucosa. The lesions may be unilateral or bilateral and can occur at any age. No sex or race predilection has been reported. Diagnosis requires visual or verbal confirmation of the nervous habit. Although morsicatio buccarum has no malignant potential, patients should be advised of the mucosal alterations. Because of the similar clinical appearance, speckled leukoplakia and candidiasis should be ruled out. Microscopy shows a normal maturing epithelial surface with a corrugated parakeratotic surface and minor subepithelial inflammation.

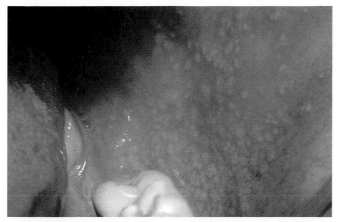

Fig. 49.1. **Fordyce's granules:** on buccal mucosa.

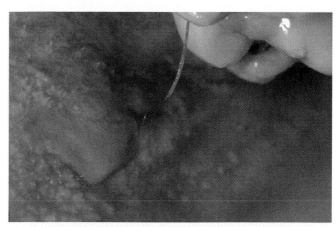

Fig. 49.2. **Fordyce's granules:** with rare intraoral hair.

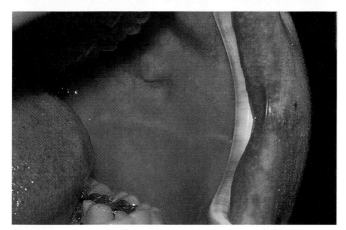

Fig. 49.3. **Linea alba buccalis:** on buccal mucosa.

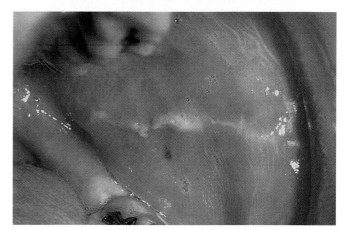

Fig. 49.4. **Prominent linea alba buccalis.**

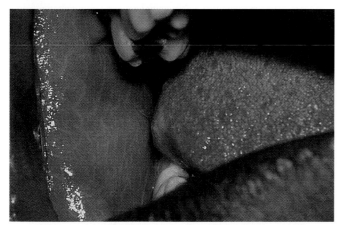

Fig. 49.5. **Leukoedema:** of buccal mucosa.

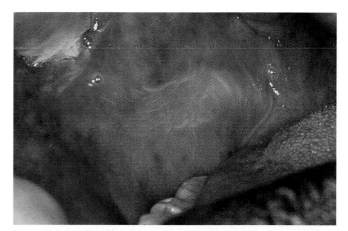

Fig. 49.6. **Leukoedema:** prominent in a smoker.

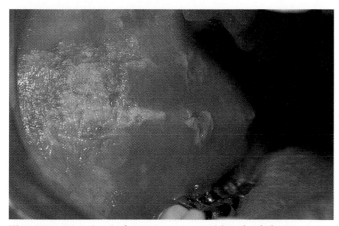

Fig. 49.7. **Morsicatio buccarum:** caused by cheek biting.

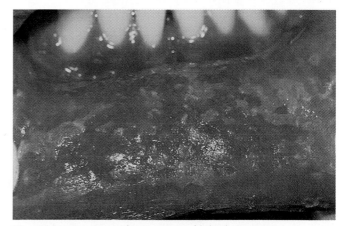

Fig. 49.8. **Morsicatio buccarum:** of labial mucosa.

White Lesions

White Sponge Nevus (Familial White Folded Dysplasia) (Figs. 50.1 and 50.2)

White sponge nevus is a relatively uncommon genodermatosis caused by point mutations in genes that regulate keratin 4 and keratin 13 production; as a result epithelial maturation and exfoliation are altered. It appears at birth or early childhood, persists throughout life and exhibits no race or sex predilection. Because it has an autosomal dominant pattern of transmission, several family members may have manifestations.

White sponge nevus produces mucosal lesions that are asymptomatic, white, folded and spongy. The lesions often exhibit a symmetric wavy pattern. The most common location is the buccal mucosa bilaterally, followed by labial mucosa, alveolar ridge, and floor of the mouth. It may involve the entire oral mucosa or be distributed unilaterally as discrete white patches. The gingival margin and dorsal tongue are almost never affected, although the soft palate and ventrolateral tongue are commonly involved. The size of the lesions vary. Extraoral mucosal sites may involve the nasal cavity, esophagus, larynx, vagina, and rectum. The oral features are remarkably similar to those of **hereditary benign intraepithelial dyskeratosis**. However, eye involvement occurs with the latter. Microscopically, white sponge nevus shows prominent parakeratosis, thickening and clearing of the spinous layer, and perinuclear tangles of keratin tonofilaments. No treatment is required.

Traumatic White Lesions (Trauma, Burns and Peripheral Scar) (Figs. 50.3–50.6)

Traumatic white lesions are caused by many physical and chemical irritants, such as frictional trauma, heat, topical use of aspirin, excessive use of mouthwash, caustic liquids, and even toothpastes. Frictional trauma is often noted on the attached gingiva. It is caused by excessive tooth brushing, movement of oral prostheses, and chewing on the edentulous ridge. With time the mucosa becomes thickened and develops a roughened white surface. Pain is characteristically absent; histologic examination reveals hyperkeratosis.

Trauma can produce a white mucosal slough if superficial layers of epithelium are lost. Underneath the white lesion is a raw, red, or bleeding surface. Acute traumatic lesions usually appear as punctate white patches with diffuse irregular borders. Moveable mucosa is more susceptible to trauma than is attached mucosa. Pain lasts several days. Treatment is removal of the cause. Another white lesion caused by trauma is a scar. It represents a fibrous healing response of the dermis. Scars are often asymptomatic, linear, whitish-pink, and sharply delineated. A thorough history may reveal previous injury, recurrent ulcerative disease, seizure disorder, self-mutilating behavior, or previous surgery.

Leukoplakia (Figs. 50.7 and 50.8)

Leukoplakia is a clinical term for a white plaque or patch on the oral mucosa that cannot be rubbed off and cannot be classified clinically as any other disease. Persons of any age may be affected, but most cases occur in men between the ages of 45 and 65 years. Recent incidence figures indicate that the male to female ratio is decreasing, with women affected almost as frequently as men.

Leukoplakias are protective reactions against chronic irritants. Tobacco, alcohol, syphilis, vitamin deficiency, hormonal imbalance, galvanism, chronic friction, and candidiasis have been implicated in causing these lesions. Leukoplakias vary considerably in size, location, and clinical appearance. The preferential sites are the lateral and ventral tongue, floor of the mouth, alveolar mucosa, lip, soft palate–retromolar trigone, and mandibular attached gingiva. The surface may appear smooth and homogeneous, thin and friable, fissured, corrugated, verrucoid, nodular, or speckled. Lesions can vary in color, from faintly translucent white, gray or brown-white.

A classification system offered by the World Health Organization recommends two divisions for oral leukoplakias: **homogeneous** and **nonhomogeneous**. Nonhomogeneous leukoplakias have been further subdivided into **erythroleukoplakia** (white lesion with large red component), **nodular** (white lesion with raised and pebbly surface), **speckled** (white lesion with small red components), and **verrucoid** (white lesion with raised corrugated surface).

Most leukoplakias (80%) are benign; the rest are dysplastic (premalignant) or cancerous. The clinical challenge lies in determining which are premalignant or malignant, since 4 to 6% of all leukoplakias progress to carcinoma within 5 years. High-risk sites of malignant transformation include the floor of the mouth, lateral and ventral tongue, uvulo-palatal complex, and lips.

Proliferative verrucous leukoplakia is a unique leukoplakia with a verrucoid appearance and malignant transformation properties. It occurs at any adult age (mean age, 62–65 years), four times more often in women than men, and mostly in smokers. The lesions have a white, corrugated or pebbly exophytic surface. A close association with human papillomavirus infection exists. Lesions are slow growing, aggressive, and often multifocal. About 70% of these leukoplakias developed into carcinoma.

Leukoplakias with localized red areas confer a high risk for carcinoma. Evidence indicates that nonhomogeneous leukoplakias, particularly oral speckled leukoplakias, represent epithelial dysplasia in about half of the cases and have the highest rate of malignant transformation among intraoral leukoplakias. *Candida albicans,* often associated with oral speckled leukoplakias, may have a role in the dysplastic changes seen.

The initial step in the treatment of leukoplakia is to eliminate any irritating and causative factors, then observe for healing. Unexplained persistent oral leukoplakias must be biopsied. Several biopsy sites may be necessary for diffuse lesions. Nonhomogeneous or reddish areas of the lesion should always be selected for biopsy because they are associated with a higher risk for dysplasia and malignant transformation.

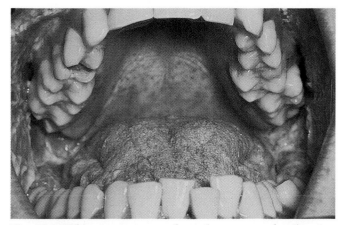

Fig. 50.1. **White sponge nevus:** buccal mucosa, soft palate.*

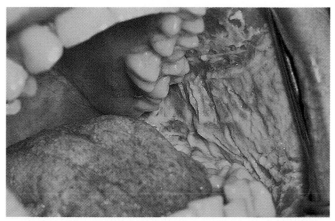

Fig. 50.2. **White sponge nevus:** of buccal mucosa.*

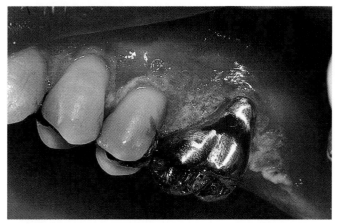

Fig. 50.3. **Traumatic white lesion:** tooth brushing associated.

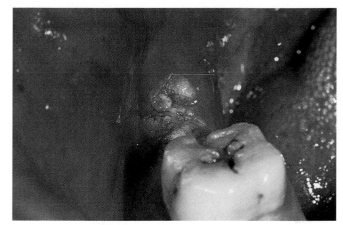

Fig. 50.4. **Traumatic white lesion:** frictional keratosis.

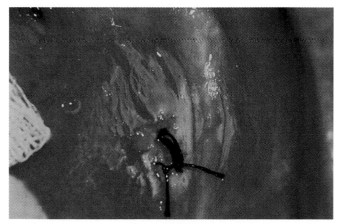

Fig. 50.5. **Traumatic white lesion:** burn from topical aspirin.

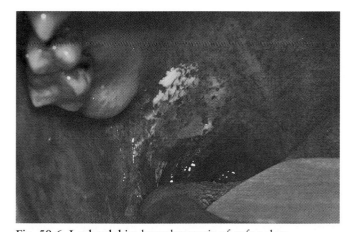

Fig. 50.6. **Leukoplakia:** hyperkeratosis of soft palate.

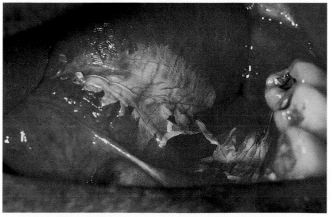

Fig. 50.7. **Leukoplakia:** of floor of mouth and ventral tongue.

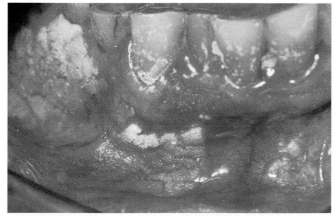

Fig. 50.8. **Proliferative verrucous leukoplakia.**

Tobacco-Associated White Lesions

Cigarette Keratosis (Figs. 51.1 and 51.2)
Cigarette keratosis is a specific reaction evident in persons who smoke nonfiltered or marijuana cigarettes to a very short length. The lesions, which approximate each other on lip closure, involve the upper and lower lips at the location of cigarette placement. These keratotic patches are about 7 mm in diameter and are located invariably lateral to the midline. Raised white papules are evident throughout the patch, producing a roughened texture and firmness to palpation. Cigarette keratoses may extend onto the labial mucosa, but the vermilion border is rarely involved. Elderly men are most commonly affected. Smoking cessation usually brings about resolution. The development of ulcer and crust formation should raise the suspicion of neoplastic transformation.

Nicotine Stomatitis (Pipe Smoker's Palate) (Figs. 51.3 and 51.4) Nicotine stomatitis is a direct response of oral mucosa to prolonged pipe and cigar smoking. Its severity is correlated with the intensity and duration of smoke exposure. It is usually found in middle-aged and elderly men, in unprotected palatal regions (not covered by a maxillary denture) that contain minor salivary glands, i.e., posterior to the palatal rugae, on the soft palate, and sometimes extending onto the buccal mucosa. Rarely, the dorsum of the tongue is affected; these tobacco-associated changes of the tongue have been termed **glossitis stomatitis nicotina.**

Nicotine stomatitis shows progressive changes with time. The irritation initially causes the palate to become diffusely erythematous. The palate eventually becomes grayish-white secondary to hyperkeratosis. Multiple discrete keratotic papules with depressed red centers develop that correspond to dilated and inflamed excretory duct openings of the minor salivary glands. The papules enlarge as the irritation persists but fail to coalesce, producing a characteristic cobblestone (parboiled) appearance of the palate. Isolated but prominent red-centered papules are common. Whether the lesion arises as a consequence of heat or of tobacco is a matter of debate. Pipe smoking and reverse cigarette smoking (lit end placed in the mouth—common to persons from India) produces similar findings. Smoking cessation usually results in regression. Biopsy is rarely needed to confirm the diagnosis.

Snuff Dipper's Patch (Tobacco Chewer's Lesion, Snuff Keratosis) (Figs. 51.5 and 51.6)
A wrinkled yellow-white area in the mucobuccal fold, or mandibular buccal or labial mucosa, suggests persistent intraoral use of unburned tobacco. The hard palate, floor of the mouth, and ventral tongue may also be affected if tobacco is placed in the maxillary vestibule or beneath the tongue. Smokeless tobacco has various forms (snuff, dip, plug, or quid) and leaves its characteristic mark at the preferential site of tobacco placement. Posterior sites are commonly used for dip, plug, or quid, whereas anterior sites are preferred for snuff. Persons who vary placement of the tobacco have multiple, less prominent oral lesions. Male teenagers are most frequently affected, largely because of intensive marketing and peer and sports associations. Higher prevalence is found in Southern and Appalachian states.

Early snuff dipper's patches are pale pink keratoses with corrugated or wrinkled surfaces. The color may progress from white and yellow-white to yellow-brown as hyperkeratosis and exogenous staining occur. Lesions are asymptomatic and often at least 1 cm in diameter.

Long-term use of smokeless tobacco is associated with periodontal recession, caries, epidermal dysplastic changes, and verrucous carcinoma. The dysplastic changes, which take many years to develop, are associated with the carcinogenic nitrosamines present in the tobacco. To achieve resolution, cessation of use is recommended. If normal appearance does not return 14 days after cessation, biopsy is necessary.

Verrucous Carcinoma (of Ackerman) (Figs. 51.7 and 51.8) Verrucous carcinoma is a variant malignant squamous cell tumor that is considered low-grade and nonmetastasizing. It is a less common form of oral cancer than squamous cell carcinoma. It most frequently arises in association with long-term use of tobacco, especially smokeless tobacco, and human papillomavirus infection (about 30% of cases).

Verrucous carcinoma appears as a warty, exophytic, white-and-red mass that is firm to palpation. Some would describe it as cauliflower-like or papulonodular. The buccal mucosa and mandibular gingiva are the most common locations. Men older than 60 years who have used smokeless tobacco for many years are most often affected. The disease is rare in persons younger than 40 years and in persons who do not use tobacco.

Verrucous carcinoma has a distinctive surface appearance. A characteristic feature is a white-gray, undulating keratotic surface with pink-red pebbly papules throughout. Lateral growth, which usually exceeds vertical growth, leads to an increase in mass and diameters of several centimeters. Large lesions can be locally destructive by invading and eroding the underlying alveolar bone. Similar-appearing lesions include verrucous epithelial hyperplasia, pyostomatitis vegetans, and proliferative verrucous leukoplakia.

Recommended treatment for verrucous carcinoma is wide surgical excision. Radiation therapy is contraindicated because of the demonstrated risk for anaplastic transformation to squamous cell carcinoma. After surgery, the long-term prognosis of affected patients is better than squamous cell carcinoma and improves when the use of smokeless tobacco is discontinued.

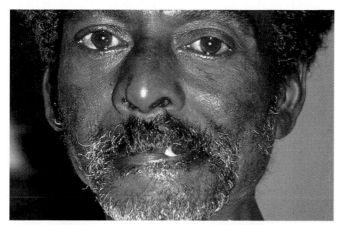

Fig. 51.1. Cigarette keratosis: user of unfiltered cigarettes.*

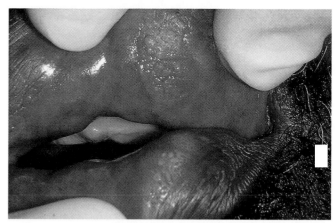

Fig. 51.2. Cigarette keratosis: on labial mucosa.*

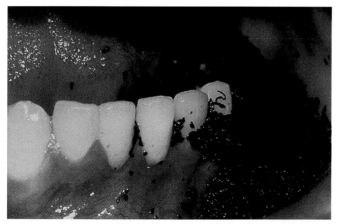

Fig. 51.3. Nicotine stomatitis: prominent on soft palate.

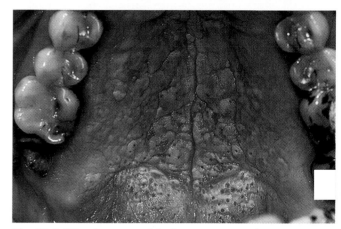

Fig. 51.4. Nicotine stomatitis: in a reverse smoker.

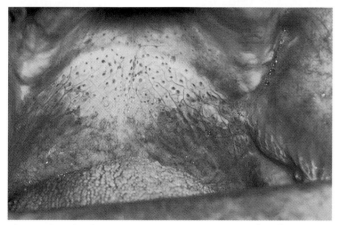

Fig. 51.5. Snuff dipper's patch: under chewing tobacco.

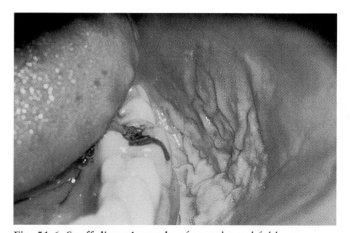

Fig. 51.6. Snuff dipper's patch: of mucobuccal fold.

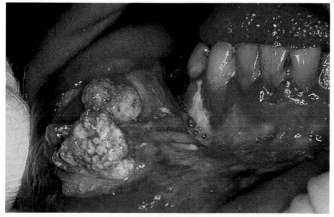

Fig. 51.7. Verrucous carcinoma: of the labial mucosa.

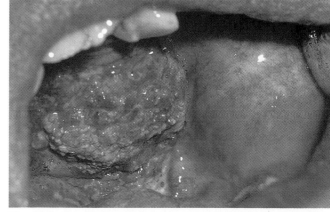

Fig. 51.8. Verrucous carcinoma: maxillary alveolar ridge.

Red Lesions

Many red lesions appear red because they have a vascular component. This page discusses red lesions associated with abnormalities of blood vessels and blood.

Purpura (Petechiae, Ecchymoses, Hematoma) (Figs. 52.1–52.4) Purpura are circumscribed regions of pooled extravasated blood in the dermis. The cause can be iatrogenic, factitial, or accidental trauma to vascular tissues contained within the dermis or submucosa. In circumstances in which trauma is not involved, quantitative or qualitative deficits in the platelets, clotting factors, capillary fragility, or infection should be suspected. Purpura initially appears bright red but tends to discolor with time, becoming purplish-blue and later brown-yellow. Because these lesions consist of extravasated blood, they do not blanch on diascopy (pressure with a glass slide).

The three types of purpura—petechiae, ecchymoses, and hematoma—are classified according to size and cause. **Petechiae** are pinpoint, nonraised circular red spots. The soft palate is the most common intraoral location for multifocal petechiae. Palatal petechiae may represent an early sign of viral infection (infectious mononucleosis), scarlet fever, leukemia, bleeding diatheses, or blood dyscrasia. They may also indicate rupture of palatal capillaries caused by coughing, sneezing, vomiting, or fellatio. Suction petechiae under a maxillary denture are not true purpura. They result from candidal infection and the resulting inflammation of the orifices of accessory salivary glands, not because of denture-created negative pressure as previously believed.

Ecchymosis (common bruise) is an area of extravasated blood usually greater than 1 cm in diameter. They range in color from red-purple to blue-green. Careful physical evaluation may reveal the cause to be mechanical trauma, hemostatic disorders, Cushing's disease, amyloidosis, neoplastic disease, primary idiopathic or secondary thrombocytopenic purpura, or use of anticoagulant drugs such as aspirin, bishydroxycoumarin, warfarin, or heparin.

Hematomas (large bruise) are large pools of extravasated blood resulting from traumatic vascular severance. They occur commonly in the oral cavity as a result of a blow to the face, tooth eruption, or rupture of the posterior superior alveolar vein during administration of local anesthesia (Figs. 48.3 and 48.4). They are usually dark red-brown and tender to palpation. Purpura fade with time and require no specific treatment. Determining the underlying cause is the prime consideration.

Varicosity (Varix) (Fig. 52.5) A varix is a red-purple fluctuant swelling frequently seen in elderly persons. The swelling represents a venous dilatation caused by reduced elasticity of the vascular wall as a result of aging or by an internal blockage of the vein. The ventrolateral surface of the anterior two thirds of the tongue is a common location. The floor of mouth, lip, and labial commissure are other common sites. Labial varices appear dark red to blue-purple. They are usually single, round, dome-shaped, and fluctuant. Palpation of the lesion disperses the blood from the vessel and causes the area to blanch; thus, the lesions are diascopy-positive.

Varices are benign and asymptomatic and require no treatment. If they are of cosmetic concern to the patient, varices can be surgically removed without significant bleeding. Varices are sometimes slightly firm because of fibrotic changes. Thrombosis is a rare complication that produces a firm nodule within the varix. When several veins on the ventral tongue are prominent, the condition is called phlebectasia linguae, or caviar tongue.

Thrombus (Fig. 52.6) The series of events that includes trauma, activation of the clotting sequence, and formation of a blood clot typically results in the cessation of bleeding. Several days later plasminogen initiates clot breakdown and normal blood flow resumes. In certain cases, if the clot does not dissolve, blood flow stagnates and a thrombus is formed.

Intraoral thrombi appear as raised red-brown or blue round nodules, typically in the labial mucosa. They are firm to palpation and may be slightly tender. No sexual predilection is evident, but thrombi are most commonly seen in patients older than 30 years. Thrombi concentrically enlarge to occlude the entire lumen of the vessel or mature and calcify to form a **phlebolith**. Phleboliths are rare oral findings that develop in the cheek, lips, or tongue. Radiographs show phleboliths to be doughnut-like, circular, radiopaque foci with a radiolucent center.

Hemangioma (Figs. 52.7 and 52.8) Hemangiomas are benign, enlarged, vascular hamartomas that may be seen in any soft tissue or bony intraoral location. They occur early in life and somewhat more commonly in women than in men. Soft tissue hemangiomas occur commonly in the dorsum of the tongue, gingiva, and buccal mucosa. On histologic examination they may be capillary or cavernous.

Hemangiomas, when situated deep within the connective tissue, do not alter the color of the mucosal surface. Superficial hemangiomas, in contrast, are red, blue, or purple; flat or slightly elevated; smooth-surfaced; and somewhat firm. Hemangiomas are positive to diascopy and may vary in size from a few millimeters to several centimeters. The borders are usually diffuse, and lobular surfaces are infrequent. Single hemangiomas are most common, whereas multiple lesions are seen in Maffucci's syndrome. Facial and oral hemangiomas form a component of Sturge-Weber's syndrome.

Large soft tissue hemangiomas present management problems. Surgical excision, sclerosing agents, cryotherapy, and radiation therapy have been used to eliminate these lesions. A hemangioendothelioma is the malignant counterpart to the hemangioma, whereas Kaposi's sarcoma is another malignant vascular tumor seen in about 25% of patients with the acquired immune deficiency syndrome (AIDS).

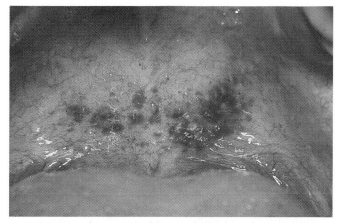

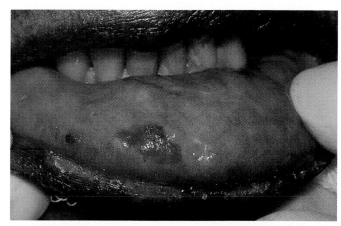

Fig. 52.1. Petechiae: caused by viral illness and coughing.

Fig. 52.2. Ecchymosis: in a patient receiving heparin.

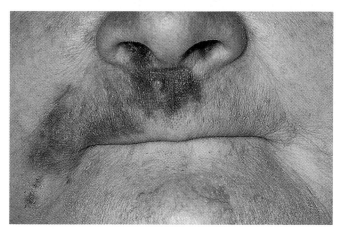

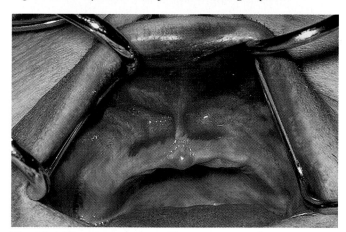

Fig. 52.3. Hematoma: after trauma from falling.*

Fig. 52.4. Hematoma: of maxillary mucosa and gingiva.*

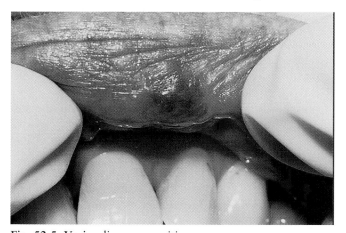

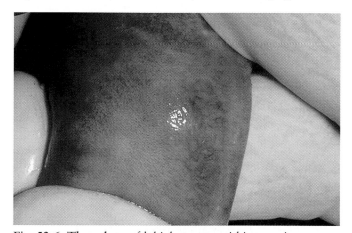

Fig. 52.5. Varix: diascopy positive.

Fig. 52.6. Thrombus: of labial mucosa within a varix.

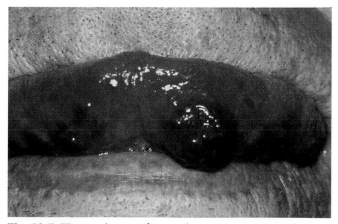

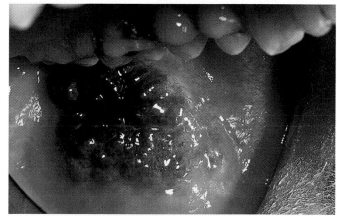

Fig. 52.7. Hemangioma: of ventral tongue.

Fig. 52.8. Hemangioma: of buccal mucosa.

Red Lesions

Hereditary Hemorrhagic Telangiectasia (Osler-Weber-Rendu Syndrome) (Figs. 53.1–53.4)

Hereditary hemorrhagic telangiectasia is a genetic disease inherited as an autosomal dominant trait. It is caused by a defect in a transmembrane protein (endoglin, activin receptor-like kinase-1) that is a component of the receptor complex for transforming growth factor beta (TGF-β). The disease is characterized by multiple telangiectasias, which are purplish red macules or slightly red papules representing permanently enlarged end capillaries of the skin, mucosa, and other tissues and organs. The lesions are usually 1 to 3 mm, lack central pulsation, and blanch on diascopy. The telangiectasias begin early in life; after puberty the size and number of lesions tend to increase with age. Men and women are affected equally. Bleeding is a prominent feature of this disease, and epistaxis is a common presenting feature.

History, clinical appearance, and histologic features are important in making the diagnosis of hereditary hemorrhagic telangiectasia, as the disease is asymptomatic in many victims. Clinically evident lesions are located immediately subjacent to the mucosa and are easily traumatized, resulting in rupture, hemorrhage, and ulcer formation. Skin lesions are less subject to rupture because of the overlying cornified epithelium. The most common locations on the skin are the palms, fingers, nail beds, face, and neck. Mucosal lesions can be found on the lips, tongue, nasal septum, and conjunctivae. The gingiva and the hard palate are less commonly involved. Vascular malformations also involve the lung, brain, and gastrointestinal tract, especially the liver. Complications include epistaxis from drying or irritation of involved nasal mucosa or from nasotracheal intubation; gastrointestinal bleeding, melena, and iron deficiency caused by rupture of telangiectasias of gastrointestinal mucosa and prolonged bleeding; and hematuria caused by rupture of telangiectasia within the urinary tract. Other complications include cirrhosis of the liver, pulmonary arteriovenous fistulae leading to pulmonary hypertension, and brain abscesses and emboli. Precautions are recommended with the use of inhalation analgesia, general anesthesia, oral surgical procedures, and hepatotoxic and antihemostatic drugs. Rupture of a telangiectasia may cause hemorrhage that is best controlled by pressure packs. Because brain abscesses form in a small percentage of patients, antibiotic prophylaxis before invasive dental treatment may be beneficial to these patients. Identification of this disorder warrants screening of family members by a physician.

Sturge-Weber Angiomatosis (Sturge-Weber or Encephalotrigeminal Syndrome) (Figs. 53.5–53.8)

Sturge-Weber angiomatosis is a rare, nonhereditary, congenital disorder that manifests venous angiomas of the leptomeninges of the brain, ipsilateral macular hemangiomas of the face, neuromuscular deficits, and oculo-oral lesions. The macular hemangioma of the facial skin, also called port-wine stain or nevus flammeus, is the most striking feature of the syndrome. The facial hemangioma is well demarcated, flat or slightly raised, and red to purple in color. It blanches under pressure. The stain is present at birth, is distributed along one or several branches of the trigeminal nerve, and typically extends to the patient's midline without crossing to the other side. The ophthalmic division of the trigeminal nerve is most frequently affected. No tenderness or inflammation is associated with the hemangioma, and it does not enlarge with age. In many patients with solitary congenital port-wine angiomas of the face, lesions regress spontaneously at puberty. Approximately 30% of persons with facial port-wine stains have Sturge-Weber angiomatosis; the remainder are free of the other features of the syndrome. Involvement of the ophthalmic branch of the trigeminal nerve appears to be most predictive of full involvement of the syndrome.

The altered venous blood flow caused by an angioma of the leptomeninges can result in cerebral cortical degeneration, seizures, mental retardation, and hemiplegia. On lateral skull radiographs, gyriform calcifications characteristically appear as double-contoured tramlines. Approximately 30% of patients have ocular abnormalities, including angiomas, colobomas, or glaucoma.

Vascular hyperplasia involving the buccal mucosa and lips is the most frequent oral finding. The palate, gingiva, and floor of the mouth may also be affected. The bright red oral patches are located on areas supplied by the branches of the trigeminal nerve. Like facial lesions, these patches stop abruptly at the midline. Involvement of the gingiva may produce edematous tissue and cause difficulty with hemostasis when surgical procedures involving these tissues are performed. Abnormal tooth eruption, macrocheilia, macrodontia, and macroglossia are sequelae of large vascular overgrowths. Gingival overgrowth may result from phenytoin therapy, which is given because these patients are subject to seizures. Careful assessment of the enlarged gingiva on the ipsilateral side, including biopsy, may be required to establish vascular involvement or drug-induced gingival overgrowth. In areas of vascular hyperplasia, oral surgery should be performed in accordance with strict hemostatic measures.

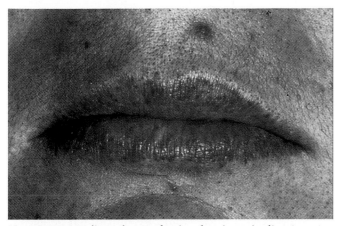

Fig. 53.1. Hereditary hemorrhagic telangiectasia: lips.*

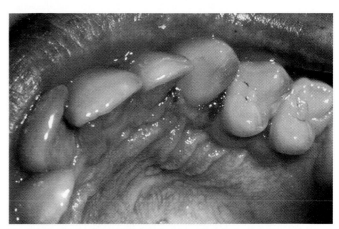

Fig. 53.2. Hereditary hemorrhagic telangiectasia: gingivi.*

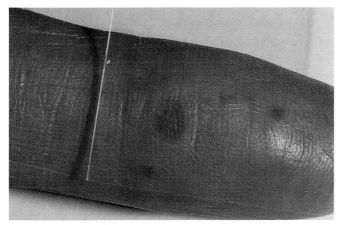

Fig. 53.3. Hereditary hemorrhagic telangiectasia.

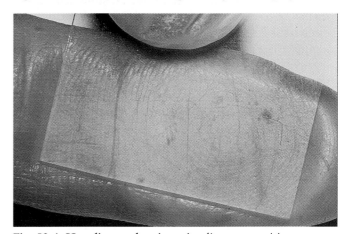

Fig. 53.4. Hereditary telangiectasia: diascopy positive.

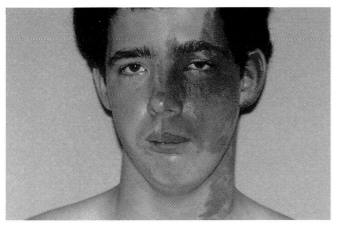

Fig. 53.5. Sturge-Weber angiomatosis.‡

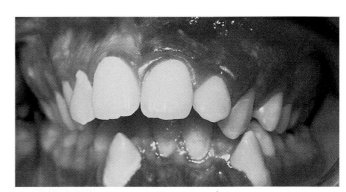

Fig. 53.6. Sturge-Weber angiomatosis.‡

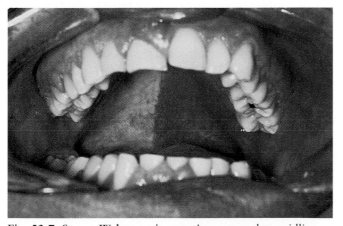

Fig. 53.7. Sturge-Weber angiomatosis: up to palate midline.

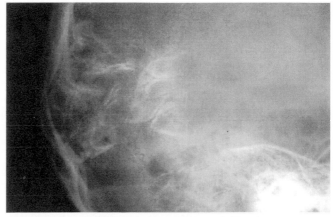

Fig. 53.8. Sturge-Weber angiomatosis: calcifications.

Red and Red-White Lesions

Erythroplakia (Figs. 54.1–54.4) Erythroplakia is defined as a persistent red patch that cannot be characterized clinically as any other condition. The term, like leukoplakia, has no histologic connotation. However, most erythroplakias are histologically diagnosed as epithelial dysplasia or worse and have a much higher propensity for progression to carcinoma than leukoplakia. Erythroplakias are most prevalent in the mandibular mucobuccal fold, oropharynx, tongue, and floor of the mouth, and are often associated with tobacco or alcohol use. They are usually asymptomatic. The redness of the lesion is a result of atrophic mucosa overlying a highly vascular (reddish) submucosa. The border is often well demarcated. There is no gender predilection, and patients older than 55 years are most commonly affected.

Three clinical variants of erythroplakia have been recognized: 1) the homogeneous form, which is completely red; 2) **erythroleukoplakia**, which mainly has red patches interspersed with occasional white areas; and 3) **speckled erythroplakia**, which contains white specks or granules scattered throughout the red lesion. Biopsy is mandatory for all types of erythroplakia because 91% represent severe dysplasia, carcinoma in situ, or invasive squamous cell carcinoma. Inspection of the entire oral cavity is required because 10 to 20% of these patients have several erythroplakic areas, a phenomenon known as **field cancerization**.

Erythroleukoplakia and Speckled Erythroplakia (Fig. 54.5)

Erythroleukoplakia and speckled erythroplakia, or speckled leukoplakia, as some prefer, are precancerous red and white lesions. Both are usually asymptomatic. Erythroleukoplakia and speckled erythroplakia have a male predilection, and most are detected in patients older than 50 years. They may occur at any intraoral site but frequently affect the lateral border of the tongue, buccal mucosa, and soft palate. Lesions are often associated with heavy smoking, alcoholism, and poor oral hygiene.

Fungal infections are common in speckled erythroplakias. *C. albicans,* the predominant organism, has been isolated in most cases; thus, management of these lesions should include analysis for candida. The cause-and-effect relationship between candidiasis and speckled leukoplakia is unknown, but erythroplakia with leukoplakic regions confers a greater risk for atypical cytologic changes. Because of the increased risk for carcinoma, biopsy of all red-white lesions is mandatory.

Squamous Cell Carcinoma (Figs. 54.6–54.8)

Squamous cell carcinoma is an invasive malignancy of oral epithelium. It is the most common type of oral cancer, accounting for more than 90% of all malignant neoplasms of the oral cavity. Oral cancer may occur at any age, but it is primarily a disease of the elderly; more than 95% of oral cancers occur in persons older than 40 years. In the past, the prevalence was much higher in men, but the male to female ratio has dramatically decreased in recent years to approximately 2:1 because of the increased number of women who smoke.

The exact cause of oral squamous cell carcinoma is unknown but appears to involve mutations of genes on chromosomes 3 and 9 (*p53, ras*) that regulate cell proliferation and apoptosis. Cytological changes occur with excessive use of tobacco and alcohol, infection by human papillomavirus, and immune compromise. Other contributory factors are those associated with aging and exposure to a variety of biologic, chemical, and physical agents, such as infection with *Treponema pallidum,* herpes simplex virus, or *C. albicans*; nutritional deficiency states; oral neglect; chronic trauma; and radiation.

In the United States, the most common site of intraoral squamous cell carcinoma is the lateral border and ventral surface of the tongue, followed by the oropharynx, floor of the mouth, gingiva, buccal mucosa, lip, and palate. The buccal mucosa is a common site in persons of developing countries who chronically use quid tobacco. The occurrence of carcinoma of the lip has decreased dramatically in the past decade because of the increased use of protective sunscreen agents. The dorsal surface of the tongue is almost never affected.

The appearance of squamous cell carcinoma is variable; more than 90% of cases are erythroplakic, and about 60% have a leukoplakic component. A combination of colors and surface patterns, such as a red and white lesion that is exophytic, infiltrative, or ulcerated, indicates instability of the oral epithelium and is highly suggestive of carcinoma. Early lesions are often asymptomatic and slow-growing. As the lesion develops, the borders become diffuse and ragged, and induration and fixation ensue. If the mucosal surface becomes ulcerated, the most frequent oral symptom is that of a persistent sore or irritation. With advancing disease, patients may report numbness or a burning sensation, swelling, or difficulty in speaking or swallowing. Lesions can extend to several centimeters in diameter if treatment is delayed; this delay permits lesions to invade and destroy vital osseous structures.

Squamous cell carcinoma spreads by local extension or by way of lymphatic vessels. Affected patients may have palpable regional (submandibular or anterior cervical) lymph nodes. These nodes can be large, firm, rubbery, and possibly fixed to underlying tissue. Staging of the tumor according to the TNM system—size (T), regional lymph nodes (N), and distant metastases (M)—allows assessment of the extent of disease. Surgery and radiation therapy have been the principal forms of treatment for oral cancer. The prognosis for oral cancer depends, in large measure, on the site involved (posterior tumors having worse prognosis), the clinical stage at the time of diagnosis and treatment, tumor diameter, the patient's access to adequate health care, and the patient's ability to cope and mount an immunologic response. Because early treatment is paramount, biopsy should be done if neoplasia is suspected.

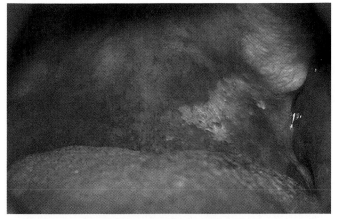

Fig. 54.1. **Erythroplakia:** must depress tongue to see.*

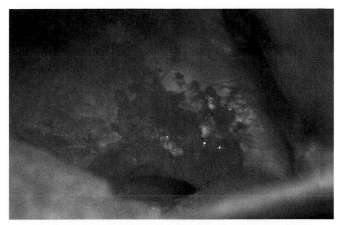

Fig. 54.2. **Erythroplakia:** soft palate tongue depressed.*

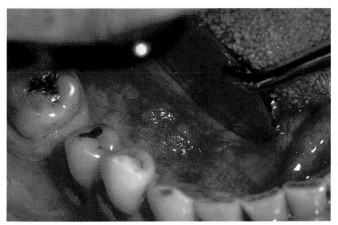

Fig. 54.3. **Erythroplakia:** of floor of mouth.

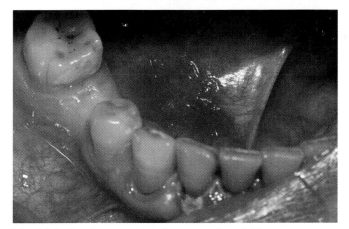

Fig. 54.4. **Carcinoma appearing as erythroplakia.**

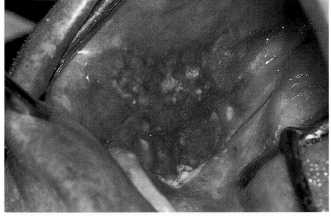

Fig. 54.5. **Erythroleukoplakia:** squamous cell carcinoma.‡

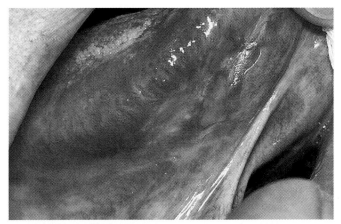

Fig. 54.6. **Squamous cell carcinoma:** of the tongue.‡

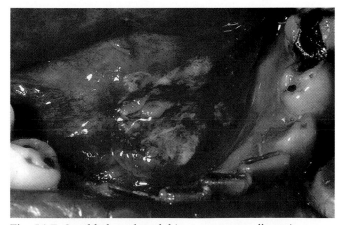

Fig. 54.7. **Speckled erythroplakia:** squamous cell carcinoma.

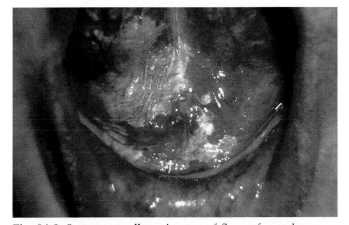

Fig. 54.8. **Squamous cell carcinoma:** of floor of mouth.

125

Red and Red-White Lesions

Lichen Planus (Figs. 55.1–55.6) Lichen planus is a common skin disease that can have mucosal manifestations. The cause and pathogenesis are unknown, although evidence suggests that lichen planus is an immunologic disorder in which T lymphocytes destroy the basal cell layer of the affected epithelium. Both CD4 and CD8 T-cell subsets have been identified in the submucosal lymphocyte population. Nervous, high-strung persons and persons infected with hepatitis C virus are predisposed to lichen planus. Most patients are women older than 40 years. The disease exhibits a protracted course with periods of remission and exacerbation.

The skin lesions of lichen planus initially consist of small, flat-topped, red papules with a depressed central area. The lesions may enlarge and become polygonal in shape or coalesce into larger plaques. The papules progressively acquire a violaceous hue and surface lichenification, which consists of fine white striae. Skin lesions usually itch and may change color to yellow or brown before resolution. Bilateral distribution on the flexor surfaces of the extremities is common, occasionally involving the fingernails, causing dystrophic changes. Patients with characteristic purple, polygonal, pruritic papules on the skin often have concurrent intraoral lesions. The vulva or glans penis are sometimes affected.

Oral lesions of lichen planus may have one of four appearances: **atrophic, erosive, striated (reticular), or plaquelike.** More than one form may affect a single patient. The most frequently affected site is the buccal mucosa. The tongue, lips, palate, gingiva, and floor of the mouth may also be affected. Bilateral and relatively symmetric lesions are common. Patients with reticular oral lichen planus characteristically have several delicate white lines and tiny papules arranged in a lacy, weblike network known as Wickham's striae. The glistening white areas are often asymptomatic but may be of cosmetic concern. They may involve large areas.

Atrophic lichen planus results from atrophy of the epithelium and predominantly appears as a red, nonulcerated mucosal patch. Wickham's striae are often present at the border of the lesion. When the attached gingiva is affected, the term desquamative gingivitis has been used.

Erosive lichen planus occurs if the surface epithelium is completely lost and erosion results. The buccal mucosa and tongue are commonly affected sites. A vesicle or bulla may initially appear; this eventually breaks down and produces an erosion. Mature lesions have irregular red borders, a yellowish necrotic central pseudomembrane, and an annular white patch, often at the periphery. The condition is intermittently painful and may develop rapidly. All of these features are helpful in differentiating oral lichen planus from other lesions with a similar clinical appearance, such as leukoplakia, erythroplakia, candidiasis, lupus erythematosus, pemphigoid, and erythema multiforme.

The least common type of lichen planus is the asymptomatic plaque form. This lesion is a solid white plaque or patch that has a smooth to slightly irregular surface and an asymmetric configuration. Lesions are commonly found on buccal mucosa or the tongue. Patients may be unaware of the lesions.

In many cases, clinical appearance alone can confirm the diagnosis of oral lichen planus, and biopsy is not necessary. Asymptomatic intraoral lesions can be left alone. Biopsy of the atrophic or erosive form should be performed at the border of the lesion, away from areas of ulceration.

The oral lesions of lichen planus tend to be more persistent than those of the skin. A vacation, change in routine, or discharge of psychologically burdensome problems can bring about abrupt and dramatic resolution of the lesions. Chronic, symptomatic, erosive lichen planus lesions are best managed with topical steroids, or short courses of systemic steroids and immunosuppressant agents. A few patients with oral lichen planus are diabetic and should be tested for glucose intolerance. Carcinomatous transformation has been reported (in fewer than 100 cases) to have an association with erosive lichen planus and tobacco use. The true cause-and-effect relationship, however, has yet to be established for squamous cell carcinoma and lichen planus.

Electrogalvanic White Lesion (Lichenoid Mucositis, Oral Lichenoid Reaction) (Figs. 55.7 and 55.8) Electrogalvanic white lesions closely resemble the hypertrophic form of lichen planus. This disorder is more apparent after 30 years of age and frequently occurs on the buccal mucosa, immediately adjacent to a metallic material (usually a restoration). Mild cases are asymptomatic, whereas erosive cases can cause a burning type of pain. The histologic features of this lesion mimic those of lichen planus. Electric microcurrents induced by dissimilar restorations is one explanation for this phenomenon. A more recent theory suggests that the disorder results from a delayed hypersensitivity reaction to antigens in various metals, particularly mercury. Interestingly, lichenoid drug reactions, which are similar in appearance to electrogalvanic white lesions, can be caused by the systemic administration or application of the same metals (mercury and gold) found in dental restorations. When systemically used drugs produce these lesions they are called oral lichenoid reactions or **lichenoid drug eruptions** (see Figs. 56.6–56.8). Treatment consists of replacing the restoration with a different restorative material, preferably gold, porcelain, glass ionomer, or composite materials. The prognosis is excellent, and healing occurs within weeks of removing the offending agent.

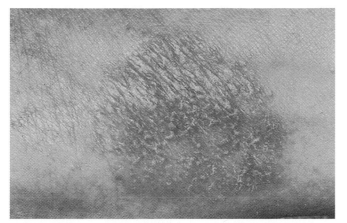

Fig. 55.1. Lichen planus: violaceous skin plaque of wrist.

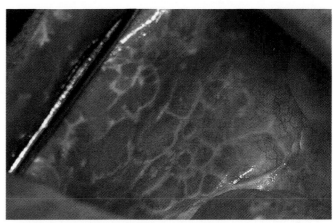

Fig. 55.2. Reticular lichen planus.

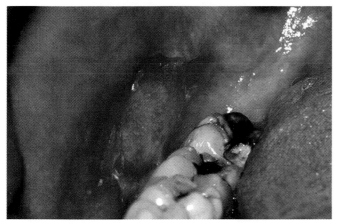

Fig. 55.3. Erosive lichen planus: of buccal mucosa.*

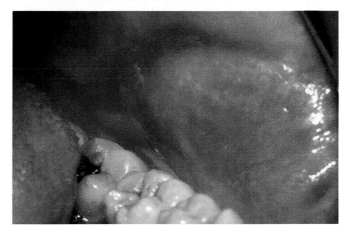

Fig. 55.4. Erosive lichen planus: opposite buccal mucosa.*

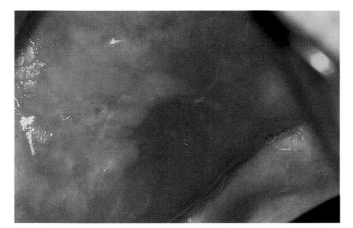

Fig. 55.5. Atrophic lichen planus: of buccal mucosa.

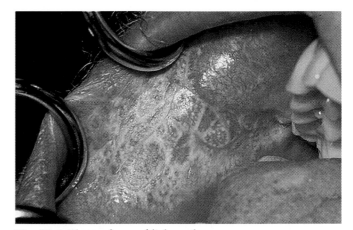

Fig. 55.6. Plaque form of lichen planus.

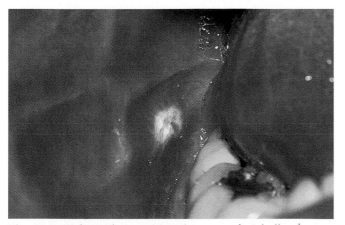

Fig. 55.7. Lichenoid mucositis: adjacent to facial alloy.‡

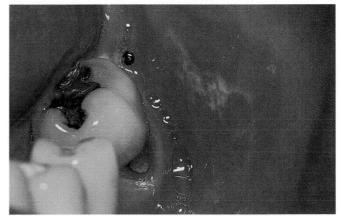

Fig. 55.8. Lichenoid mucositis: opposite buccal mucosa.‡

127

Red and Red-White Lesions

Lupus Erythematosus (Figs. 56.1–56.4) Lupus erythematosus is an autoimmune collagen disease characterized by the production of antinuclear antibodies (ANA) and anti-DNA antibodies that participate in immunologically mediated tissue injury. Three forms exist: chronic discoid lupus erythematosus, also known as chronic cutaneous lupus erythematosus, which only involves the skin; systemic lupus erythematosus, in which multiple organ systems are involved; and subacute cutaneous lupus erythematosus, a cutaneous variant with mild systemic symptoms. The cause of all three types is unknown.

Chronic discoid lupus erythematosus, the benign form of the disease, is a purely mucocutaneous disorder. It may appear at any age but predominates in women older than 40 years. The condition is classically characterized by the appearance of a red butterfly rash symmetrically distributed on the cheeks across the bridge of the nose. Other prominent photosensitive areas of the face, including the malar areas, forehead, scalp, and ears, may be involved.

The lesions of lupus erythematosus are chronic, with periods of exacerbation and remission. Mature lesions exhibit three zones: an atrophic center lined by a hyperkeratotic margin, which is surrounded by an erythematous periphery. As the center heals, hypopigmentation results from melanocyte damage at the epidermal–dermal junction and the ensuing collagen deposition. Telangiectasias, blackheads, a fine scale, and hair loss at sites of involvement are common dermal findings. The lesions are usually limited to the upper portion of the body, particularly the head and neck.

Twenty to 40% of patients with lupus erythematosus have oral lesions. These lesions may develop before or after skin lesions develop. Lip lesions are red with a white to silvery, scaly margin. A sun-exposed lower lip at the vermilion border is a common site, whereas the upper lip is usually involved as a result of direct extension of dermal lesions. Intraoral lesions are frequently diffuse erythematosus plaques, with erosive, ulcerative, and white components.

Chronic discoid lupus erythematosus sometimes appears as isolated red-white plaques. The buccal mucosa is the most frequent intraoral site, followed by the tongue, palate, and gingiva. The oral lesions are characterized by a central, red atrophic area sometimes covered by a fine stippling of white dots. The peripheral margins are irregular and are composed of alternating red and keratotic white lines extending for a short length up to about 1 cm in a radial pattern. These lesions may mimic lichen planus, but concurrent ear involvement helps to exclude the diagnosis of lichen planus. Ulcerative lesions are painful and require treatment. Avoidance of emotional stress, cold, sunlight, and hot spicy foods is necessary. The use of sunscreens, topical steroids, systemic steroids, and antimalarial and immunosuppressive agents have proven effective. Patients using antimalarial agents require close ophthalmologic follow-up.

Systemic manifestations of the disease often begin with complaints of fatigue, fever, and joint pain. Generalized nontender lymphadenopathy is often present. Hepatomegaly, splenomegaly, peripheral neuropathy, and hematologic abnormalities may also be seen. Strict avoidance of sun exposure is necessary because sunburn can trigger acute exacerbations. Involvement of the kidneys and heart is a common occurrence that may prove fatal. Skin and oral lesions may accompany the condition, but there is little chance of conversion from discoid to systemic lupus. Patients with systemic lupus erythematosus often have other concurrent autoimmune collagen-vascular diseases, such as Sjögren's syndrome and rheumatoid arthritis. Allergic mucositis, candidiasis, leukoplakia, erythroleukoplakia, and lichen planus must be considered in the differential diagnosis of oral lupus erythematosus lesions. Biopsy and histologic examination with immunofluorescence confirm the diagnosis. Precautions are advised in the dental treatment of patients with lupus erythematosus, who may be taking high doses of systemic steroids, because of their predisposition to delayed wound healing, their risk for infection, and the possibility of stress-induced adrenal crisis characterized by cardiovascular collapse. These patients are also at risk for cardiomyopathy, which if severe requires antibiotic prophylaxis.

Lichenoid and Lupuslike Drug Eruption (Figs. 56.5–56.8) Stomatitis medicamentosa is a general term for an oral hypersensitivity reaction to drugs. Two subcategories of oral hypersensitivity, called lichenoid drug eruption and lupuslike drug eruption, produce reticular or erosive lesions similar in appearance to lichen planus and lupus erythematosus. Although the appearance may vary, white linear plaques with red margins are common. The lesions may erupt on immediate use or after prolonged use of a drug. Persistent inflammatory changes may result in large erythematous areas, eventual mucosal ulceration, and pain. Drug-induced lupus erythematosus is often associated with arthritis, fever, and renal disease. Hydralazine and procainamide are the most common instigators of lupuslike drug eruptions. Other drugs known to cause lupuslike eruptions include gold, griseofulvin, isoniazid, methyldopa, penicillin, phenytoin, procainamide, streptomycin, and trimethadione. Drugs known to induce lichenoid eruptions include the following: chloroquine, dapsone, furosemide, gold, mercury, methyldopa, palladium, penicillamine, phenothiazines, quinidine, thiazides, certain antibiotics, and heavy metals. Consultation with a physician and withdrawal of the offending medication leads to regression of the lesion. A substitute drug is usually selected to manage the patient's systemic problem.

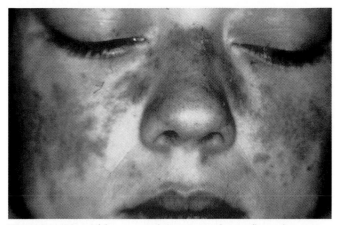

Fig. 56.1. Discoid lupus erythematosus: butterfly rash.

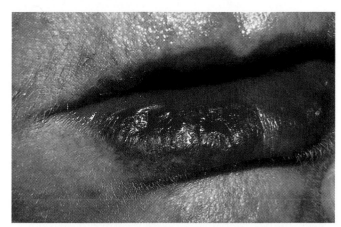

Fig. 56.2. Discoid lupus erythematosus: lip lesion.

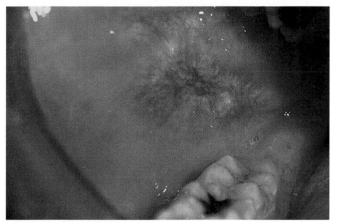

Fig. 56.3. Alternating red-white lines of lupus erythematosus.

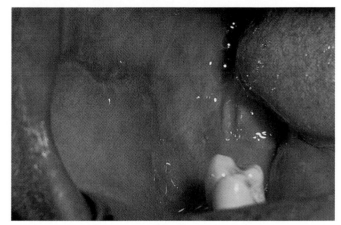

Fig. 56.4. Atrophic lesion of lupus erythematosus.

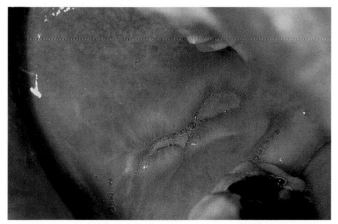

Fig. 56.5. Lupuslike drug eruption: with amitriptyline use.*

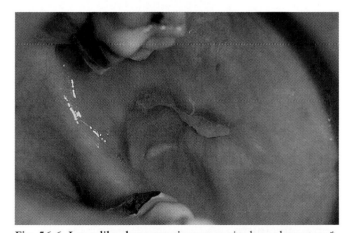

Fig. 56.6. Lupuslike drug eruption: opposite buccal mucosa.*

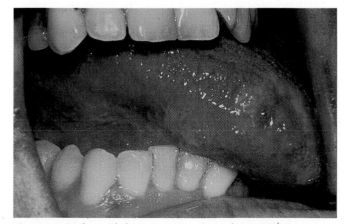

Fig. 56.7. Lichenoid drug eruption: lateral tongue.‡

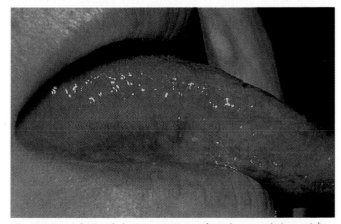

Fig. 56.8. Lichenoid drug eruption: after drug withdrawal.‡

Red and Red-White Lesions

Acute Pseudomembranous Candidiasis (Thrush) (Figs. 57.1 and 57.2) Acute pseudomembranous candidiasis, an opportunistic infection, is caused by an overgrowth of the superficial fungus C. albicans. It appears as diffuse, curdy, or velvety white mucosal plaques that can be wiped off, leaving a red, raw, or bleeding surface. The organism is a common inhabitant of the oral cavity, gastrointestinal tract, and vagina. Infants whose mothers have vaginal thrush at the time of birth and adults who have experienced an upset in the normal oral microflora because of antibiotics, steroids, or systemic alterations such as diabetes, immunodeficiency, or chemotherapy are frequently affected. There is no racial or gender predilection. Acute pseudomembranous candidiasis is usually found as white plaques with red borders on the buccal mucosa, tongue, and soft palate. In patients with asthma who use a steroid inhaler, the pattern appears as a circular or oval reddish-white patch at the site of aerosol contact on the palate. Diagnosis is made by clinical examination, fungal culture, or direct microscopic examination of tissue scrapings. A cytologic smear treated with potassium hydroxide, Gram's, or periodic acid–Schiff stain will reveal budding organisms with branching pseudohyphae. Topical application of antifungal medication for 2 weeks usually produces resolution.

Chronic Hyperplastic Candidiasis (Figs. 57.3 and 57.4) Chronic hyperplastic candidiasis is caused by candidal organisms that penetrate the mucosal surface and stimulate a hyperplastic response. Chronic irritation, poor oral hygiene, and xerostomia are predisposing factors; thus, smokers and denture wearers are commonly affected. Systemic diseases such as diabetes mellitus and HIV infection can also be involved.

Chiefly affected are the dorsum of the tongue, palate, buccal mucosa, and labial commissures. The lesion invariably has a distinctive raised border, a white or grayish pebbly surface and an occasional red area caused by destruction of the mucosal cell layer. Thus, the condition may resemble leukoplakia, erythroleukoplakia, or verrucoid growths.

The white patch of chronic hyperplastic candidiasis cannot be peeled off; thus, the diagnosis must be made by biopsy. On microscopy, the organisms may be identified by routine hematoxylin and eosin stain or, more appropriately, by the periodic acid–Schiff stain. With adequate topical application of an antifungal agent, the condition usually resolves. In some instances surgical stripping may be required. All patients with chronic keratotic candidiasis should be followed closely because this form may be related to speckled erythroplakia, a lesion that is often premalignant or worse.

Acute Atrophic Candidiasis (Antibiotic Sore Mouth) (Fig. 57.5) The use of broad-spectrum antibiotics, particularly tetracyclines, or topical steroids can result in acute atrophic candidiasis. This fungal infection is the result of an imbalance in the oral ecosystem between *Lactobacillus acidophilus* and *C. albicans*. Antibiotics taken by the patient reduce the *Lactobacillus* population and permit candidal organisms to flourish. The infection produces desquamated areas of surface mucosa that appear as diffuse, nonelevated red patches. Burning pain is the most frequent symptom. The distribution of the patches sometimes indicates the cause. Lesions affecting the buccal mucosa, lips, and oropharynx often suggest the systemic administration of antibiotics, whereas redness of the tongue and palate are more common after the use of antibiotic troches. When the tongue is affected, a surface devoid of filiform papillae is common. Candidiasis rarely affects the attached gingiva; if this is the clinical finding, severe immunosuppression is a distinct possibility. The diagnosis is confirmed by demonstration of budding organisms or hyphal forms on a stained cytologic smear. Treatment should be withdrawal of offending antibiotics and use antifungal drugs.

Angular Cheilitis (Fig. 57.6) Angular cheilitis, or *perleche*—meaning to lick—is a chronic painful condition involving the labial commissures caused by C. albicans, lip-licking, and pooling saliva. On clinical examination, angular cheilitis appears red, fissured, and centrally ulcerated. Erythema, crusting, and brownish granulomatous nodules may occur along the peripheral margins. Discomfort caused by opening the mouth may limit normal oral function. Predisposing factors include nutritional deficiency, loss of vertical dimension, and high sucrose intake. Treatment involves antifungal agents, correction of predisposing factors, and habit cessation.

Chronic Atrophic Candidiasis (Denture Stomatitis) (Figs. 57.7 and 57.8) Chronic atrophic candidiasis is the most common form of chronic candidiasis. It is present in 15 to 65% of complete and partial denture wearers, particularly elderly women who wear their dentures at night; rarely, dentate patients may also be affected. The mandible, however, is rarely involved. Misnomers for this disease are denture sore mouth and denture base allergy.

Chronic atrophic candidiasis is caused by candidal organisms under the denture base. There are three stages of mucosal alterations. The earliest lesions are red pinpoint areas of hyperemia limited to the orifices of the palatal minor salivary glands. Progression produces a diffuse erythema of the hard palate that is sometimes accompanied by epithelial desquamation. **Papillary hyperplasia**, consisting of multiple fibromalike papules, is the third stage. It may be generalized or restricted to relief areas. With time, the papules may enlarge to form red nodules on the palate. Effective therapy requires antifungal treatment of the mucosa and denture base. Traumatic influences, such as the rocking action of the denture, should be eliminated to expedite healing. Occasionally surgical removal is required.

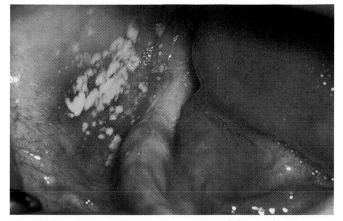

Fig. 57.1. **Acute pseudomembranous candidiasis:** diabetic.

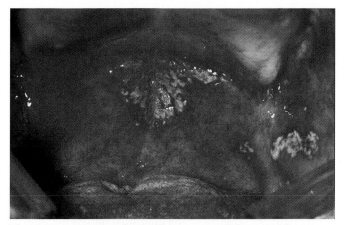

Fig. 57.2. **Acute pseudomembranous candida:** steroid user.

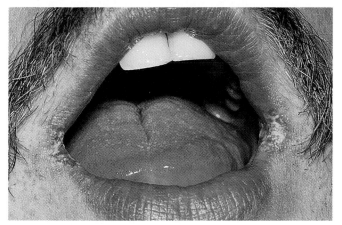

Fig. 57.3. **Chronic hyperplastic candidiasis:** at commissures.

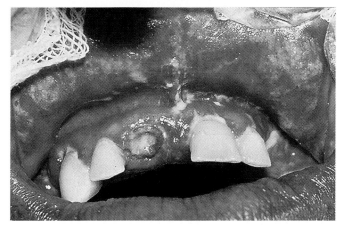

Fig. 57.4. **Chronic hyperplastic candidiasis:** of labial mucosa.

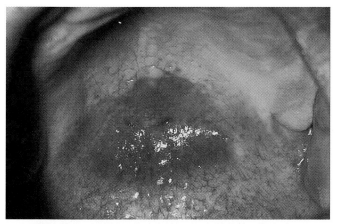

Fig. 57.5. **Acute atrophic candidiasis:** inhaled steroid use.

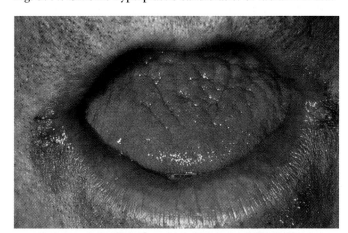

Fig. 57.6. **Angular cheilitis:** after antibiotic therapy.

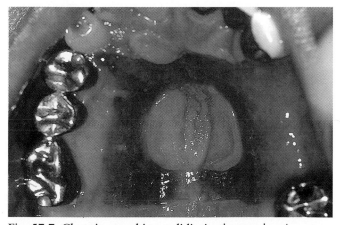

Fig. 57.7. **Chronic atrophic candidiasis:** denture-bearing area.

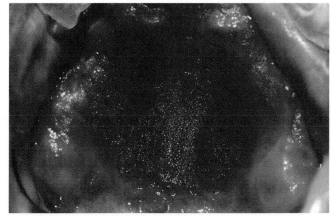

Fig. 57.8. **Papillary hyperplasia:** third stage.

131

Pigmented Lesions

Melanoplakia (Fig. 58.1) Melanoplakia is a generalized and constant dark pigmentation of the oral mucosa, commonly seen in dark-skinned persons (melanoderms). The condition is physiologic, not pathologic, and results from increased amounts of melanin, an endogenous pigment, that are deposited in the basal layer of the mucosa and lamina propria. The most common site for observing melanoplakia is the attached gingiva. It often appears as a diffuse, ribbonlike, dark band with a well-demarcated and curvilinear border that separates it from the alveolar mucosa. The region is characteristically symmetric and asymptomatic. The degree of pigmentation varies from light brown to dark brown and infrequently may appear blue-black. Other sites of occurrence are the buccal mucosa, hard palate, lips, and tongue. At these sites the deposition of pigment is often multifocal and diffuse. Melanoplakia should be differentiated from similar-appearing conditions that produce oral pigmentations, such as Addison's disease, Albright's syndrome, Peutz-Jeghers syndrome, heavy metal pigmentation, and use of antimalarial drugs.

Tattoo (Figs. 58.2–58.5) Tattoos are caused by intentional or accidental implantation of exogenous pigments into the mucosa. The most common intraoral type is the **amalgam tattoo,** which has been referred to as focal argyrosis. The amalgam tattoo appears as a blue-black, nonelevated discoloration that is usually irregular in shape and variable in size. It results from the entrapment of amalgam in a soft tissue wound such as an extraction socket or a gingival abrasion from a rotating bur. Deterioration of the silver compounds of the amalgam impart the characteristic blue-black color. Focal discolorations may occasionally appear green to dark gray because of the deposition of high copper alloys.

Amalgam tattoos are usually seen in the gingiva in posterior areas adjacent to a large amalgam restoration or gold casting. These lesions are not limited to the gingiva and may also be seen on the edentulous ridge, vestibular mucosa, palate, buccal mucosa, and floor of the mouth. The clinical diagnosis of an amalgam tattoo can be confirmed by finding radiographic evidence of the foreign metal in the paradental tissue. The radiographic appearance may vary from the absence of demonstrable particles to pinpoint or globular radiopacities several millimeters in diameter. If radiographs fail to demonstrate suspected metallic particles, a biopsy is required to rule out more serious pigmented lesions.

Other types of tattoos seen in the oral cavity are the graphite pencil wound and India ink tattoos. The graphite pencil wound appears after trauma as a focal, slate-gray macule. Sites frequently affected are the lip and the palate. The nature of the lesion can be easily ascertained by questioning the patient. Ordinary India ink tattoos are occasional findings on the labial mucosa of the lower lip. In general, tattoos are harmless and of no clinical significance; however, they may be indistinguishable from more potentially ominous lesions.

Ephelis (Freckle) (Fig. 58.6) An ephelis is a light to dark-brown macule that appears on the lip or skin after active deposition of melanin triggered by exposure to sunlight. Unlike some pigmentations, this lesion remains essentially unchanged in size with time, darkens in response to sunlight, and has a predilection for light-skinned or red-headed persons. A single freckle is clinically distinguished from an oral melanotic macule by the history of a traumatic or inflammatory episode that precedes the development of the latter condition. On microscopic examination, an ephelis shows an increase in melanin pigment without an increase in the number of melanocytes. Multiple freckles on the lip should be distinguished from the identical lip ephelides seen in conjunction with palmar pigmentations and intestinal polyposis of Peutz-Jeghers syndrome. Ephelides may be of cosmetic concern and require surgical removal; otherwise, observation is normally recommended.

Smoker's Melanosis (Tobacco-Associated Pigmentation) (Figs. 58.7 and 58.8) Smoking tobacco imparts smoker's melanosis, a characteristic change in color to exposed mucosal surfaces. The condition is not a normal physiologic process but instead results primarily from the deposition of melanin in the basal cell layer of the mucosa. The relationship of smoker's melanosis and inflammatory changes that result from heat, smoke inhalation, and the absorption of exogeous pigments has not been determined.

Smoker's melanosis affects older persons who are heavy smokers. It appears as a diffuse brown patch up to several centimeters in size. The mandibular anterior gingiva and buccal mucosa are the most frequently affected sites; other susceptible sites include the labial mucosa, palate, tongue, floor of the mouth, and lips. The degree of pigmentation ranges from light to dark brown and appears to be directly related to the amount of tobacco consumed. Dark-brown foci are usually distributed asymmetrically throughout an ill-defined, light-brown patch. Brown-stained teeth and halitosis usually accompany the condition. Smoker's melanosis itself is not premalignant; however, the clinician should closely inspect the adjacent tissues for other tobacco-induced lesions, which may be more significant.

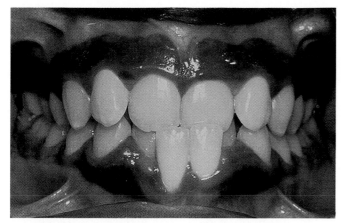

Fig. 58.1. **Melanoplakia:** along the attached gingiva.

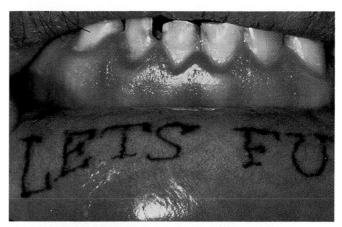

Fig. 58.2. **India ink tattoo.**

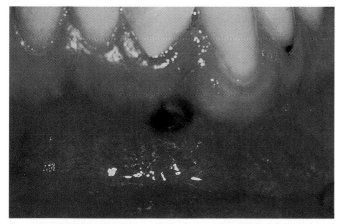

Fig. 58.3. **Amalgam tattoo:** in attached gingiva.*

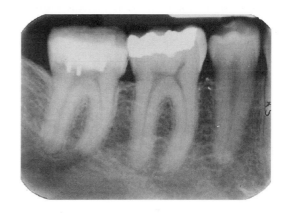

Fig. 58.4. **Radiograph of amalgam tattoo.***

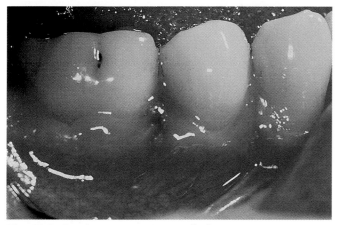

Fig. 58.5. **Focal argyrosis:** after silver-point endodontics.

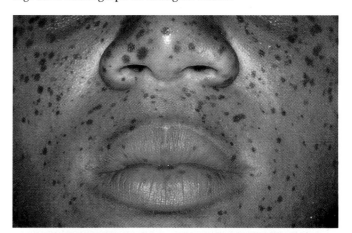

Fig. 58.6. **Ephelides:** multiple freckles of the face and lips.

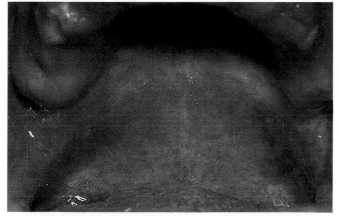

Fig. 58.7. **Smoker's melanosis:** in lateral soft palate.

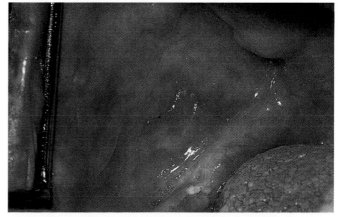

Fig. 58.8. **Smoker's melanosis:** of the buccal mucosa.

133

Pigmented Lesions

Oral Melanotic Macule (Focal Melanosis) (Figs. 59.1 and 59.2) An oral melanotic macule is a flat circumscribed pigmentation of the lip or mouth. It results from focal deposition of melanin along the basal layer of epithelium. These asymptomatic pigmentations are usually single, less than 1 cm in diameter, and common in light-skinned persons between the ages of 25 and 45 years. They probably represent posttraumatic or inflammatory pigmentation, a condition analogous to postinflammatory hypermelanosis of skin. The most common site is the lower lip close to the midline. Other sites include the gingiva, buccal mucosa, and palate. The color is uniform and may be blue, gray, brown, or black. Biopsy is recommended unless it has been present for many years without visible change and periodic observation is provided.

Nevus (Figs. 59.3–59.6) The nevus is a mucocutaneous lesion comprised of a collection of nevus cells (called theques) in the epithelium or dermis. It is commonly seen on the skin and occasionally occurs in the mouth. There are many types of nevi, which are broadly classified as either congenital or acquired. Congenital nevi are present at birth and are also known as birthmarks or garment trunk nevi. They are usually larger than acquired nevi and have a higher incidence of malignant transformation.

Acquired nevi, or moles, occur later in life and usually appear as dark, slightly raised papules or dome-shaped nodules. They vary in pigment and can be brown, grayish, or black. Occasionally nevi are amelanotic and appear pink. In the mouth, nevi are rare. They are usually asymptomatic, small, pigmented, well-circumscribed, dome-shaped papules or macules that occur on the palate and buccal mucosa mainly of women. Their size tends to remain constant after puberty.

Benign nevi have been classified into four subtypes according to the histologic appearance and location of the nests of nevus cells. The intramucosal nevus is the most common nevus in the mouth and the body followed by the blue nevus, compound nevus, and junctional nevus.

The **intramucosal nevus** has ovoid nevus cells located in the connective tissue only. This entity is analogous to the intradermal nevus, which appears as a dark, raised papule on the skin, often seen with a hair growing from it. It is rare, however, to find a hair associated with the intramucosal nevus of the mouth. The intramucosal nevus is usually brown and raised and ranges from 0.4 to 0.8 cm in diameter.

The second most common intraoral nevus is the **blue nevus.** The name originates from the typical blue or blue-black color imparted by the spindle-shaped nevus cells located deep in the connective tissue. These cells are derivatives of neural crest cells that fail to migrate from the region. A small, focal blue macule is the typical appearance, although the nevus often fades with age. The palate is the most common location. Malignant transformation of intraoral blue nevi has never been reported.

The **compound nevus,** as the name implies, is composed of nevus cells located in the epithelium and the lamina propria. The compound nevus rarely undergoes malignant transformation. The **junctional nevus** is a subtype of acquired nevus in which nevus cells are located at the junctional layer of the epithelium and the lamina propria. These lesions are the rarest type of oral nevus and usually appear flat and brown and have a diameter less than 1 cm. The palate and buccal mucosa are common locations.

On rare occasions the **melanotic freckle of Hutchinson** (lentigo maligna) is found in the mouth. The melanotic freckle is usually seen on the face of persons older than 50 years. This lesion is flat, irregularly shaped, and dirty gray-brown. It may spread superficially in a horizontal direction and undergo malignant transformation.

Nevi may be difficult to distinguish from their malignant counterparts; thus, all intraoral pigmented lesions should be biopsied.

Melanoma (Figs. 59.7 and 59.8) Melanomas are malignant neoplasms of melanocytes that occur primarily in sun-exposed skin surfaces, and infrequently in the oral cavity. The tumors occur twice as frequently in men as women and mostly in light-skinned persons between 20 and 50 years of age. Mucosal lesions often appear after age 50. There is no sex predilection. About 30% of melanomas arise from previously existing pigmented lesions, such as moles, particularly ones with a history of trauma. They may appear flat or raised, nonpigmented or pigmented. Pigmented lesions are usually deep brown, gray, blue, or jet black. The most frequent oral sites are the maxillary alveolar ridge, palatal tissues, anterior gingivae, and labial mucosa. Malignant changes appear associated with a defect of *CDKN2A* located on chromosome 9 and *BRAF* gene mutations.

Melanoma begins as a small superficial or slightly raised patch that grows slowly and laterally over several months. Early recognizable signs are A, asymmetrical lesion; B, border irregularity; C, color variegation within the lesion; and D, diameter enlarging. Eventually a prominent, nonmovable, dark lesion develops. The clinician should be alert to features that include multiple colors (the combination of red together with blue-black and white is particularly ominous); change in size; satellite lesions arising at the periphery of the lesion; and signs of inflammation, such as a peripheral zone of erythema. Late signs include bleeding and ulceration, firmness, and firm regional lymph nodes. Intraoral melanomas are extremely dangerous and more serious than their cutaneous counterpart because of early and wide metastasis, which results in poor prognosis. Early diagnosis when tumors are less than 1.5 mm in size and complete resection are critical to long-term survival. The 5-year survival rate of oral melanoma is only about 20%.

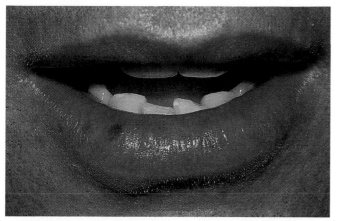

Fig. 59.1. **Oral melanotic macule:** in the lower lip.

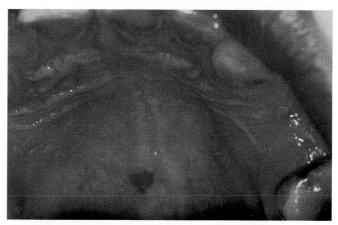

Fig. 59.2. **Oral melanotic macule:** of the hard palate.

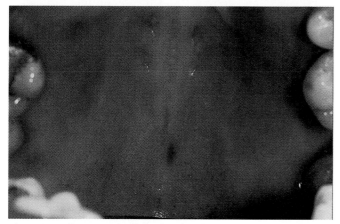

Fig. 59.3. **Blue nevus:** of the hard palate.

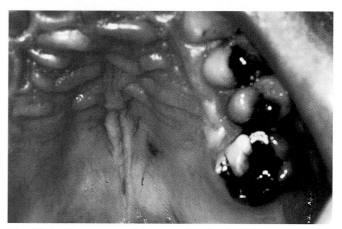

Fig. 59.4. **Blue nevus:** of the lateral palatal vault.

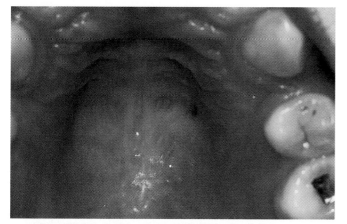

Fig. 59.5. **Compound nevus:** on the anterior palate.

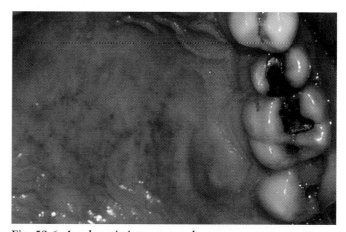

Fig. 59.6. **Amelanotic intramucosal nevus:** next to upper molar.

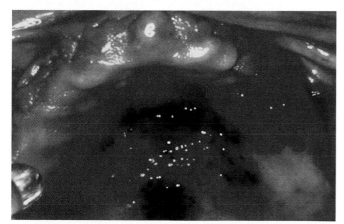

Fig. 59.7. **Melanoma:** satellite lesions of palate.

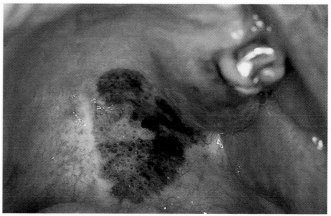

Fig. 59.8. **Melanoma:** of the soft palate.

Pigmented Lesions

Peutz-Jeghers Syndrome (Hereditary Intestinal Polyposis) (Figs. 60.1 and 60.2) Peutz-
Jeghers syndrome is an autosomal dominant condition associated with multiple melanotic macules and gastrointestinal polyposis. It appears to be caused by a germ-line mutation in the *LKB1* gene of chromosome 19 that encodes a multifunctional serine-threonine kinase. The macules are distributed on the skin around the eyes, nose, mouth, lips, perineum, oral mucosa, gingiva, and palmar and plantar surfaces of the hands and feet. The multiple benign intestinal polyps are hamartomatous tissue growths that usually occur in the ileum but also are found in the stomach and colon. Symptoms such as intermittent colicky pain and reports of obstruction may be concurrent. The perioral pigmentations must be distinguished from multiple ephelides and lentigenes of the LEOPARD syndrome.

The most common intraoral locations for the macules are the lips and buccal mucosa. Characteristically, the density of macules is higher on the vermilion than the adjacent skin. The macules are asymptomatic, small, flat brown ovals that do not darken with exposure to the sun, as freckles do. In contrast to their cutaneous counterparts, the intraoral spots tend to persist into adulthood, whereas the dermal macules may fade with age. No treatment is necessary for the macules, which on microscopic examination are shown to contain hyperpigmentation of the basal cell layer and lamina propria. Although the macules are benign, they are of considerable clinical significance because a small percentage of affected patients are prone to develop gastrointestinal (colorectal) adenocarcinoma and are at an increased risk for tumors of the reproductive system. The diagnosis of Peutz-Jeghers syndrome therefore necessitates prompt medical evaluation.

Addison's Disease (Adrenal Cortical Insufficiency, Hypoadrenocorticism) (Figs. 60.3 and 60.4) Addison's disease most commonly results from autoimmune-induced destruction of the adrenal gland. Other causes include infectious diseases, adrenalectomy, Gram-negative sepsis, pituitary insufficiency, and tumor invasion. Progression of the disease results in anemia, anorexia, diarrhea, hypotension, lethargy, nausea, and weight loss.

A complication associated with this disorder is failure of the feedback loop from the adrenal gland to the pituitary gland. This causes an increase in adrenocorticotrophic hormone, which induces melanocyte-stimulating hormone and the deposition of melanin in the skin, especially in sun-exposed areas. Classically the skin acquires a bronze tan that persists after sun exposure. Darkening may be initially noted on the knuckles, elbows, palmar creases, and intraoral mucosa.

In the mouth, the disease is characterized by hypermelanosis that is similar in appearance to melanoplakia. The pattern is not unique and may consist of multiple focal brown-bronze to blue-black spots or generalized, diffuse streaks of dark-brown pigmentation. The pigmented areas are usually macular, nonraised, brown, and varied in shape. The buccal mucosa and gingiva are most commonly affected, but the pigmentation may also extend onto the tongue and lips. Biopsy is not diagnostic, and serum cortisol tests are recommended. Replacement therapy with corticosteroids produces a gradual diminution of the hyperpigmentation; thus, the degree of oral pigmentation is a sensitive indicator of therapeutic effectiveness. Transient changes in pigmentation in a treated patient may indicate inadequate therapy.

Heavy Metal Pigmentation (Figs. 60.5–60.8)
Excessive ingestion of heavy metals (bismuth, lead, mercury, silver) and certain drugs (cis-platinum, antimalarial agents, antipsychotic agents, birth control pills) can produce mucocutaneous pigmentations. Bismuth is commonly found in diarrhea medications, which if used for a long term results in diffuse deposition of the metal in the gingiva. The discoloration is confined to the marginal gingiva, particularly in areas where inflammation is present. The bismuth line usually appears blue to black in a linear distribution along the gingival sulcus. A metallic taste and burning mucosa are common symptoms.

Lead poisoning, or plumbism, is usually a result of occupational exposure to excessive doses of lead used in paints, batteries, or plumbing. The most prominent intraoral change and early diagnostic sign is a gray-black lead line that occurs from the deposition of lead sulfide in the marginal gingiva. Spotty gray macules on the buccal mucosa, a coated tongue, neurologic deficits (tremor of the extended tongue), and hypersalivation are other intraoral findings. The condition is reversible if exposure to lead is eliminated.

Mercury poisoning, or acrodynia, can be acquired by absorption, inhalation, or ingestion. Although uncommon today, acrodynia was the result of treatment for syphilis earlier in the century. Inadequate mercury hygiene measures, such as handling mercury, breathing mercury vapors, and spilling mercury, place dental personnel at risk for acrodynia. Like bismuth and lead intoxication, mercury poisoning produces a dark mercury gingival line. In addition, the disease is often accompanied by many signs and symptoms, including abdominal pain, anorexia, headaches, insomnia, psychological symptoms, vertigo, oral ulcerations, hemorrhage, a metallic taste, sialorrhea, burning mouth, and periodontal destruction.

Silver pigmentation, or argyria, is a rare occurrence that most often results from prolonged exposure to silver-containing ocular, nasal, or oral medications. Asymptomatic pigmentations accumulate in the sun-exposed areas of the skin, along with the hair, fingernails, and oral mucosa. A blue-gray pigmentation is characteristic; once evident, the pigmentation is irreversible. Nasal inhalation of solutions containing silver salts have a propensity to deposit in the palatal mucosa, imparting a color similar to that seen on the skin. Treatment is immediate withdrawal of the medication.

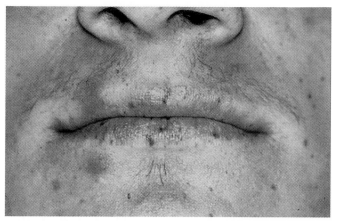

Fig. 60.1. Peutz-Jeghers syndrome: lips and perioral skin.

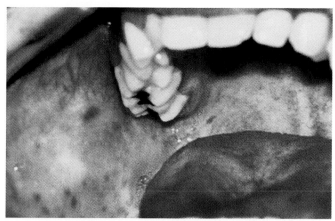

Fig. 60.2. Peutz-Jeghers syndrome: of the buccal mucosa.

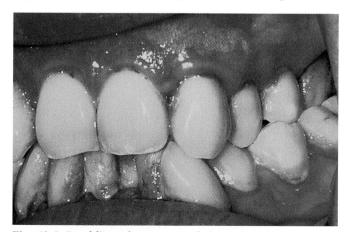

Fig. 60.3. Addison's disease: pigmentation of the lips.*

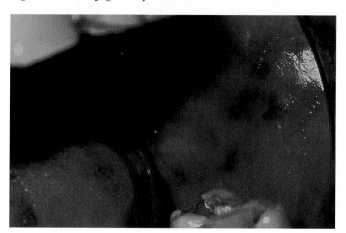

Fig. 60.4. Addison's disease: of the buccal mucosa.*

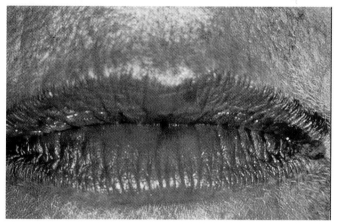

Fig. 60.5. Lead line: along marginal gingiva.

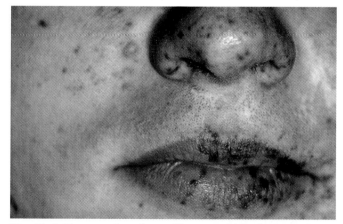

Fig. 60.6. Pigmentation: from silver acetaldehyde detonation.

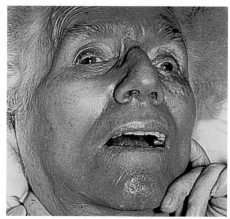

Fig. 60.7. Argyria: chronic use of silver-containing nose drops.‡

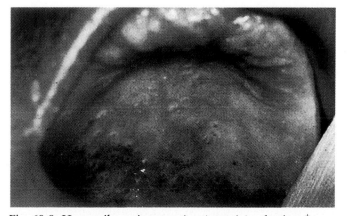

Fig. 60.8. Heavy silver pigmentation (argyria): of palate.‡

Intraoral Findings by Surface Change

Nodules

Retrocuspid Papilla (Figs. 61.1 and 61.2) Not all persons have a retrocuspid papilla. This particular growth appears as a firm, round, fibroepithelial papule about 1 to 4 mm in diameter. It is located on the lingual surface of the attached gingiva of the mandibular cuspids just below or several millimeters below the marginal gingiva. The surface mucosa is pink, soft, and smooth. Rarely, the structures may be pedunculated and the stalk can be lifted off the gingiva by a periodontal probe. The retrocuspid papilla is a variation of normal and is frequently found bilaterally. Some authorities state that it is a developmental anomaly that represents a variant form of fibroma. The retrocuspid papilla seems to be present in most children but regresses with maturity; thus, the incidence and size decrease with increasing age. The retrocuspid papilla has no gender predilection, and no treatment is necessary unless interference with a removable prosthesis is anticipated.

Oral Lymphoepithelial Cyst (Figs. 61.3 and 61.4) The oral lymphoepithelial cyst is an encapsulated dermal or submucosal papule that arises from epithelium entrapped in lymphoid tissue that has undergone cystic transformation. The cyst is benign and asymptomatic, but may enlarge and spontaneously fistulate. Most appear in children and young adults. No sex predilection has been demonstrated.

When the lymphoepithelial cyst is derived from degenerative tissue of the second branchial arch, it is referred to as a **cervical lymphoepithelial cyst** or a **branchial (cleft) cyst**. This cyst appears on the lateral aspect of the neck just anterior and deep to the superior third of the sternocleidomastoid muscle near the angle of the mandible. The cyst may occur in the proximity of the parotid gland. The extraoral lymphoepithelial cyst is a well-circumscribed, soft, fluctuant mass that is rubbery to the touch. They may enlarge to 1 or 2 cm and can drain externally.

Common sites for the oral lymphoepithelial cyst are the floor of the mouth, lingual frenum, ventral tongue, posterior lateral border of the tongue, and, rarely, the soft palate. These small swellings, rarely exceeding 1 cm in diameter, are characteristically well circumscribed, soft, doughy, yellow when superficial, and pink when deeper. Palpation yields a slightly moveable nodule. When located in the anterior floor, the lesion may resemble a mucous-retention cyst. Infrequently, multiple lymphoepithelial cysts can be found.

Histologic examination shows that lymphoepithelial cysts are usually lined with stratified squamous epithelium; occasionally, pseudostratified, columnar, or cuboidal epithelium is found. A fibrous connective tissue wall surrounds the lesion. More centrally located are dark-staining lymphoid aggregates with prominent germinal centers. The luminal fluid is yellow and viscous because of a cheesy keratinaceous content. Excisional biopsy should be performed to provide histologic confirmation. Lymphoepithelial cysts rarely recur.

Torus, Exostosis, and Osteoma (Figs. 61.5–61.8; also see Figs. 27.1 and 27.2) Tori, exostoses, and peripheral osteomas are readily recognizable bony hard nodules that appear histologically identical. The term used depends on location, appearance, and systemic associations.

Tori are bony protuberances of the jaws, localized to the palatal midline or mandibular lingual attached gingiva. They are the most common intraoral lesions that are exophytic by nature. Women are more frequently affected. Tori have smooth, rounded contours, normal-appearing or slightly pale mucosa, and a sessile base. Tori are often found to have a lobulated surface. Internally they are composed of cortical bone with an occasional central core of spongy bone. Hereditary factors contribute to the development of tori.

Exostoses are bony outgrowths in alternate locations of tori. The facial aspect of the maxillary and mandibular alveolar ridge are common sites. Infrequently, the palatal alveolar ridge adjacent to maxillary molars is affected. Most exostoses are multiple hard nodules that demonstrate creaselike folds between distinct nodules. The surface mucosa is firm, taut, and white to pale pink.

Tori and exostoses tend to increase slowly in size with advancing age but remain asymptomatic unless traumatized. After a traumatic incident, patients may be concerned about neoplasia and state that the bony mass is enlarging or that it was not present before the injury. Removal is generally unnecessary unless prompted by cosmetic, prosthodontic, psychological, or traumatic considerations.

Osteomas are considered to be neoplastic growths that are distinct from the developmental lesions, tori and exostoses, because osteomas have more growth potential, tend to be larger, and may rarely be confined to soft tissue. Those that arise on the surface of bone are known as **periosteal osteomas**, whereas those arising within bone are **endosteal osteomas**. Patients with osteomas should be examined radiographically for multiple impacted supernumerary teeth and odontomas, which may indicate the presence of **Gardner's syndrome**. This autosomal dominant condition, associated with a gene abnormality on chromosome 5, is characterized by osteomas, dermal cysts, multiple impacted and supernumerary teeth, odontomas, and intestinal polyposis that have a high propensity for malignant transformation. Most patients with Gardner's syndrome demonstrate malignant polyposis by 40 years; thus, all patients with this condition require close medical management.

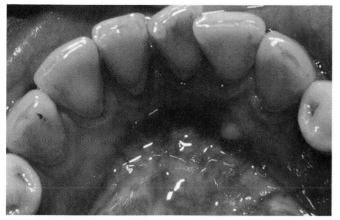

Fig. 61.1. **Retrocuspid papilla.**

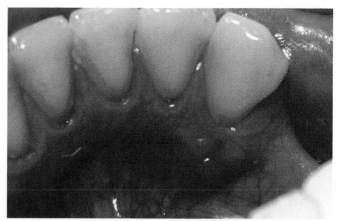

Fig. 61.2. **Retrocuspid papilla:** with unusual clefting.

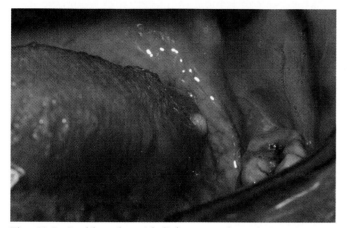

Fig. 61.3. **Oral lymphoepithelial cyst:** on lateral tongue.

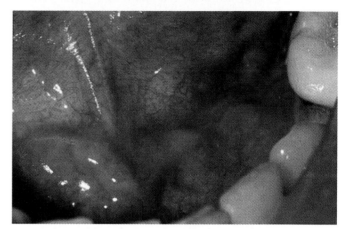

Fig. 61.4. **Oral lymphoepithelial cyst:** in floor of mouth.

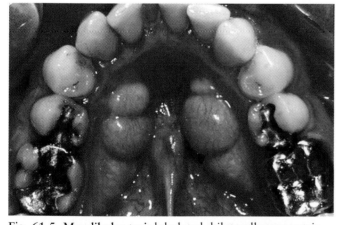

Fig. 61.5. **Mandibular tori:** lobulated, bilaterally symmetric.

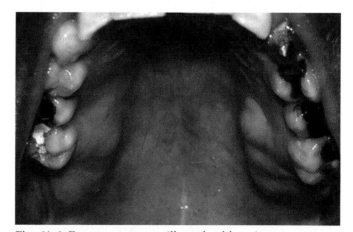

Fig. 61.6. **Exostoses:** on maxilla, palatal location.

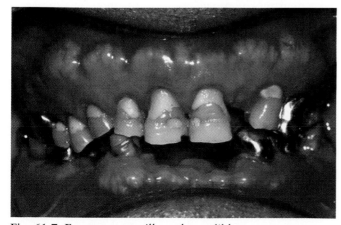

Fig. 61.7. **Exostoses:** maxilla and mandible.

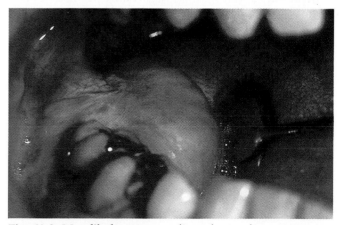

Fig. 61.8. **Mandibular osteoma:** lingual to molars.

Nodules

Irritation Fibroma (Fig. 62.1) The irritation fibroma is one of the most common benign lesions of the oral cavity. It results from reactive hyperplasia caused by a chronic irritant; thus, this lesion is not a true neoplasm as the term implies. True intraoral neoplastic fibromas are rare. The irritation fibroma typically appears as a well-defined, pale pink papule that slowly enlarges to form a nodule. This smooth and symmetrically round lesion is firm and painless to palpation. Infrequently, a white, roughened, or ulcerated surface is present because of repeated trauma. The growth arises usually from a sessile base of the buccal mucosa, labial mucosa, gingiva, or tongue. Histologic examination shows an interlacing mass of dense collagenous tissue subjacent to thinned epithelium. Fibromas are treated by removing the source of the irritation together with conservative surgical excision. Fibromas occur mostly in adults. They recur infrequently if treated properly. Multiple intraoral (angio)fibromas are associated with **tuberous sclerosis**, an autosomal dominant disorder characterized by seizures, mental deficiency, and angiofibromas of the face.

Peripheral Odontogenic Fibroma The peripheral odontogenic fibroma is clinically similar to the irritation fibroma but characterized by its unique location and tissue of origin—arising from cells of the periodontal ligament. Accordingly, it is generally found in the region of the interdental papilla. An example is shown in Figure 32.7.

Giant Cell Fibroma (Fig. 62.2) The giant cell fibroma is a pink papule or nodule that has a sessile base and smooth or slightly pebbly surface. It represents a variant of the irritation fibroma and is distinguished mostly by its histologic appearance. The giant cell fibroma has many large, polynucleated stellate-shaped fibroblasts scattered among a loosely arranged vascular connective tissue; the irritation fibroma does not. Most giant cell fibromas occur before 35 years of age; the mandibular gingiva, tongue, and palate are common sites. Excision is recommended, and recurrence is rare.

Lipoma (Fig. 62.3) The lipoma is a common benign dermal tumor, but a rare intraoral finding. This slow-growing neoplasm is composed of mature fat cells surrounded by a thin, fibrous connective tissue wall. Adults older than 30 years of age are commonly affected, and no gender predilection exists. In the mouth, lipoma appears as a well-circumscribed, smooth-surfaced, dome-shaped, or diffusely elevated nodule that is yellow to pale pink. Lipomas are sometimes polypoid, pedunculated, or lobulated. They occur on the buccal mucosa, tongue, floor of the mouth, alveolar fold, and lip. The palate is a rare site of involvement. Palpation reveals a soft, movable, and compressible submucosal mass that has a slightly doughy consistency. Therapy consists of surgical removal, which includes the base of the lesion. Lipomas rarely recur.

Lipofibroma (Fig. 62.4) The lipofibroma is a rare benign intraoral neoplasm of mixed connective tissue origin. It is a well-demarcated submucosal mass consisting of mature lipid-containing cells with a significant fibrous connective tissue component. Clinical examination shows a blend of a fibroma and lipoma. It is generally found on labial and buccal mucosa. The lesion is nonindurated, movable, painless, and soft or firm depending on the lipoid-to-collagen content. They grow slowly but can obtain several centimeters in diameter.

Traumatic Neuroma (Figs. 62.5 and 62.6) A neuroma is a benign tumor of neural tissue. It arises de novo or as a result of trauma (amputation or traumatic neuroma). The **traumatic neuroma** results from a hyperplastic response to nerve damage after severance of a large nerve fiber. In the mouth, the traumatic neuroma is frequently encountered in the mandibular mucobuccal fold in the region adjacent to the mental foramen. It also arises facial to the mandibular incisors, lingual to the retromolar pad, and in ventral tongue. Size of the lesion depends on the degree of insult and hyperplastic response.

Traumatic neuromas are usually small nodules, measuring less than 0.5 cm in diameter. Visualization may be difficult if the lesion is located deep below normal oral mucosa. Neuromas are painful when palpated. Pressure applied to the neuroma elicits a response often described as an electric shock. Multiple neuromas discovered on the lips, tongue, or palate may indicate the possibility of **multiple endocrine neoplasia type III**, also known as MEN IIb—an autosomal dominant condition characterized by numerous mucosal neuromas, marfanoid habitus, and endocrine neoplasms. Treatment of the traumatic neuroma is surgical excision or intralesional injection with corticosteroids. Excision may further damage the nerve and lead to recurrence.

Neurofibroma (Figs. 62.7 and 62.8) Neoplastic proliferation of peripheral nerve, including the sheath of Schwann, results in neurofibroma. Neurofibromas are benign tumors that commonly appear as sessile, firm, pink nodules. They may be solitary or diffuse, or exceed 1,000 in number. Solitary nodules are rare. More commonly, multiple large neurofibromas are encountered, with **neurofibromatosis** (von Recklinghausen's disease). See "Swellings of the Face" (Fig. 47.6).

Intraoral neurofibromas may be located on the dental arches, buccal mucosa, tongue, and lips. Most soft tissue neurofibromas are asymptomatic, but those arising within deeper tissues or bone may produce pain and paresthesia. Diffuse neurofibromas are striking for their firmness and irregular nodular surface, which results in physical deformity. In some cases, neurofibromas undergo sarcomatous change, which necessitates close follow-up. Solitary neurofibromas not associated with von Recklinghausen's disease have no tendency for malignant transformation.

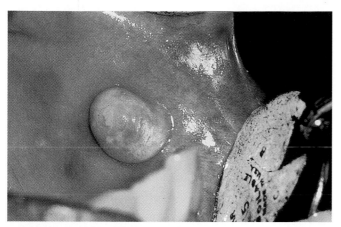

Fig. 62.1. **Irritation fibroma:** on buccal mucosa.

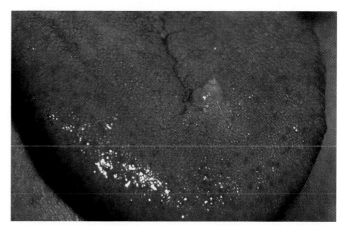

Fig. 62.2. **Giant cell fibroma:** on dorsum of tongue.

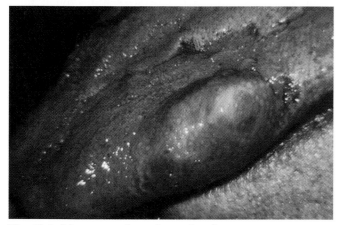

Fig. 62.3. **Lipoma:** on lateral margin of tongue.

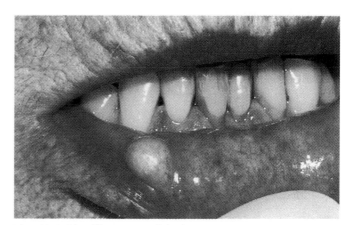

Fig. 62.4. **Lipofibroma:** on labial mucosa.

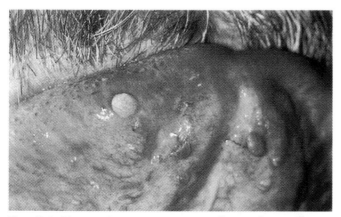

Fig. 62.5. **Traumatic neuroma:** near midline and a papilloma.

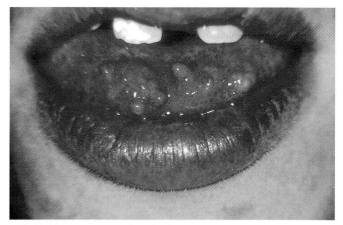

Fig. 62.6. **Neuromas of multiple endocrine neoplasia.**

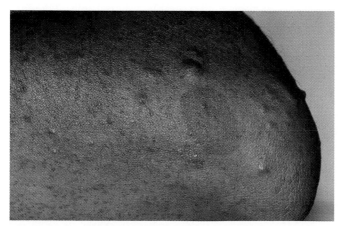

Fig. 62.7. **Neurofibromas:** and café-au-lait spot.

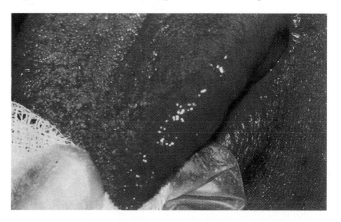

Fig. 62.8. **Neurofibroma:** on lateral margin of tongue.

Papulonodules

Oral Squamous Papilloma (Papilloma) (Figs. 63.1 and 63.2)
Papillomas are the most common benign epithelial neoplasm of the oral cavity. They appear as small, pink-white, exophytic masses that are usually less than 1 cm in diameter. The surface of the papule may be smooth, pink, and pebbly (vegetative) or have numerous small fingerlike projections. The base is pedunculated and well circumscribed. Intraoral lesions are typically soft, whereas keratin-producing lesions are rough or scaly. Lesions are generally solitary, but multiple lesions are occasionally seen. Human papillomavirus (HPV) types 6 and 11 have been detected in more than 50% of papillomas examined and are generally accepted as the cause of this disease.

The mean age of occurrence of papilloma is 35 years; both sexes are affected equally. The most common location is the uvulopalatal complex, followed by the tongue and frenum, lips, buccal mucosa, and gingiva. Other HPV-induced lesions, such as the condyloma acuminatum, focal epithelial hyperplasia (Heck's disease), and verruca vulgaris, share similar clinical features but are microscopically distinct. Histologic features include fingerlike epithelial projections and a fibrovascular core. Treatment is complete excision, including the base. Recurrence is rare. Malignant transformation has not been reported; thus, any rapidly advancing papillomatous lesion should be suspected to be a more aggressive lesion.

Verruca Vulgaris (Fig. 63.3)
Verruca vulgaris is the common skin wart that seldom occurs intraorally. The etiologic agents are HPV types 2, 4, 6, and 11. Virally induced cellular changes result in the characteristic clinical findings. The lesional surface is typically rough and raised, with white fingerlike projections. The whiteness of intraoral verrucae varies depending on the amount of surface keratinization. Pink areas are not unusual at the lesional base. Verrucae are commonly located on the skin, commissure, vermilion border, labial and buccal mucosa, tongue, and attached gingiva. The base of the lesion is broad, but the size is usually less than 1 cm. On clinical examination it may appear identical to a papilloma, although the clefts are more shallow and the mass more sessile. Viral inclusion bodies are frequently seen on histologic examination. Patients with skin verrucae are more likely to have oral lesions as a result of autoinoculation. A lesion may sometimes regress spontaneously. If not, treatment is complete excision or ablation with a carbon dioxide laser using high-speed evacuation. Recurrence is possible.

Focal Epithelial Hyperplasia (Heck's Disease) (Fig 63.4)
Focal epithelial hyperplasia is a virus-induced disease associated with multiple asymptomatic, papulonodular growths of the oral mucosa, particularly the tongue and labial and buccal mucosa. It was first described in Native Americans and Eskimos but now has been reported in many populations. The etiologic agents have been identified as HPV types 13 and 32. The virus is transmitted during kissing. Virus replication in epithelial cells produces soft papular growths in children and teenagers. Lesions are initially small, discrete, flat papules that are pink or whitish-pink. Later lesions enlarge, become papillary or cobblestoned, and can coalesce. Some lesions undergo spontaneous regression; surgical excision can be performed for those that do not regress.

Condyloma Acuminatum (Venereal Wart) (Figs. 63.5 and 63.6)
The condyloma acuminatum is a transmissible papillomatous growth that occurs orally much less frequently than the papilloma. It is seen more commonly in sexually active persons and is much more likely to be multiple. The warm, moist, intertriginous areas of the anogenital skin and mucosa are frequent sites of growth. In more than 85% of condyloma acuminata, HPV types 6 and 11 DNA is present in the epithelium.

Condyloma acuminata are usually small and pink to dirty gray. The surface may be flat but is more often pebbly and resembles a cauliflower. The base is sessile and the borders are raised and rounded. Contagious spread may occur between sexual partners. When multiple lesions are present, proliferation of adjacent condylomas can form extensive clusters that may appear as a single mass. Any oral mucosal surface may be affected, but the labial mucosa is the most common site. Other sites include the tongue, lingual frenum, gingiva, and soft palate. Histologic examination shows parakeratosis, cryptic invagination of cornified cells, and koilocytosis. Wide excision or antiviral agents are used in treatment, as condylomata have a high rate of recurrence. Occasional oncogenic transformation of long-standing anogenital growths has been reported, but this is not the case with oral lesions.

Lymphangioma (Figs. 63.7 and 63.8)
Lymphangiomas are benign hamartomas of lymphatic channels that develop early in life with no sex predilection. They may occur on the skin or mucous membrane. In the oral cavity, they occur commonly in the dorsal and lateral surface of the anterior portion of the tongue, lips, and labial mucosa.

Small superficial lymphangiomas have irregular papillary projections that resemble a papilloma. They are soft and compressible and vary from normal pink to whitish, slightly translucent, or blue. Deep-seated lesions cause diffuse enlargement and stretching of the surface mucosa. A diffuse lymphangioma in the tongue causes macroglossia, in the lips it causes macrocheilia, and in the neck it is called a **cystic hygroma**. Aspiration or diascopy is mandatory before surgical excision of a lymphangioma to prevent complications associated with the similar-appearing hemangioma. Patients with a large, diffuse lesion often require hospitalization to monitor postoperative edema and possible airway obstruction. Lymphangiomas do not undergo malignant change. Some lymphangiomas, especially congenital types, regress spontaneously during childhood.

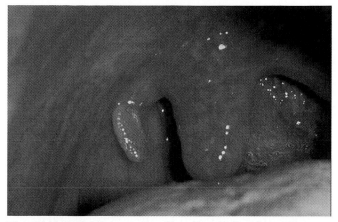

Fig. 63.1. Oral squamous papilloma: on soft palate.

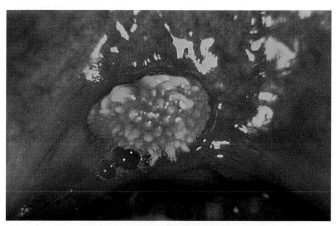

Fig. 63.2. Papilloma: with finger-like projections.

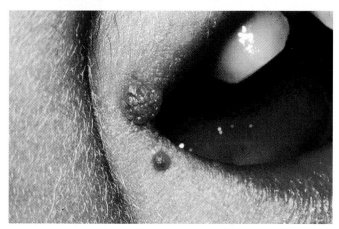

Fig. 63.3. Verruca vulgaris: autoinoculation from fingers.

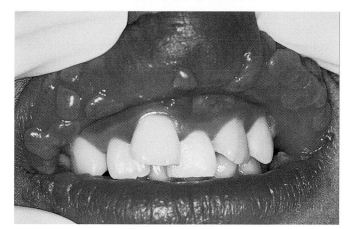

Fig. 63.4. Focal epithelial hyperplasia: on labial mucosa.

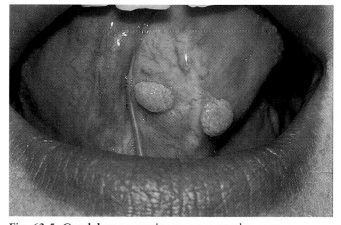

Fig. 63.5. Condyloma acuminata: on ventral tongue.

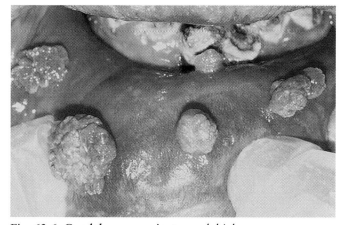

Fig. 63.6. Condyloma acuminata: on labial mucosa.

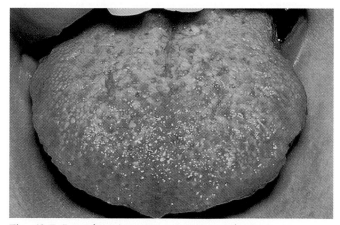

Fig. 63.7. Lymphangioma: causing macroglossia.*

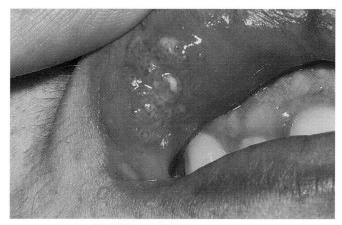

Fig. 63.8. Lymphangioma: of lip.*

Vesiculobullous Lesions

Primary Herpetic Gingivostomatitis (Figs. 64.1–64.3)

Herpes simplex virus (HSV) types 1 and 2 belong to the family Herpesviridae, which includes eight viruses (cytomegalovirus, varicella-zoster virus, Epstein-Barr, and human herpes virus VI, VII, and VIII). Approximately 75 to 90% of the adult human population have been infected with HSV. Transmission occurs by direct mucocutaneous contact of infected oral secretions. In most cases, HSV-1 is the causative organism; however, HSV-2, which has a propensity to infect the skin below the waist, can cause herpetic gingivostomatitis by oral-genital or oral-oral contact.

The manifestations of the primary infection may be trivial or fulminating. Trivial infections are the norm, producing subclinical signs that go unrecognized or may produce flulike symptoms. When symptomatic, the infection is called primary herpetic gingivostomatitis. It occurs most commonly in children younger than 10 years, and second most commonly in young adults. The acute inflammatory response of the primary HSV infection usually follows a 2- to 10-day incubation period. Infected patients report fever, malaise, and irritability. Focal areas of the marginal gingiva initially become fiery red and edematous. The swollen interdental papillae bleed after minute trauma because of capillary fragility and increased permeability. Widespread inflammation of the marginal and attached gingiva develops, and small clusters of vesicles rapidly erupt throughout the mouth. The vesicles burst, forming yellowish ulcers that are individually circumscribed by a red halo. Coalescence of adjacent lesions forms large ulcers of the buccal mucosa, labial mucosa, gingiva, palate, tongue, and lips. Shallow erosions of the perioral skin and hemorrhagic crusts of the lips are characteristic. Headache, lymphadenopathy, and pharyngitis are usually present, with some reports indicating preferential pharyngeal involvement in young adults, especially with HSV-2 infection.

A significant problem in patients with primary herpetic gingivostomatitis is the pain. Mastication and deglutition may be impaired, resulting in dehydration and subsequent elevation of temperature. Viral culturing, serum antibody levels, and results of cytologic testing are confirmatory. Treatment is supportive and should include antiviral agents in severe cases. Patients with a high temperature (exceeding 101°F) should receive nonaspirin antipyretic drugs and antibiotics.

Primary herpetic gingivostomatitis is a contagious disease that usually regresses spontaneously within 12 to 20 days without scarring. Complications associated with the primary infection include autoinoculation of other epidermal sites, producing keratoconjunctivitis and herpetic whitlow; extensive epidermal infection in the atopic patient, which is called Kaposi's varicelliform eruption; and meningitis, encephalitis, and disseminated infections in immunosuppressed patients. Immunity to HSV is relative, and patients previously infected with the virus may be reinfected with a different strain of HSV.

Recurrent Herpes Simplex (Figs. 64.4–64.7)

After the initial infection, HSV infects sensory nerve fibers, migrates to a regional neuronal ganglia, and becomes stably associated with the nucleus of the infected cell in a latent and undetectable manner. Reactivation of virus, replication of progeny particles, and clinical recurrence occurs in approximately 40% of persons who harbor latent virus. Recurrences are often precipitated by sunlight, heat, stress, trauma (dental procedures), or immunosuppression. Normal immune mechanisms are required to eliminate reactivated HSV. Asymptomatic shedding of virus into saliva in the absence of oral lesions occurs in 10% of any given HSV-infected population.

Recurrent herpes simplex produces clusters of vesicles that ulcerate. The vesicles repeatedly develop at the same site, following the distribution of the infected nerve. Recurrences on the vermilion border of the lip (recurrent herpes labialis) are clinically more apparent than intraoral recurrences (recurrent herpetic stomatitis). The lesions of recurrent herpes labialis appear as a small cluster of vesicles that erupt, coalesce, ulcerate, form a scab, and heal without scarring. Spread to perioral skin is common, especially with use of greasy lip ointments that permit horizontal weeping of vesicular fluid. Contact of vesicular fluid at other epidermal sites can result in spread of the infection. In relatively healthy persons, recurrent herpetic stomatitis produces small ulcers with red halos that are limited to periosteal-bound, keratinized mucosa (i.e., the attached gingiva and hard palate). Recurrences on the buccal mucosa and tongue are infrequent unless the patient is immunosuppressed.

Most patients with recurrent herpes simplex report pain and tenderness of affected tissues. Prodromal neurogenic symptoms such as tingling, throbbing, and burning often precede the eruption of lesions by 6 to 24 hours. Sunscreens are effective in the prevention of lip and skin recurrences. Management also includes lysine, vitamin C, and antiviral agents (acyclovir, famciclovir, penciclovir, and valacyclovir). Patients should be informed that lesions are contagious and that the saliva is contaminated with virus.

Herpangina (Fig. 64.8)

Herpangina is a highly contagious but self-limiting infection involving the oral cavity that is caused by group A and sometimes group B coxsackie viruses. The disease is spread by infected saliva. It is seen mainly in children during the warmer months of summer. Young adults are occasionally affected. Herpangina produces light-gray papillary vesicles that rupture to form multiple, discrete, shallow ulcers. The ulcers have an erythematous border and are limited to the anterior pillars of the fauces, soft palate, uvula, and the tonsils. Diffuse pharyngeal erythema, dysphagia, and sore throat are common features, as are fever, malaise, headache, lymphadenitis, abdominal pain, and vomiting. Convulsions rarely occur. Treatment is palliative, and spontaneous healing occurs within 1 to 2 weeks.

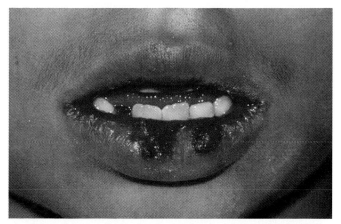

Fig. 64.1. Primary herpetic gingivostomatitis: in a 7-year-old.*

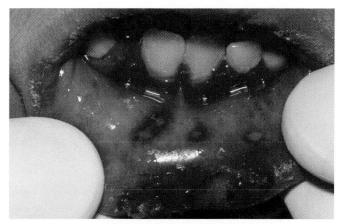

Fig. 64.2. Primary herpetic gingivostomatitis.*

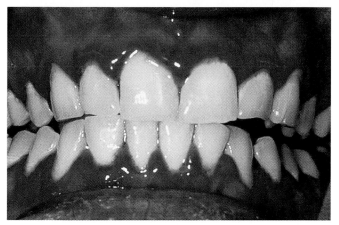

Fig. 64.3. Primary herpetic gingivitis: a 27-year-old man.

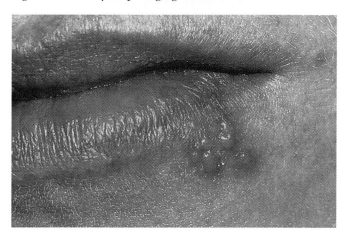

Fig. 64.4. Recurrent herpes labialis: clustered vesicles.

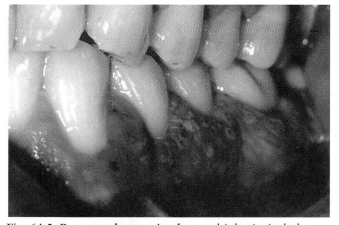

Fig. 64.5. Recurrent herpes simplex: multiple gingival ulcers.

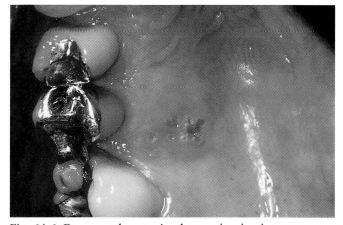

Fig. 64.6. Recurrent herpes simplex: on hard palate.

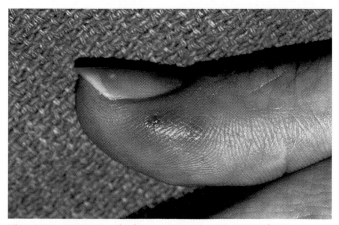

Fig. 64.7. Herpetic whitlow: caused by autoinoculation.

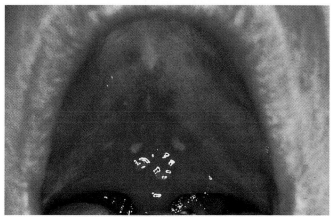

Fig. 64.8. Herpangina: soft palate ulcers and redness.

147

Vesiculobullous Lesions

Varicella (Chickenpox) (Figs. 65.1 and 65.2)

Varicella and herpes zoster are caused by the same herpetic virus, varicella-zoster. Varicella is the highly contagious primary infection, whereas herpes zoster is the recurrent neurodermal infection. Typically, young children become infected with the virus during the late winter and spring months. After exposure to the virus and a 2- to 3-week incubation period, mild prodromal features appear.

Fever, malaise, and a distinctive red and very itchy rash on the trunk are the first recognizable signs of this disease. The pruritic rash quickly spreads to the neck, face, and extremities and is followed shortly by the eruption of papules that form vesicles and pustules. On bursting, the pus-laden vesicles have the appearance of a dewdrop on a rose petal. The first and largest skin lesion is called the herald spot. It is often located on the face and, if scratched, may heal with scarring.

Intraoral lesions of varicella are few and often go unnoticed. They appear as vesicular lesions that break down and form ulcers with an erythematous halo. The soft palate is the predominant site, followed by the buccal mucosa and mucobuccal fold. Anorexia, chills, fever, nasopharyngitis, and musculoskeletal aches may accompany the course of the disease. Complications such as pneumonitis and encephalitis are infrequent. Vesicles typically crust over and resolve spontaneously within 7 to 10 days. Infection during pregnancy poses a significant risk to the fetus. A live-attenuated vaccine (Varivax) is recommended to prevent the development of chickenpox.

Herpes Zoster (Shingles) (Figs. 65.3 and 65.4)

Herpes zoster is the recurrent infection of chickenpox. Unknown factors associated with aging, cancer, and immunosuppression result in reactivation of dormant varicella virus from sensory ganglia and migration of virus along the affected sensory nerves. Viral recrudescence usually affects adults older than 50 years but may be seen in young adults or children. Before eruption, prodromal signs of itching, tingling, burning, pain, or paresthesia occur. Lesions are characterized by acutely painful vesicular eruptions of the skin and mucosa that are unilaterally distributed along nerve pathways and stop abruptly at the midline. Two areas are affected the most: 1) the trunk between vertebrae T3 and L2; and 2) the face along the ophthalmic division of the trigeminal nerve.

Cutaneous lesions of shingles begin as pruritic, erythematous macules that are followed by vesicular and pustular eruptions. Crust formation occurs within 7 to 10 days and persists for several weeks. Pain is intense but usually dissipates when the crusts fall off.

The intraoral lesions are vesicular and ulcerative with an intense red, inflammatory border. Ulcers may bleed; within several days, a large yellowish surface slough may form. The lips, tongue, and buccal mucosa may have unilateral ulcerative lesions if the mandibular branch of the trigeminal nerve is affected. Involvement of the second division of the trigeminal nerve typically produces unilateral palatal ulcerations that extend up to but not beyond the palatal raphe. Considerable malaise, fever, and distress accompany herpes zoster. Patients often present with intense pain 1 to 2 days before the viral vesicles erupt.

Herpes zoster usually heals without scar formation in about 3 weeks. However, scarring can occur, and many patients may experience persistent pain after the lesions have faded. This condition, called **postherpetic neuralgia,** may continue for 6 months to 1 year before regressing. Immunosuppressed patients are particularly susceptible to shingles and have a high morbidity rate. In the past the rare occurrence of bilateral shingles was called the death sign because these victims inevitably died. Varicella-zoster virus infection is occasionally associated with the **Ramsay Hunt syndrome** (herpes zoster, unilateral facial paralysis, and ear eruptions) and **Reye's syndrome** (high fever, cerebral edema, liver degeneration, high mortality, and salicylate use in children). The antiviral agents, famciclovir (Famvir) and valacyclovir (Valtrex), are highly effective in blocking replication of varicella-zoster virus.

Hand-Foot-and-Mouth Disease (Figs. 65.5–65.8)

Hand-foot-and-mouth disease is a mildly contagious disease caused by many coxsackie A and B viruses. It usually affects children but may be seen in young adults. It typically occurs in spring and summer. As the name implies, it produces small ulcerative lesions in the mouth together with an erythematous and vascular rash on the dorsal and ventral surface of the hands, fingers, and soles of the feet. Multiple pinpoint vesicles that ulcerate and crust are characteristic. Patients may have several to more than 100 pinpoint lesions with distinctive erythematous halos.

Oral lesions of hand-foot-and-mouth disease are scattered mainly on the tongue, hard palate, and buccal and labial mucosa. In time they coalesce to form large eroded areas. The oropharynx is usually unaffected. The total number of intraoral lesions is usually fewer than 20. Pain is a common symptom, along with elevated temperature, malaise, and lymphadenopathy. The diagnosis can be made by viral culture and serum antibody studies; however, the classic distribution of lesions on the palms of hands, soles of feet, and oral mucosa is diagnostic in most instances. Healing occurs regardless of treatment in approximately 10 days.

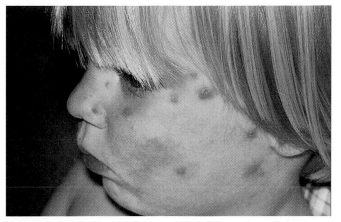

Fig. 65.1. Varicella (chickenpox): herald spot lateral to eye.

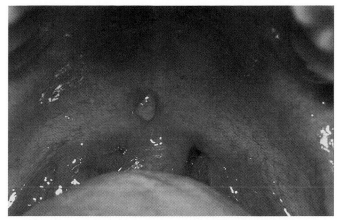

Fig. 65.2. Varicella (chickenpox): vesicle in common location.

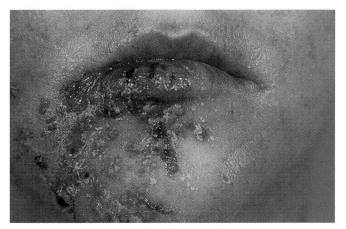

Fig. 65.3. Herpes zoster (shingles): mandibular eruption.*

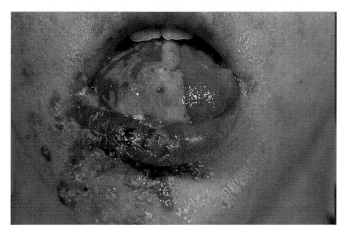

Fig. 65.4. Herpes zoster (shingles): painful oral lesions.*

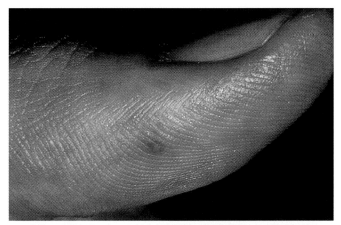

Fig. 65.5. Hand-foot-and-mouth disease: a young adult.‡

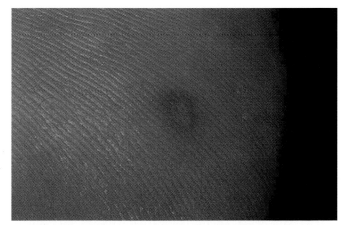

Fig. 65.6. Hand-foot-and-mouth disease: foot ulcer.‡

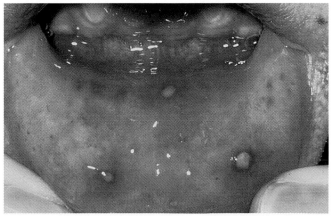

Fig. 65.7. Hand-foot-and-mouth disease: of labial mucosa.¶

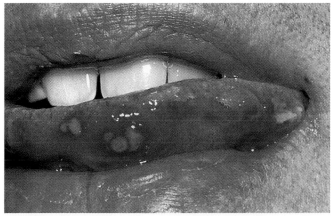

Fig. 65.8. Hand-foot-and-mouth disease: painful vesicles.¶

Vesiculobullous Lesions

Allergic Reactions (Figs. 66.1–66.8) Allergy is a condition of hypersensitivity to certain substances acquired by repeated exposure to an allergen. These reactions usually produce inappropriate tissue damage as a result of antigen-antibody reactions. Manifestations may be generalized or localized and may occur at any age. A genetic predisposition to allergy and persistent sensitivity are common features.

Hypersensitivity reactions are classified into several types according to the following factors: the speed with which the symptoms occur (immediate or delayed); clinical appearance; and cellular and tissue response (**type I:** IgE-mediated immediate hypersensitivity; **type II:** antibody-dependent cytotoxic hypersensitivity; **type III:** complex-mediated hypersensitivity; and **type IV:** cell-mediated, or delayed, hypersensitivity). Reactions of dental significance include immediate hypersensitivity type I reactions (anaphylactic shock, urticaria, angioneurotic edema, allergic stomatitis) and delayed hypersensitivity type IV reactions (contact allergy).

Localized Anaphylaxis (Figs. 66.1 and 66.2)
Localized anaphylaxis is an immediate allergic response mediated by IgE and histamine that occurs within minutes of exposure to an antigen. The localized condition produces vasodilation and increased permeability of superficial blood vessels, tissue swelling, and pruritis. The localized form manifests as wheals, urticaria, or hives that arise after the ingestion of such foods as shellfish, citrus fruits, peanuts, chocolate, or systemically administered drugs.

Generalized Anaphylaxis
Generalized anaphylaxis is an immediate and potentially life-threatening (type I) hypersensitivity reaction. It results from an antigen-antibody (IgE) interaction that produces mast cell degranulation and the release of vasoactive amines and mediators such as histamine. In fulminant cases, a generalized increase in vascular permeability and smooth-muscle contraction causes urticaria, dyspnea, hypotension, laryngeal edema, and vascular collapse. Mild localized immediate hypersensitivity reactions are treated with antihistamines. Epinephrine 1:1000 (0.3–0.5 mL, subcutaneously) is required to effectively manage severe generalized anaphylactic reactions. Treatment should always include the elimination of the causative allergen.

Allergic Stomatitis (Fig. 66.3)
Allergic stomatitis, also called allergic mucositis, is an oral type I hypersensitivity reaction to a systemically administered drug or food. The oral manifestations of drug-related eruptions are varied and may be clinically similar to erythema multiforme, lichen planus, or lupus erythematosus. In the mouth, a dry, glistening, red area is usually apparent. Focal white areas may be adjacent. The formation of multiple vesicles that break down and produce fibrin-covered ulcers eventually results. An erythematous, inflammatory border and a painful, burning sensation are common. The response may be limited to the buccal mucosa, gingiva, labial mucosa, lips, or tongue or may involve the entire oral cavity. Concurrent dermal lesions are possible. Treatment requires withdrawal of the allergen and administration of antihistamines.

Angioedema (see Figs. 42.1, 42.2, and 48.1)
Angioedema is a hypersensitivity reaction characterized by accumulation of serum within tissues, usually brought about by histamine-mediated vasodilation. Hereditary and acquired forms exist. The former, caused by a deficiency in C1 esterase inhibitor, is more serious because of possible visceral involvement. Swelling is the most prominent feature. It appears rapidly and lasts for 24 to 36 hours. Sensations of warmth, tenseness, and itchiness are concurrent. The perioral and periorbital tissues are commonly affected. See Conditions Peculiar to the Face for full discussion.

Delayed Hypersensitivity (Figs. 66.4 and 66.5)
Delayed hypersensitivity or type IV hypersensitivity is a response of the immune system to a locally or systemically introduced allergen that usually develops slowly and reaches its maximum 24 to 48 hours after antigenic exposure. Topically applied allergens such as latex gloves or chemical disinfectants may produce a delayed hypersensitivity response evident as itchy, erythematous skin lesions (contact dermatitis) that eventually become inflamed and ulcerated at the site of contact. Delayed hypersensitivity is treated with corticosteroids and avoidance of the allergen.

Contact Stomatitis (Figs. 66.6 and 66.7)
Contact stomatitis is a form of delayed hypersensitivity that may occur intraorally. It produces mucosal erythema at the site of contact with the allergen. Reactions to lipstick or sunscreens may cause the lips to appear red, swollen, fissured, or dry; a sensation of burning may be present. Antiseptics, antibiotic lozenges, topical anesthetics, eugenol preparations, and mouthwashes may produce similar burning lesions. These appear on the alveolar mucosa, dorsum of the tongue, or palate as erythematous ulcers that are covered by a gray-white pseudomembrane. Cast alloy restorations and partial denture frameworks that contain heavy metals (cobalt, mercury, nickel, or silver) can also induce delayed hypersensitivity reactions of the mucosa adjacent to the restored area. The area is usually red and ulcerated and often burns. Allergy to the free monomer in dentures, once thought to be common, is a rare occurrence.

Plasma Cell Gingivitis (Fig. 66.8)
Plasma cell gingivitis affects the gingiva, producing diffusely edematous and fiery red gingiva because of the flavoring ingredients (such as cinnamon) in some toothpastes and chewing gums. The lips and commissures are frequently involved, resulting in cheilitis. Microscopy shows that the tissue is infiltrated with plasma cells, a type of differentiated B cell that produces antibodies. Withdrawal of the causative agent is curative.

Fig. 66.1. Immediate (type 1) hypersensitivity: facial wheal.

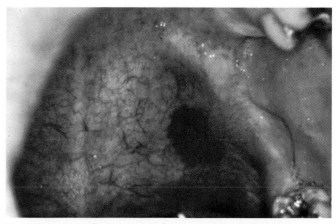

Fig. 66.2. Immediate (type 1) hypersensitivity: bee sting.

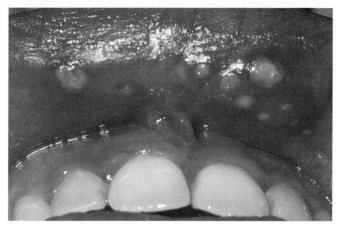

Fig. 66.3. Immediate (type 1) hypersensitivity: penicillin.

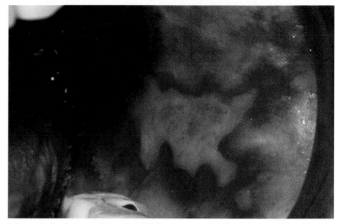

Fig. 66.4. Delayed (type IV) hypersensitivity: from thiazide.

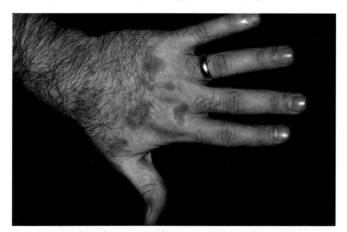

Fig. 66.5. Delayed (type IV) hypersensitivity: latex allergy.

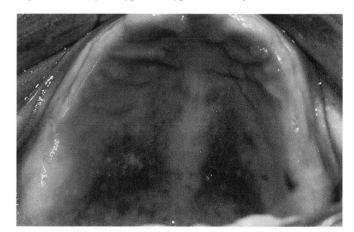

Fig. 66.6. Delayed (type IV) hypersensitivity: benzocaine.

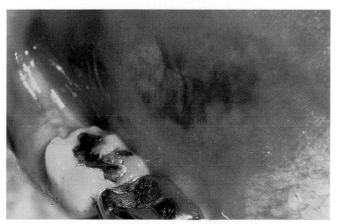

Fig. 66.7. Delayed (type IV) hypersensitivity: alloy contact.

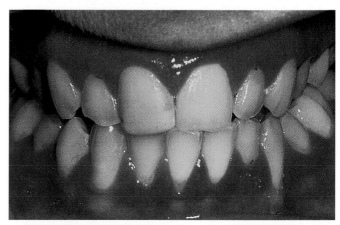

Fig. 66.8. Plasma cell gingivitis: type IV hypersensitivity.

Vesiculobullous Lesions

Erythema Multiforme Erythema multiforme is a vesiculobullous disease of varied involvement of the skin and mucous membranes. It commonly affects young adults, particularly men, but may affect children and the elderly. Low-grade fever, malaise, and headache typically precede the emergence of lesions by 3 to 7 days. The cause is unknown. However, accumulating evidence suggests that circulating immune complexes that provoke complement-mediated cytopathic effects, combined with lymphocyte-stimulated and neutrophil-stimulated vascular injury, play a pathogenic role. Precipitating factors include infections with bacterial, fungal, and viral organisms such as herpes simplex and *Mycoplasma pneumoniae*; emotional stress; and allergy, especially to drugs containing sulfa or barbiturates. In about 50% of cases herpes simplex virus DNA has been identified in diseased tissue.

Erythema multiforme can be classified into four types according to its spectrum of clinical presentations. An association between ingested drugs and increasing severity of erythema multiforme has been recognized.

Oral Erythema Multiforme (Fig. 67.1) Oral erythema multiforme is the minimal manifestation of erythema multiforme. It is usually limited to the gingiva, but eruptions may also affect the tongue, lips, or palate. A history of infection or drug therapy is common. Constitutional symptoms such as anorexia, malaise, and low-grade fever may or may not be present. As the name multiforme suggests, the lesions have a varied appearance. Affected gingiva appears fiery red, similar to the appearance of desquamative gingivitis, whereas mucosal surfaces of the tongue and lips often show several discrete irregular and bilateral ulcers. The borders of lesions are erythematous but seldom hemorrhagic, as is seen in pemphigoid, pemphigus, and other forms of erythema multiforme.

Erythema Multiforme (Figs. 67.2–67.4) The hallmarks of classic erythema multiforme are the red-white, concentric, ringlike macules termed target, bull's-eye, or iris lesions that rapidly appear on the extensor surfaces of the arms, legs, knees, and palms of the hands. The trunk of the body is classically exempt from lesions, except in the most severe cases. The skin lesions are initially small, red, circular macules that vary in size from 0.5 to 2.0 cm in diameter. The macules then enlarge and develop a pale white or central clear area. Shortly thereafter the lesions form vesicles and bullae. The vesicles may go unnoticed until they rupture and become confluent, forming large, raw, and shallow ulcers with erythematous borders. A necrotic slough and a fibrinous pseudomembrane typically cover the ulcers. Urticarial plaques that do not break down may also be present.

In the mouth, red macular areas, multiple ulcerations, and erosions with a gray-white fibrinous surface may be seen. These are generally limited to the buccal mucosa, labial mucosa, or tongue or involve all of those areas. The gingiva and palate are sometimes involved. Dark red-brown, hemorrhagic crusts are characteristically present on the lips, which helps establish the diagnosis. Lesions are usually short-lived and last about 2 weeks. Erythema multiforme rarely persists for more than 1 month. Recurrent and chronic forms exist but are rare.

Pain is the most common symptom. Oral hygiene may be neglected, resulting in secondary bacterial infection. Treatment consists of topical palliative rinses and, in some instances, low-dose systemic steroids. Complications resulting from erythema multiforme are uncommon unless the disease progresses to its major form, Stevens-Johnson syndrome.

Stevens-Johnson Syndrome (Erythema Multiforme Major) (Figs. 67.5–67.7) A severe form of erythema multiforme is termed erythema multiforme major or Stevens-Johnson syndrome, named for the two investigators who first described the clinical appearance of the disease in the early 1920s. It frequently affects children and young adults, predominantly men. The oral signs of Stevens-Johnson syndrome are similar to those of erythema multiforme; however, the former is characterized by more widespread involvement of cutaneous and stomatologic structures, and more constitutional signs such as fever, malaise, headache, cough, chest pain, diarrhea, vomiting, and arthralgia.

The classic clinical triad of Stevens-Johnson syndrome consists of eye lesions (conjunctivitis), genital lesions (balanitis, vulvovaginitis), and stomatitis. Other features include the characteristic target skin lesions on the face, chest, and abdomen that later develop into painful weeping vesiculobullous lesions. Like erythema multiforme, the gingiva is less commonly affected by desquamating bullae than is the nonkeratinized mucosa. Extensive ulcerative and hemorrhagic lesions of the lips and denuded areas of oral mucosa are intensely painful and usually prevent affected patients from eating and swallowing. Inadequate nutritional intake, dehydration, and debilitation are common sequelae that necessitate hospitalization. Healing takes about 6 weeks.

Toxic Epidermal Necrolysis (Fig. 67.8) Toxic epidermal necrolysis is the most severe form of erythema multiforme. Its occurrence is rare, and most cases are associated with drug therapy. Unlike other forms of erythema multiforme, older persons are most commonly affected, especially women. The condition primarily affects the skin, eyes, and oral mucosa; the skin manifestations are especially severe. Large areas of the skin form coalescing bullae that eventually slough, leaving huge areas of denuded skin. Management is similar to that of a burn patient. Significant morbidity will occur if supportive therapy is not provided. Treatment consists of intravenous fluid, nutritional therapy, corticosteroids, anesthetic and antiseptic rinses, and prevention of secondary infection with antibiotics. Affected areas take weeks to heal, and permanent eye damage is a frequent outcome. Both Stevens-Johnson syndrome and toxic epidermal necrolysis have been fatal.

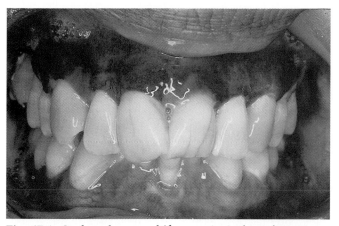

Fig. 67.1. **Oral erythema multiforme:** gingival involvement.

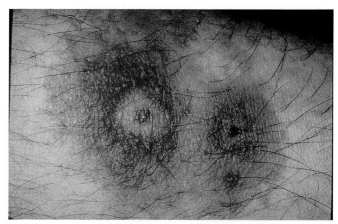

Fig. 67.2. **Erythema multiforme:** classic target skin lesions.

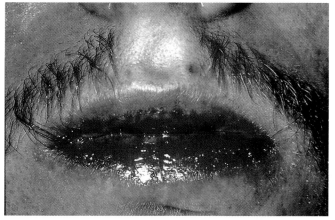

Fig. 67.3. **Erythema multiforme:** hemorrhagic lip crusts.

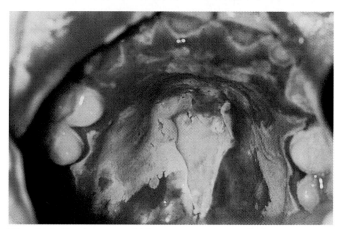

Fig. 67.4. **Erythema multiforme:** extensive oral ulceration.

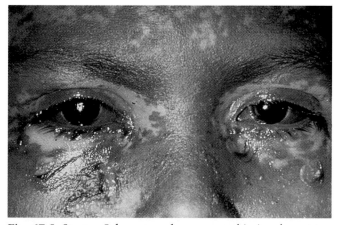

Fig. 67.5. **Stevens-Johnson syndrome:** eye, skin involvement.

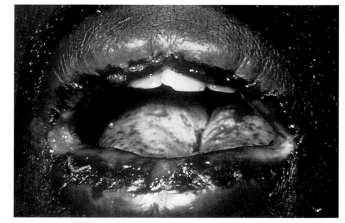

Fig. 67.6. **Stevens-Johnson syndrome:** hemorrhagic, crusted lips.

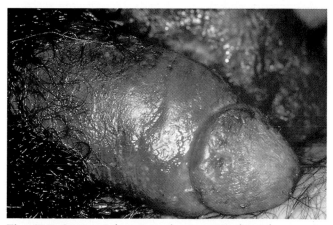

Fig. 67.7. **Stevens-Johnson syndrome:** genital involvement.*

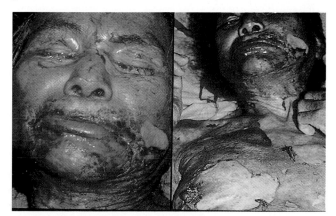

Fig. 67.8. **Toxic epidermal necrolysis:** life threatening.

Vesiculobullous Lesions

Pemphigus Vulgaris (Figs. 68.1–68.4) Pemphigus is a potentially fatal, autoimmune, vesiculobullous disease of epithelium. Four types have been described: **vulgaris** and **vegetans,** which have intraoral manifestations, and **foliaceous** and **erythematosus,** which generally do not. Pemphigus vulgaris, the most common intraoral type, usually develops between 40 and 60 years of age; less commonly it occurs in children and the elderly. It occurs more often in women and is usually encountered in light-pigmented patients of Jewish or Mediterranean origin. Acute and chronic forms exist; the slow chronic form is more common.

Pemphigus vulgaris is caused by autoantibody destruction of critical adhesion proteins (desmogleins) of epithelium that comprise the desmosome. Desmosomes are the intercellular glue-like substance that hold epithelial cells together. Desmogleins are the extracellular domain of the desmosomal cadherin proteins. Their destruction causes cell-to-cell separation (acantholysis), particularly the basal cell layer from the stratum spinosum. Events that induce autoantibody production (anti-desmoglein 3 IgG) are unknown, but occasionally are induced by drugs. Destruction of the attachments produces multiple intraepithelial blisters (bullae) that rupture quickly leaving painful erosions of skin and oral mucosa. Lesions develop rapidly and form weeping bullae or clear gelatinous plaques (a collapsed bulla). The bullae are extremely fragile and rapidly disintegrate, bleed, and crust. They tend to recur and spread to adjacent regions. Light lateral pressure applied to a bulla causes the blister to enlarge by extension (**Nikolsky's sign**). A characteristic mucosal finding is the appearance of a whitish superficial covering, which is the roof of a collapsed bulla that can be easily stripped away.

Pemphigus may appear as sloughing or folded epithelium, as an ulcer, or as multiple, large irregular ulcers. It most frequently involves the buccal mucosa, gingiva, palate, floor of the mouth, and lips. Less frequently the tongue and oropharynx are involved. Individual lesions have circular or serpiginous borders, whereas extensive erosions of the buccal mucosa appear red and raw and have diffuse irregular borders. New eruptions may superimpose over healing lesions so periods of remission are absent. Fetor oris is characteristic. Hemorrhagic lip crusts and severe pain are common of extensive disease.

The diagnosis of pemphigus is made by positive Nikolsky's sign, biopsy, and immunofluorescent staining. Early recognition of oral lesions, which precede skin involvement by several months in more than half the cases, is important because early diagnosis greatly enhances the initiation of treatment and the prognosis. Remission and control are gained with use of corticosteroid and immunosuppressive agents. Dehydration and septicemia are potentially fatal complications. A small percentage of cases are associated with an underlying neoplasm (i.e., **paraneoplastic pemphigus**).

Pemphigoid (Bullous and Cicatricial [Benign Mucous Membrane]) (Figs. 68.5–68.8) Pemphigoid is a chronic, self-limiting, autoimmune disease of adults and the elderly that involves the oral cavity in about 90% of cases. It is more common intraorally than pemphigus, but associated with much less morbidity and mortality. Pemphigoid is caused by separation of the epithelium from the basement membrane. Two types of pemphigoid (bullous and cicatricial) and several subgroups exist. They produce identical oral lesions and are distinguished by clinical and immunohistologic features.

Bullous pemphigoid, the less common of the two, affects both the skin and the oral cavity and has no sex or racial predilection. Skin folds of the axilla, inguinal, and abdominal regions are commonly affected. **Cicatricial pemphigoid,** also called **benign mucous membrane pemphigoid,** is characterized by lesions predominantly of mucous membranes, particularly the ocular and oral mucosa. It occurs twice as frequently in women as men and usually develops after 50 years of age. There is no racial predilection. Pemphigoid occurs when autoantibodies (IgG, IgM, or IgA) bind and destroy the anchoring filament complex of the basement membrane. Bullous pemphigoid targets the 180-kilodalton basement protein (bullous pemphigoid antigen II [BP180]) at sites within the upper lamina lucida. In contrast, cicatricial pemphigoid targets basement membrane proteins, laminin 5 or a BP180, at epitopes near the lamina densa. The detached epithelium separates at the level of the lamina lucida, thus exposing the underlying connective tissue.

Pemphigoid skin lesions usually precede oral lesions, tend to be desquamative and localized, and heal spontaneously. The lips are rarely affected. Intraoral bullae are usually small, yellow or hemorrhagic blebs. They form slowly and favor the palate, gingiva, and buccal mucosa. Because pemphigoid bullae result from subepithelial separation (Nikolsky positive), they are thicker-walled, less fragile, and longer-lasting than those of pemphigus. Rupture leads to patchy ulcers that coalescence. The ulcers are symmetric, curvilinear, and surrounded by an erythematous ring and may heal with scarring.

When limited to the gingiva, the clinical term **desquamative gingivitis** has been used to describe the bright red, burning, and denuded tissue. Desquamative gingivitis is a descriptive term and may represent several clinically similar vesicolobullous conditions.

Cicatricial pemphigoid may affect the anal, vaginal, and pharyngeal mucosa, but the most severe complication is ocular involvement, producing conjunctivitis, occasional bullae, clouding of the cornea, and fibrous scarring. Blindness is a serious sequela of protracted eye disease. Although the condition is rarely fatal, close follow-up is suggested because rare reports of carcinoma of the rectum and uterus have been associated with pemphigoid. Moderate doses of dapsone and corticosteroids, alone or in conjunction with immunosuppressive agents such as azathioprine, have provided effective management.

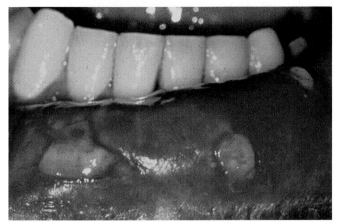

Fig. 68.1. **Pemphigus vulgaris:** lip and nose crusts.

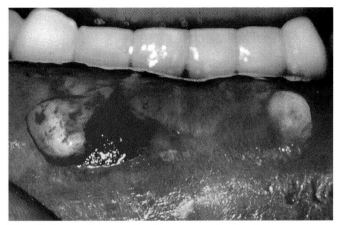

Fig. 68.2. **Pemphigus vulgaris:** hemorrhagic lip crusts.

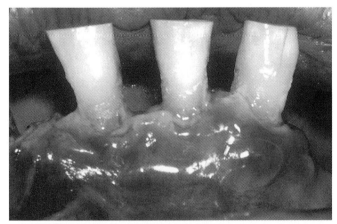

Fig. 68.3. **Pemphigus vulgaris:** rare, intact bullae on mucosa.*

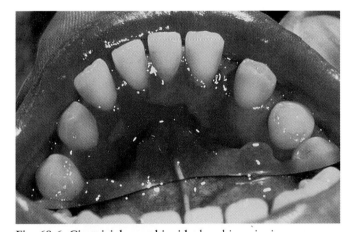

Fig. 68.4. **Pemphigus vulgaris:** ruptured bullae.*

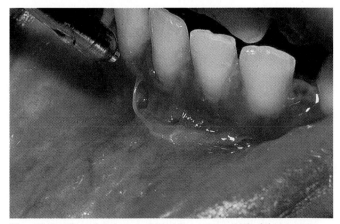

Fig. 68.5. **Cicatricial pemphigoid:** intact bulla.

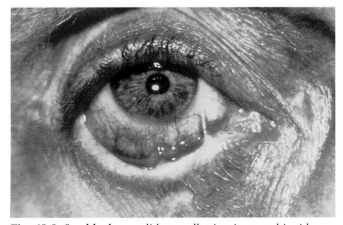

Fig. 68.6. **Cicatricial pemphigoid:** sloughing gingiva.

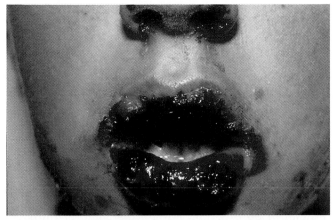

Fig. 68.7. **Cicatricial pemphigoid:** positive Nikolsky's sign.

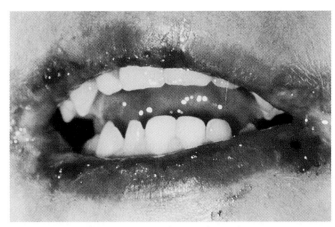

Fig. 68.8. **Symblepharon:** lid-eye adhesion in pemphigoid.

Ulcerative Lesions

Traumatic Ulcer (Figs. 69.1–69.3)

Recurrent oral ulceration is a common condition caused by several factors, primarily trauma. Ulcers may occur at any age and in either sex. Likely locations for traumatic ulcers are the labial mucosa, buccal mucosa, palate, and peripheral borders of the tongue.

Traumatic ulcers may result from chemicals, heat, electricity, or mechanical force and are often classified according to the exact nature of the insult. Pressure from an ill-fitting denture base or flange or from a partial denture framework is a source of a decubitous or pressure ulcer. Trophic, or ischemic, ulcers occur particularly on the palate at the site of a previous injection. Dental injections have also been implicated in the traumatic ulcerations seen on the lower lip by children who chew their lip after dental appointments. In addition to factitial injury, young children and infants are prone to traumatic ulcers of the soft palate from thumb sucking, called **Bednar's aphthae.**

Ulcers may be precipitated by contact with a fractured tooth or restoration, a partial denture clasp, or inadvertent biting of the mucosa. The palate is often burned by food or drinks that are too hot. Other traumatic ulcers are caused by factitial injury from inappropriate use of fingernails or other objects on the oral mucosa. The diagnosis of these conditions is simple and is often established from a careful history and examination of the physical findings.

The appearance of a mechanically induced traumatic ulcer varies according to the intensity and size of the agent. The ulcer usually appears slightly depressed and oval. An erythematous zone is initially found at the periphery; the zone progressively lightens because of the keratinization process. The center of the ulcer is usually yellow-gray. Chemically damaged mucosa, such as that seen with an aspirin burn, is less well defined and contains a loosely adherent, coagulated, white surface slough. After removal of the traumatic influence, the ulcer should heal within 2 weeks; if healing does not occur, other causes should be suspected and a biopsy should be performed.

Recurrent Aphthous Stomatitis (Minor Aphthae, Aphthous Ulcer) (Figs. 69.4–69.6)

Recurrent aphthous stomatitis is classified into three categories according to size: minor aphthae, major aphthae, and herpetiform ulcers. Approximately 20% of the population is afflicted with minor aphthae, or canker sores as they are commonly called. They may be seen in anyone, but women and young adults are slightly more susceptible. Familial patterns have been demonstrated, and persons who smoke are less frequently affected than nonsmokers. Factors that precipitate aphthae include atopy, trauma, endocrinopathies, menstruation, nutritional deficiencies, stress, and food allergies. Although the cause is unknown, studies suggest an immunopathic process involving T cell-mediated cytolytic activity and tumor necrosis factor in response to human leukocyte antigen or foreign antigens. Factors that promote thinned mucosa also are contributory as this allows for presentation of antigens to the Langerhans' cells.

Minor aphthae have a propensity for movable mucosa that is situated over minor salivary gland tissue. The labial, buccal, and vestibular mucosa are frequently affected, as are the fauces, tongue, and soft palate. In contrast, ulcers are rarely seen on heavily keratinized mucosa such as the gingiva and hard palate. Prodromal symptoms of paresthesia or hyperesthesia are sometimes reported. The lesions appear as shallow, yellow-gray, oval ulcers usually about 3 to 5 mm in diameter. A prominent erythematous border surrounds the fibrinous pseudomembrane. No vesicle formation is seen in this disease, a distinctive diagnostic feature. Ulcers that occur along the mucobuccal fold often appear more elongated. Burning is a preliminary symptom that is followed by intense pain lasting a few days. Tender submandibular, anterior cervical, and parotid lymph nodes are sometimes present, particularly when the ulcer becomes secondarily infected.

Aphthae are recurrent, and the pattern of occurrence varies. Most persons exhibit single ulcers once or twice a year, beginning during childhood or adolescence. The ulcers occasionally appear in crops, but usually fewer than five occur at one time.

Minor aphthae usually heal spontaneously without scar formation within 14 days. Some patients have multiple ulcers during a period of several months. In these cases, ulcers are in various stages of erupting and healing and produce constant pain. Although no medication has been totally successful for treating aphthous stomatitis, patients have responded to 5% amlexanox (Aphthasol), topical corticosteroids, and coagulating and cauterizing agents.

Pseudoaphthous (Figs. 69.7 and 69.8)

Pseudoaphthae, a term coined by Binney, refers to recurrent, aphthouslike mucosal ulcers of the mouth that are associated with nutritional deficiency states. Studies indicate that 20% of patients with recurrent aphthous stomatitis are deficient in folic acid, iron, or vitamin B_{12}. Pseudoaphthae are frequently seen with inflammatory bowel disease, Crohn's disease, gluten intolerance (celiac disease), and pernicious anemia.

Pseudoaphthae resemble both minor and major aphthous stomatitis but are characteristically more persistent. There is a slight predilection for women between 25 and 50 years of age. The ulcers are depressed, rounded, and painful and are sometimes multiple in number. The borders may be raised, firm, and irregular. Occasionally lesions are accompanied by mucosal fissures and nodules. Alterations of the tongue papillae may suggest an underlying nutritional deficiency state. Healing is slow, and patients may report that they are rarely free of ulceration. Chronic and persistent presence of aphthae necessitates evaluation for nutritional deficiencies, including hematologic studies. If the laboratory results are abnormal, a medical referral is required.

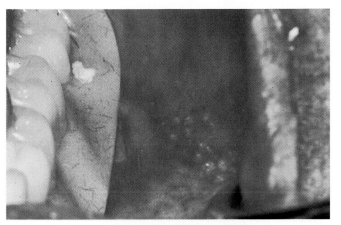

Fig. 69.1. **Traumatic ulcer:** denture flange-induced.*

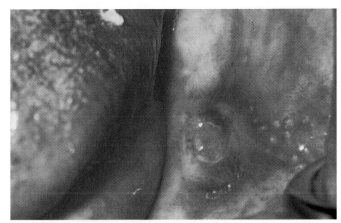

Fig. 69.2. **Traumatic ulcer:** molar region.*

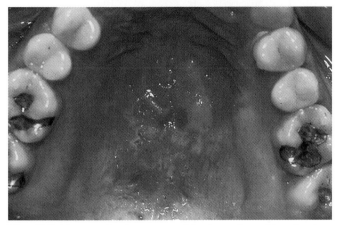

Fig. 69.3. **Traumatic ulcer:** caused by ingestion of hot food.

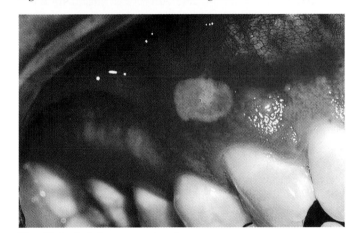

Fig. 69.4. **Aphthous:** on alveolar mucosa.

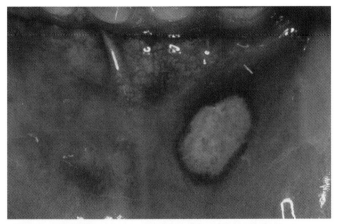

Fig. 69.5. **Aphthous:** prominent red border on labial mucosa.

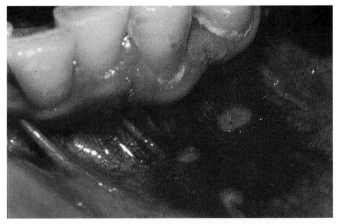

Fig. 69.6. **Aphthae:** a cluster of ulcers with typical shapes.

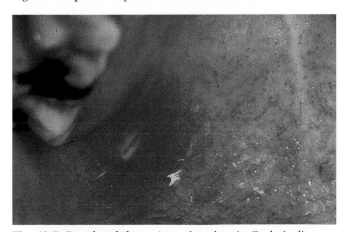

Fig. 69.7. **Pseudoaphthous:** irregular ulcer in Crohn's disease.

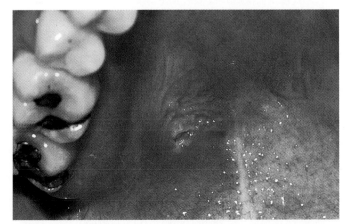

Fig. 69.8. **Pseudoaphthae:** corrugated ulcers, Crohn's disease.

Ulcerative Lesions

Major Aphthous (Periadenitis Mucosa Necrotica Recurrens, Sutton's Disease, Scarifying Stomatitis, Recurrent Scarring Aphthous) (Figs. 70.1–70.4) Major aphthous is a severe form of minor aphthous that produces larger (>1 cm), more destructive, and deeper ulcers that last longer and recur more frequently. The cause is the same as for minor aphthae, namely, an immune defect in T-lymphocyte function. Young women with anxious personality traits and HIV-seropositive persons are commonly affected.

Major aphthae are usually multiple. They involve the soft palate, tonsillar fauces, labial and buccal mucosa, and tongue and occasionally extend onto the attached gingiva. Characteristically, the ulcers are crateriform, asymmetric, and unilateral. The most prominent feature is the large size together with a depressed, necrotic center. A red, raised inflammatory border is common. Depending on size, traumatic influences, and secondary infection, ulcers may last from several weeks to months. Because the ulcers erode deep into the connective tissue, they may heal with scar formation and tissue distortion after repeated recurrences. Muscle destruction can result in tissue fenestration. If the periodontium is involved, loss of tissue attachment may occur. Extreme pain and lymphadenopathy are common symptoms.

Use of steroids (topical, intralesional, or systemic) can accelerate healing and reduce scarring. Ulcers similar to those of major aphthae are seen with some frequency in association with cyclic neutropenia, agranulocytosis, and gluten intolerance. Ulcers located on the tongue may strongly resemble carcinoma. The presence of scarring is of diagnostic importance to rule out a malignant condition.

Herpetiform Ulceration (Figs. 70.5 and 70.6)

Herpetiform ulceration is a type of recurrent focal ulceration of the oral mucosa that clinically resembles the ulcers seen in primary herpes (hence the name herpetiform). This condition, however, is a variant form of recurrent aphthous stomatitis. The prominent feature of the disease is the numerous, pinhead-sized, gray-white erosions that enlarge, coalesce, and become irregular ulcers. Initially, ulcers are 1 to 2 mm in diameter and occur in clusters of 10 to 100. The mucosa adjacent to the ulcer is erythematous, and pain is a predictable symptom.

Any part of the oral mucosa may be affected by herpetiform ulcerations, but the anterior tip of the tongue, margins of the tongue, and labial mucosa are particularly affected. The smaller size of these ulcerations distinguishes them from minor aphthae, and the absence of vesicles and gingivitis together with their frequent and recurrent nature distinguishes them from primary herpes and other oral viral infections. Virus cannot be cultured from these lesions, and the ulcers are not contagious.

The first episode of herpetiform ulceration usually occurs in patients in their late twenties and thirties, 10 years after the peak incidence of minor aphthae. The duration of recurrent attacks is variable and unpredictable. Most patients experience healing within 2 weeks; however, some patients have constant lesions for months. The trigger of this disease has yet to be determined. Recurrent herpetiform ulcerations respond especially well to tetracycline suspensions, both topically and systemically, and the condition often regresses spontaneously after several years.

Behçet's Syndrome (Oculo-Oral-Genital Syndrome) (Figs. 70.7 and 70.8) Behçet's syndrome, named for the Turkish physician who first described the ulcerative disorder, principally involves the oral cavity, eye, and genitals. For this reason it has been categorized as a triple-symptom complex with ulcerative manifestations. In the fully developed state of this disorder, cutaneous lesions, arthritis of the major joints, gastrointestinal ulcerations, cardiovascular and neurologic manifestations (headaches), and thrombophlebitis can be seen, although rarely are all components present in the same patient. The syndrome appears to be the result of a delayed hypersensitivity reaction, immune complexes, and vasculitis triggered by the presentation of human leukocyte antigens (HLA-B51) or environmental antigens, such as viruses, bacteria, chemicals, and heavy metals.

Behçet's syndrome is two to three times more prevalent in men than in women and develops between 20 and 30 years of age. Persons from Asia, the Mediterranean coast, and Great Britain are most commonly affected.

Eye manifestations of Behçet's syndrome include photophobia, conjunctivitis, and chronic recurrent iritis with hypopyon that occasionally leads to blindness. Ocular manifestations may be concurrent with or occur years after oral and genital ulcers. Skin changes are characterized by subcutaneous nodules and macular and papular eruptions that vesiculate, ulcerate, and encrustate. Genital ulcers may involve the mucosa or skin and tend to be smaller and less common than the oral lesions.

Oral ulcers, the most prevalent lesion of Behçet's syndrome, may be the initial sign of the disease. One, a few, or crops of aphthouslike ulcers on the buccal or labial mucosa are characteristic, but any oral mucosal site may be affected. Similar to aphthous, the ulcers are flat, shallow, oval, and variable in size. Small lesions tend to occur more frequently than larger lesions. A serofibrinous exudate covers the surface, and the margins are red and well demarcated. Patients frequently report pain, and recurrent periods of exacerbation and remissions are characteristic. Topical and systemic steroids are used to treat the symptoms of patients with limited mucocutaneous involvement. Protracted disease involving the neuro-ocular structures requires the care of a physician. Azathioprine, cyclophosphamide, thalidomide, and colchicine have been used successfully in select cases. All of these agents have potentially serious side effects.

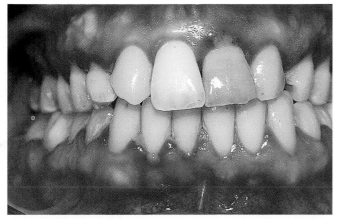

Fig. 70.1. **Major aphthous:** persistent ulcers on gingiva.*

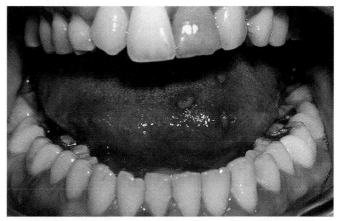

Fig. 70.2. **Major aphthous:** multiple, irregular tongue ulcers.*

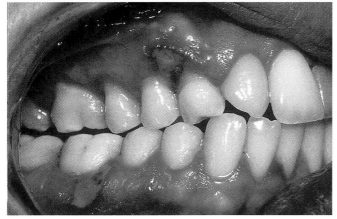

Fig. 70.3. **Major aphthous:** deep, painful gingival ulcers.*

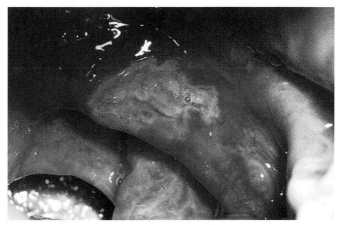

Fig. 70.4. **Major aphthous:** large irregular ulcer soft palate.*

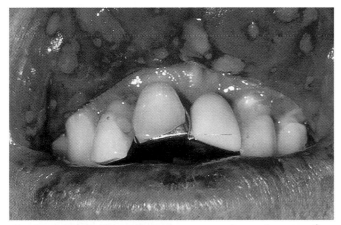

Fig. 70.5. **Herpetiform ulceration:** many ulcers of mucosa.‡

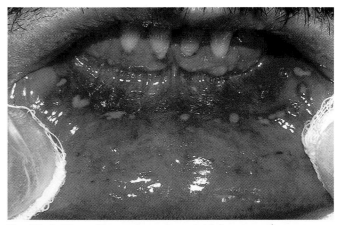

Fig. 70.6. **Herpetiform ulcerations:** labial mucosa.‡

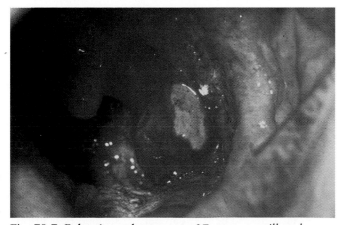

Fig. 70.7. **Behçet's syndrome:** man 27-years, tonsillar ulcer.

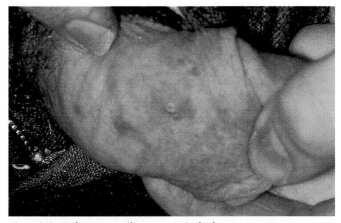

Fig. 70.8. **Behçet's syndrome:** genital ulcers.

Ulcerative Lesions

Granulomatous Ulcer (Figs. 71.1 and 71.2) Two granulomatous infections that may produce oral ulcers are **tuberculosis** and **histoplasmosis**. These two infections exhibit primary, secondary or reactivated states. Although the oral lesions are relatively uncommon, they occur with frequency when infected respiratory secretions are implanted into oral mucosa following trauma. Adults with advanced pulmonary disease and younger adults with acquired immune deficiency syndrome (AIDS) are affected. Pulmonary lesions usually precede oral lesions; thus, symptoms of persistent cough, fever, night sweats, weight loss, and chest pain are important historic findings.

Dissemination of organisms (*Mycobacterium tuberculosis or Histoplasmosis capsulatum*) from the lungs via infected sputum is the primary mode of oral infection. The classic oral manifestation of tuberculosis and histoplasmosis infection is a chronic nonhealing ulcer. These ulcers may occur on any mucosal surface; however, tuberculous lesions occur preferentially on the dorsum of the tongue, labial mucosa at the commissure, gingiva and palate. The clinical picture varies. The ulcer may resemble a traumatic ulcer or epidermoid carcinoma, particularly when the location is on the lateral tongue border. Lesions on the alveolar ridge often resemble a granulating extraction site. The center of the granulomatous ulcer is necrotic, yellow-gray and depressed. The periphery of the ulcer is undulating or lumpy and cobblestoned. The margin of the lesion is irregular, well demarcated, and undermined. Nodular and vegetative components are often seen in conjunction with the ulcers of histoplasmosis. Cervical lymphadenopathy is a common finding. Some patients report pain; in these patients the discovery may be an incidental finding. Other patients experience severe, unremitting discomfort or bony involvement. Tuberculous and histoplasmosis lesions are contagious, and active organisms can be transmitted by coughing and aerosols.

A biopsy or culturing is required to confirm the diagnosis. Histologic features and special stains (Ziehl-Neelsen for TB) demonstrate the presence of the causative organisms. Treatment of the primary lung problem is with specific long-term antibiotics. For tuberculosis, isoniazid, rifampin, rifapentine, ethambutol, streptomycin, and pyrazinamide are administered. Drug combinations are selected based on drug resistance exhibited by the infecting organism. For histoplasmosis, amphotericin B is administered with ketoconazole or fluconazole. The lung disease should be effectively treated before initiating dental treatment.

Squamous Cell Carcinoma (Figs. 71.3–71.6) Squamous cell carcinoma often appears as a chronic, nonhealing ulcer. In early stages, the lesion is usually small, nonpainful, and nonulcerative. However, the persistent nature of the disease results in neoplastic proliferation that soon exhausts the blood supply, resulting in surface telangiectasia and eventual ulcer formation. Older ulcers tend to be large and crateriform, covered by a central yellow-gray necrotic slough. Red, raw foci are frequent; the borders are firm, raised, irregular and sometimes fungating or rolled.

Carcinomas may occur anywhere in the mouth. The most common sites are the posterior third of the lateral margin of the tongue and the floor of the mouth. The retromolar trigone, soft palate and tonsillar fauces are also frequently affected. Associated features may include pain, numbness, leukoplakia, erythroplakia, induration, fixation, and regional lymphadenopathy. Metastatic lymphadenopathy is characterized by nonpainful rubbery or hard nodes that are fixed at the base and matted together. Excessive use of alcohol and tobacco heighten suspicion of oral carcinoma when a persistent ulcer does not heal within 14 days. Biopsy should be performed by the clinician, who provides the definitive treatment. Treatment involves surgery and radiation therapy. Gene therapy for squamous cell carcinoma is in its formative stages.

Chemotherapeutic Ulcer (Figs. 71.7 and 71.8) Patients receiving immunosuppressant drugs for a variety of serious illnesses, including organ transplantation, autoimmune conditions, and neoplasia, may develop oral ulcerations and stomatitis. Side effects of the chemotherapeutic drug may be directly or indirectly harmful to the oral mucosa. Antimetabolites such as methotrexate inhibit the replication of rapidly reproducing cells, including the oral epithelium, whereas alkaloids such as cyclophosphamide induce leukopenia and secondary ulcer formation.

The chemotherapeutic ulcer, an early sign of drug toxicity, appears during the second week of therapy and usually persists for 2 weeks. These ulcers may occur on any oral mucosal site, but more commonly affect nonkeratinized mucosa (lips, buccal mucosa, tongue, floor of the mouth, and soft palate) before keratinized mucosa (gingival, hard palate and dorsal tongue). The affected area initially turns red and burns. The surface epithelium is lost and a large, deep, necrotic, and painful ulcer then forms. The margins of the ulcer are irregular, and the characteristic red inflammatory border is often not present because of the lack of an inflammatory response by the host. If the pain becomes severe and the intake of adequate nutrition and fluids is impaired, a reduction in drug dose may be necessary.

Culturing is highly recommended for all lesions because of their propensity for infection with Gram-negative organisms and fungi and because of the likelihood that the ulcers may represent recrudescence of latent herpes simplex virus. Topical anesthetics and benadryl mouthrinses are used to minimize symptoms, whereas oral hygiene measures, including antimicrobial agents such as chlorhexidine, are critical to prevent secondary infection, soft tissue necrosis, and osseous necrosis. Consultation and open communication between the physician and the dentist can help reduce complications and promote oral comfort.

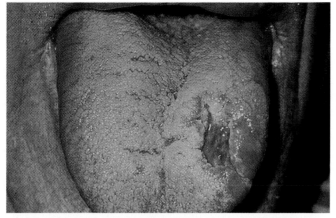

Fig. 71.1. **Granulomatous ulcer:** caused by *M. tuberculosis*.

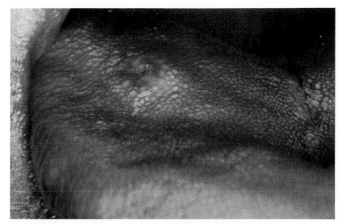

Fig. 71.2. **Granulomatous ulcer:** cause: histoplasmosis.

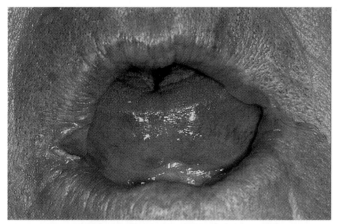

Fig. 71.3. **Squamous cell carcinoma:** indurated and raised.

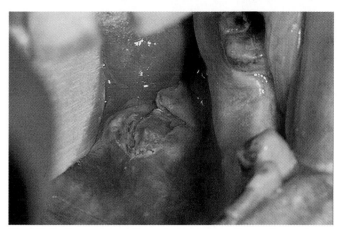

Fig. 71.4. **Squamous cell carcinoma:** ulcer floor of mouth.

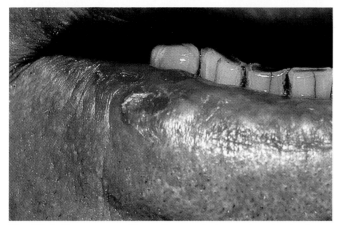

Fig. 71.5. **Squamous cell carcinoma:** at labial commissure.*

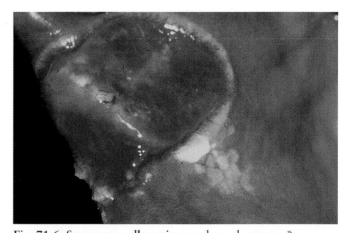

Fig. 71.6. **Squamous cell carcinoma:** buccal mucosa.*

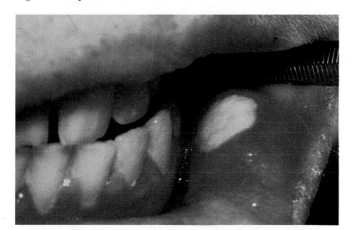

Fig. 71.7. **Chemotherapy-induced ulcer:** in leukemia.

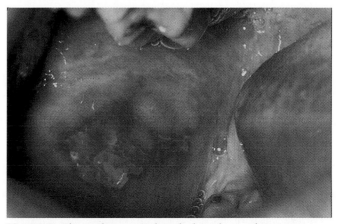

Fig. 71.8. **Chemotherapy-induced ulcer:** by methotrexate.

Section XI

Sexually Related and Sexually Transmissible Conditions

Sexually Related and Sexually Transmissible Conditions

Traumatic Conditions (Figs. 72.1 and 72.2)

Injury to the lingual frenum and soft palate are common oral conditions associated with sexual activity. Ulceration of the lingual frenum may occur when the tongue is mechanically abraded against the incisal edge of the mandibular incisors during orogenital sexual activity. A gray-white fibrinous exudate and an erythematous border are commonly seen. A history of cunnilingus confirms the diagnosis, and abstinence is recommended to permit healing. Chronic irritation may lead to secondary bacterial infection, development of leukoplakia, or a traumatic fibroma, or it may permit ingress of the human papillomavirus. Fellatio can traumatize oral soft tissues and produce erythema and submucosal hemorrhage of the soft palate. Isolated bright red petechiae initially appear. They eventually become a confluent patch that bridges the palatal midline. The purpuric lesion is painless and does not blanch on diascopy. It clinically resembles the petechial patch produced by infectious mononucleosis. However, lymphadenopathy and fever are characteristically absent. The petechiae darken and fade away in about a week.

Sexually Transmitted Pharyngitis (Figs. 72.3 and 72.4)

Venereal organisms such as herpes simplex virus (HSV) type 2, *Neisseria gonorrhoeae*, and *Chlamydia trachomatis* may cause pharyngitis by transmission from direct contact with infected genital or oral secretions or lesions. These infections occur most often in sexually active persons between 15 and 35 years of age. When primary HSV type 2 infection manifests in the oral cavity, it produces a prominent pharyngotonsillitis and fever, whereas inflammation of the gingivae may be less severe than HSV type 1 primary infection. Multiple small vesicles are usually apparent in the early stages; the vesicles collapse to form ulcers that resolve in 10 to 21 days. Antiviral agents are the treatment of choice.

N. gonorrhoeae infects nonkeratinized mucosal epithelium, producing a diffuse erythematosus pharyngitis, small tonsillar pustules, or an erythematous and edematous patch involving the throat, tonsillar area, and uvula. Burning is the initial symptom, followed by increased salivary viscosity and halitosis. Other oral manifestations include painful, discrete ulcerations of the oral mucosa; fiery red and tender gingiva with or without necrosis of the interdental papilla; tongue ulcerations; and glossodynia. A single dose of cefixime or ceftriaxone or a quinolone regimen is effective in managing this condition. *C. trachomatis* may also cause a sore throat, mild pharyngitis, and tonsillar inflammation with pustule formation. Treatment is with azithromycin or doxycycline.

Infectious Mononucleosis (Figs. 72.5 and 72.6)

Infectious mononucleosis is a relatively benign lymphocytic infection characterized by fatigue, fever, malaise, sore throat, stomatitis, and occasional hepatosplenomegaly. It is most commonly caused by the Epstein-Barr virus and occurs chiefly in adolescents and young adults. The disease is of low contagiousness, and transmission is probably through exchange of virus-contaminated saliva during deep kissing. Oral lesions are often the earliest manifestations of infectious mononucleosis. Multiple red petechiae located at the junction of the hard and soft palate occur during the first few weeks of infection. These lesions turn brown and fade after several days. Acute ulcerative gingivitis, pharyngeal ulcerations, and erythematous exudative tonsillitis frequently develop during the acute phase of the infection. Bilateral, posterior, painful cervical lymphadenopathy is a consistent finding. Blood analysis reveals modest lymphocytosis, atypical lymphocytes, heterophile antibodies, and mildly elevated transaminase levels. Treatment in most cases is supportive and includes bed rest, soft diet, analgesics, and antipyretic agents. Recovery usually occurs within 1 to 2 months.

Syphilis (Figs. 72.7 and 72.8)

Syphilis is a venereal disease caused by *Treponema pallidum*, an anareobic spirochete. The hallmark of primary oral syphilis is the nonpainful **chancre**, which represents a granulomatous reaction to vascular obliteration. Chancres may affect any oral soft tissue; however, the lips are the most common site of involvement, followed by the tongue, palate, gingiva, and tonsillar areas. Oral syphilis is more often observed in sexually active young men.

The syphilitic chancre initially appears as a small solitary papule that elevates, enlarges, erodes, and ulcerates. The lesion is usually punched-out, indurated, and 2 or 3 cm in diameter and lacks a red inflammatory border. The surface is covered by a yellowish, highly infectious serous discharge. Palatal erythema or an asymptomatic, reddish ulcer may be the initial lesion, along with swollen, nontender, firm, anterior cervical lymph nodes. Chancres typically persist for 2 to 4 weeks and heal spontaneously, causing patients to erroneously believe that treatment is not necessary. After a latent period of 4 weeks to 6 months, the secondary stage of syphilis appears; during this stage, the patient may report headaches, lacrimation, nasal discharge, sore throat, and generalized arthralgia, together with lymphadenopathy, elevated temperature, and weight loss. A painless, symmetric nonpruritic skin rash with notable maculopapular palmar-plantar eruptions soon follows. Concurrent oral lesions of secondary syphilis appear as oval red macules, pharyngitis, or isolated or multiple mucous patches (painless, shallow, highly infectious ulcers surrounded by an erythematous halo). The borders are often irregular and resemble snail tracks. Tertiary syphilis occurs in infected persons many years after nontreatment of secondary syphilis. It is primarily characterized by palatal perforation and neurologic symptoms. Parenteral penicillin G remains the drug of choice for treating all stages of syphilis.

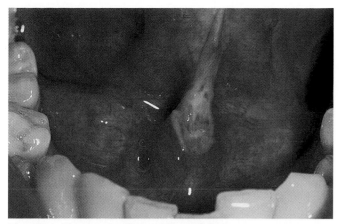

Fig. 72.1. **Traumatic ulcer:** of lingual frenum.

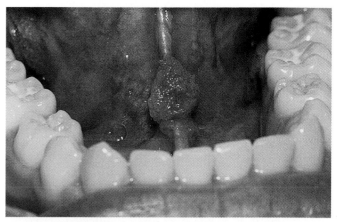

Fig. 72.2. **Condyloma acuminatum:** of lingual frenum.

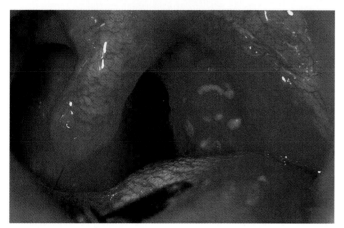

Fig. 72.3. **Sexually transmitted HSV 2 pharyngitis.***

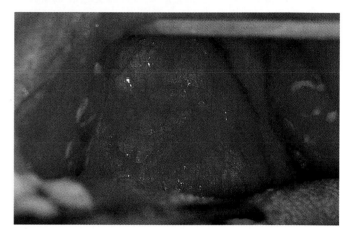

Fig. 72.4. **Primary HSV 2 infection.***

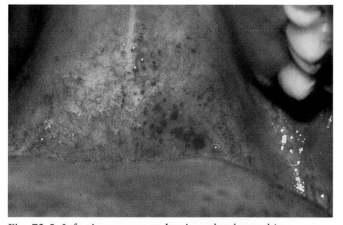

Fig. 72.5. **Infectious mononucleosis:** palatal petechiae.

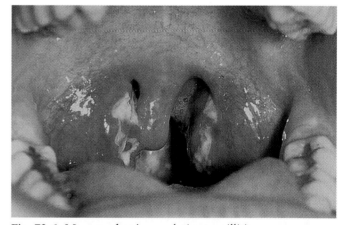

Fig. 72.6. **Mononucleosis:** exudative tonsillitis.

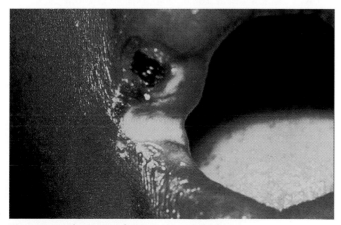

Fig. 72.7. **Chancres of primary syphilis.**

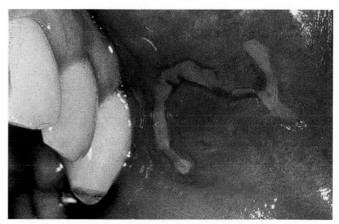

Fig. 72.8. **Mucous patch of secondary syphilis.**

HIV Infection and AIDS

Acquired Immunodeficiency Syndrome (AIDS) is a communicable disease caused by the human immunodeficiency virus (HIV) first reported by the Centers for Disease Control in 1981. HIV is an RNA virus harbored in the blood, tears, saliva, breast milk, and other bodily fluids of infected persons. It is predominantly spread by sexual contact, blood or blood products, or perinatally. Infection results by exposure to virus through participation in high-risk activities such as sharing needles with injecting drug users; having unprotected sex with one or more partners; receiving infected blood or blood products; or being accidentally exposed to infected materials.

In most cases, flulike symptoms develop 2 to 6 weeks after the initial infection; persistent generalized lymphadenopathy then occurs, followed by a latent phase. Initially the latent phase is asymptomatic; later lymphadenopathy, respiratory infections, weight loss, fever, chronic diarrhea, fatigue, skin anergy, oral candidiasis, hairy leukoplakia, parotid enlargement, and recurrent herpes virus infections develop. AIDS is defined as immune deficiency caused by HIV infection when CD4$^+$ T-cell counts decrease to less than 200 cells/mm^3 or when one of 30 opportunistic infections or certain forms of cancer develop. Treatment involves the use of highly active antiretroviral agents, such as nucleoside analogs and protease inhibitors, used in combination to block virus replication and maturation. These drugs have extended the lives of infected patients to more than 15 years. Oral manifestations of HIV infection are often numerous, concurrent, and recurrent. Recognition of the oral features warrants patient referral to a physician.

Oral Bacterial Infections (Figs. 73.1–73.4) Oral bacterial infections in patients infected with HIV often involve periodontal tissues. These infections include acute necrotizing ulcerative gingivitis, linear gingival erythema (previously called HIV gingivitis), and necrotizing ulcerative periodontitis (previously called HIV periodontitis).

Necrotizing Ulcerative Gingivitis (Figs. 73.1 and 73.2) Necrotizing ulcerative gingivitis is common in HIV-infected and immunocompromised patients. It is characterized by sudden onset of fiery red, swollen, painful, bleeding gingiva and a fetor oris. The interdental papillae appear punched-out, ulcerated, and covered by a grayish necrotic slough. Fusiform and spirochetal organisms and immunosuppression are contributing causes. Debridement is combined with metronidazole therapy when constitutional signs such as fever, malaise, anorexia, and lymphadenopathy are present.

Linear Gingival Erythema (Fig. 73.3) Linear gingival erythema is characterized by chronic gingival erythema in the absence of apparent local factors such as plaque. The maxilla and mandible are equally affected. Small, red, punctate, multifocal petechiae of the attached labial gingiva initially appear; these later form noncoalescing, distinctive red linear bands of the marginal and attached gingiva. Spontaneous gingival bleeding and lack of response to conventional therapy are common. The condition is associated with candidal infection and white blood cell abnormalities.

Necrotizing Ulcerative Periodontitis (NUP) (Fig. 73.4) Necrotizing ulcerative periodontitis is an extremely rapid and destructive process that produces rapid loss of periodontal attachment. It initially manifests in the anterior periodontal tissues, radiates to the posterior areas with time, and has a distinct propensity for the incisor and molar teeth. This bacterial infection (caused by typical and atypical pathogens) is associated with pronounced immunosuppression. It is characterized by pain and spontaneous gingival bleeding, interdental papilla necrosis and cratering, gingival edema, intense erythema, rapid gingival recession, extremely rapid and irregular bone loss, delayed wound healing, and spread to adjacent mucosa. Aggressive periodontal measures and antibiotics are required for control.

In HIV-infected patients, bacterial flora uncommon to the oral cavity can be found. The most commonly isolated bacteria are respiratory and coliform flora, *Klebsiella* species, and *Escherichia coli*. Infections by these organisms often produce diffuse, erythematous, and ulcerated changes of the tongue that result in symptoms of glossitis.

Oral Fungal Infections (Figs. 73.5–73.8) Candidiasis is the most common oral mucosal infection of patients with AIDS and is often the first oral manifestation. Candidal infections are usually chronic and may appear red, white, flat, raised, or nodular. Any oral mucosal surface may be infected, but the palate, tongue, and buccal mucosa are most frequent sites. Symptoms include mild discomfort, burning, or altered taste. The different types of candidiasis are discussed below and in Section IX, page 130.

Pseudomembranous Candidiasis This form of candidiasis is characterized by creamy-white plaques that on scraping reveal a red, raw, or bleeding mucosal surface. The organisms when smeared and stained with potassium hydroxide or cultured reveal hyphal forms typical of *Candida albicans*. The **erythematous (atrophic)** form of candidiasis appears clinically as a diffuse red area, usually located on the dorsum of the tongue. At this location it is associated with the loss of filiform papillae and is called **median rhomboid glossitis**. A diffuse, erythematous contact lesion corresponding in size and shape to the tongue lesion may be apparent on the palate. **Chronic hyperplastic candidiasis**, a late stage of candidal infection, appears as diffuse white keratotic plaques on the buccal mucosa. The plaques cannot be wiped off. HIV-infected patients require systemic therapy with antifungal drugs (Appendix II). The disease is often chronic and recurrent and may predict esophageal candidiasis.

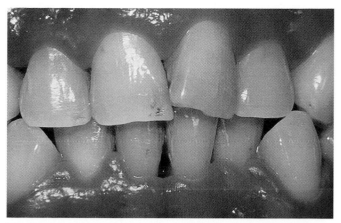

Fig. 73.1. HIV-associated necrotizing ulcerative gingivitis.

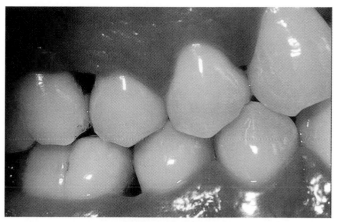

Fig. 73.2. HIV-associated necrotizing ulcerative gingivitis.

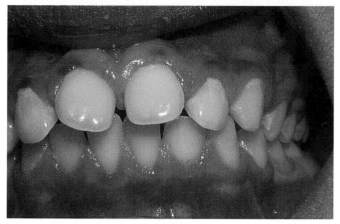

Fig. 73.3. Linear gingival erythema: above marginal gingival.

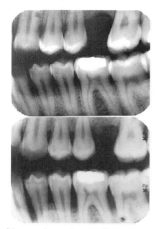

Fig. 73.4. NUP: films taken 6 months apart.

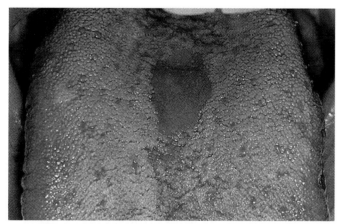

Fig. 73.5. Median rhomboid glossitis.*

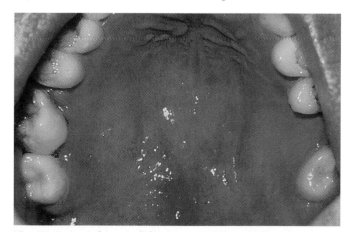

Fig. 73.6. Atrophic candidiasis: contact lesion on palate.*

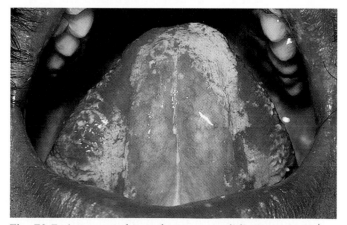

Fig. 73.7. Acute pseudomembranous candidiasis: in AIDS.‡

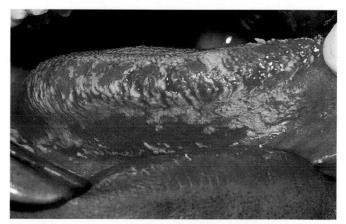

Fig. 73.8. Acute pseudomembranous candidiasis.‡

HIV Infection and AIDS

Oral Viral Infections (Figs. 74.1–74.6) The human herpes viruses (HSV types 1 and 2, varicella-zoster, cytomegalovirus, Epstein-Barr virus, human herpesvirus types 6, 7, and 8) figure prominently in acute and chronic oral disease in AIDS. **HSV infections** usually appear on the lips as herpes labialis or in the mouth on keratinized epithelium. Recurrent infection forms small vesicles that rapidly erupt, leaving shallow yellow ulcers bordered by a red halo. Coalescence of adjacent vesicles into large ulcers is common. Unlike patients with normal immune function, patients with AIDS may have herpetic infections on mucosal surfaces typically ascribed to aphthous stomatitis such as the tongue and buccal mucosa. Recurrent infections are more frequent, more persistent, and more severe in immunosuppressed patients.

Varicella-Zoster Virus Varicella-zoster virus recrudesces more frequently in HIV-positive patients than the ordinary population. The clinical appearance is similar in both groups, but the prognosis is worse for immune suppressed patients. This virus produces multiple vesicles that are commonly located on the trunk or face and are usually self-limiting and unilateral. Vesicles are typically found along a branch of the trigeminal nerve; inside or outside the mouth. Vesicle eruption, coalescence, pustule and ulcer formation, and scabbing are characteristic of the condition. Deep, searing pain is the premiere symptom and may persist as postherpetic neuralgia. Antiviral agents are used to accelerate healing and alleviate symptoms.

Cytomegalovirus The prevalence of cytomegalovirus infection is nearly 100% in HIV-positive men who have sex with men and is approximately 10% in children with AIDS. The virus has a predilection for salivary tissue and, like HSV, can be recovered from the saliva of persons infected with HIV. Inflammatory changes associated with cytomegalovirus and HIV infections include unilateral and bilateral parotid gland swelling and xerostomia. Cytomegalovirus-induced oral ulcerations resemble aphthous and can occur on periosteal-bound and non–periosteal-bound oral mucosa.

Human Papillomavirus Oral manifestations of human papillomavirus are frequently found in persons infected with HIV. So far, more than 85 serotypes of this virus have been identified. A variety of benign mucocutaneous lesions are induced by the virus, including squamous papilloma, verruca vulgaris, focal epithelial hyperplasia (Heck's disease), and condyloma acuminatum. These entities are discussed below and in Section X.

Condyloma Acuminatum The condyloma acuminatum, or venereal wart, is a slow-growing human papillomavirus–induced benign growth. It appears as a small, soft, pink to dirty gray papule that has a cauliflower-like surface. Lesions are often multiple and recurrent and coalesce to form large, sessile, pebbly growths. Condyloma acuminata can be found on any mucosal surface, particularly the ventral tongue, gingiva, labial mucosa, and palate. Transmission is by 1) direct contact that results in contagious spread from anal or genital sites or 2) self-inoculation. Treatment consists of local excision or antiviral therapy together with simultaneous eradication of all lesions of infected partners.

Hairy Leukoplakia Hairy leukoplakia is a raised, corrugated, poorly demarcated white lesion on the lateral border of the tongue that is associated with the Epstein-Barr virus and immunosuppression. Early lesions appear as discrete, white, vertical-oriented plaques on the lateral borders of both sides of the tongue. Mature lesions may cover the entire lateral and dorsal surface of the tongue and extend onto the buccal mucosa and palate. The lesions are asymptomatic, cannot be rubbed off, and may pose an esthetic problem to the patient. Histologic features are hyperkeratotic hairlike projections, koliocytosis, minimal inflammation, and candidal infection. Electron microscopic examination shows Epstein-Barr virus particles. Treatment is with antiviral agents.

Oral Malignancies (Figs. 74.7 and 74.8) Kaposi's sarcoma is the most common cancer associated with HIV infection. It is a tumor of vascular (endothelial) proliferation that affects the cutaneous and mucosal tissue. It is strongly associated with human herpesvirus type 8, a virus capable of promoting angiogenesis. Approximately 20% of all patients with AIDS are affected; with a higher prevalence in HIV-infected men who have sex with men.

Kaposi's sarcoma is characterized by three clinical stages. Initially it appears an asymptomatic red macule. The tumor then enlarges into a red-blue plaque. Advanced lesions appear as lobulated, violet nodules that ulcerate and cause pain. The hard palate is the most common location, followed by the gingiva and buccal mucosa. Lesions are frequently multifocal, uncomfortable, and esthetically displeasing. Similar-appearing lesions such as erythroplakia, hemangiomas, purpura, and bacillary angiomatosis should be ruled out by biopsy. Localized radiation therapy and direct injection of chemotherapeutic drugs (vinblastine) or sclerosing agents have proven beneficial.

Non-Hodgkin's B-cell Lymphoma and Squamous Cell Carcinoma Non-Hodgkin's B-cell lymphoma and squamous cell carcinoma are associated with HIV infection, probably as a result of viral control over apoptosis and abnormal immune surveillance. Non-Hodgkin's lymphoma often appears as a diffuse, rapidly proliferating, purplish mass of the palatal-retromolar complex. Squamous cell carcinoma is most frequently found as a reddish-white or ulcerated lesion on the posterolateral border of the tongue. Although many of the usual cofactors, such as advanced age, alcohol abuse, and poor oral hygiene, are absent in HIV-infected persons with oral cancer, Epstein-Barr virus and human papillomavirus have been detected with increasing frequency in patients with B-cell lymphomas and patients with squamous cell carcinomas, respectively.

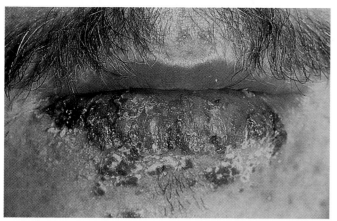

Fig. 74.1. Recurrent herpes labialis: in AIDS.

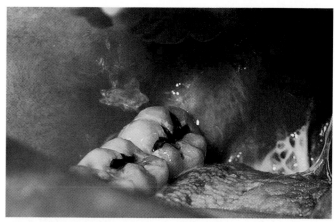

Fig. 74.2. HIV-associated recurrent herpes simplex.

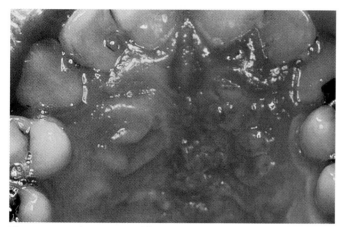

Fig. 74.3. HIV-associated herpes zoster: up to midline.

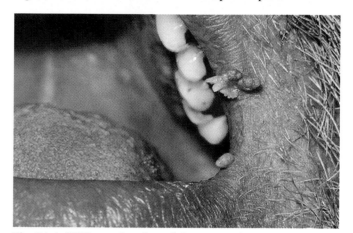

Fig. 74.4. HIV-associated condyloma acuminata.

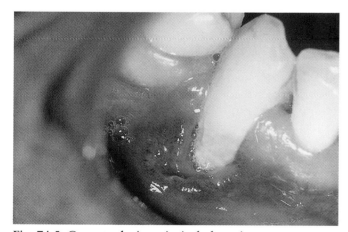

Fig. 74.5. Cytomegalovirus gingival ulceration.

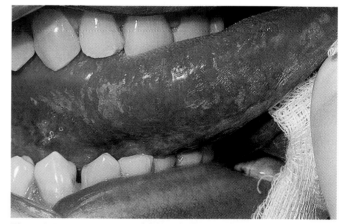

Fig. 74.6. HIV-associated hairy leukoplakia: lateral tongue.

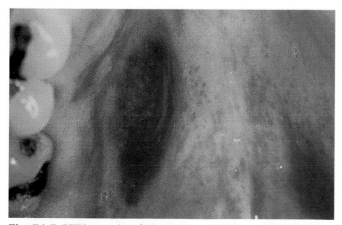

Fig. 74.7. HIV-associated Kaposi's sarcoma: purple macule.

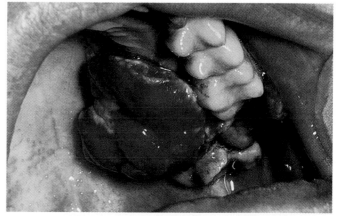

Fig. 74.8. HIV-associated non-Hodgkin's lymphoma.

Appendix I

Rx Abbreviations

Rx Abbreviations

ABBREVIATION	ENGLISH	LATIN DERIVATIVE
ad lib	at pleasure	ad libitum
a.c.	before meals	ante cibum
p.c.	after meals	post cibum
aq.	water	aqua
d.	a day, daily	dies
b.i.d	twice a day	bis in die
t.i.d.	three times a day	ter in die
q.i.d	four times a day	quater in die
h.	hour	hora
h.s.	at bedtime	hora somni
q.h.	every hour	quaque hora
q.3h.	every three hours	quaque tertia hora
q.4h.	every four hours	quaque quarta hora
q.6h.	every six hours	quaque sexta hora
n.r.	do not repeat	non repetatur
p.r.n.	as needed	pro re nata
stat.	immediately	statim
Sig.	label	signetur
c.	with	cum
gtt.	drops	guttae
tab	tablet	tabella
caps.	capsule	capsula
q.d.	every day	quaque die
p.o.	orally	per os

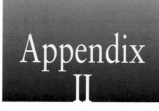

Appendix
II

Therapeutic Protocols

ANALGESICS

For Relief of Mild to Moderate Pain

Rx   Acetaminophen (Tylenol) 325 mg [OTC]

Disp.: 25 Tablets

Sig: Take 2 tablets q.4h. p.r.n. for pain; not to exceed 12 tablets in 24 hours.

Rx   Aspirin 325 mg [OTC]

Disp.: 25 Tablets

Sig: Take 2 tablets q.4h. p.r.n for pain.

Rx   Ibuprofen (Motrin) 400 mg

Disp.: 25 Tablets

Sig: Take 2 tablets q.4h. p.r.n for pain.

Rx   Propoxyphene napsylate 50 mg, and acetaminophen 325 mg (Darvocet-N 50)

Disp.: 25 Tablets

Sig: Take 2 tablets q.4h. p.r.n. for pain.

Rx   Naproxen sodium (Aleve) 220 mg [OTC] Naprosyn 375 mg

Disp.: 50 Tablets

Sig: Take 2 tablets b.i.d p.r.n. for pain.

Rx   Rofecoxib (Vioxx) 25 mg

Disp.: 50 Tablets

Sig: Take 1 tablet q.d. for pain.

ANALGESICS

For Relief of Moderate Pain

Rx   Acetaminophen 300 mg, with codeine 30 mg (Tylenol with Codeine No. 3)

Disp.: 30 Tablets

Sig: Take 2 tablets q.4h. p.r.n. for pain.

Rx   Aspirin 325 mg, with codeine 30 mg (Empirin with Codeine No. 3)

Disp.: 30 Tablets

Sig: Take 2 tablets q.4h. p.r.n. for pain.

Rx   Aspirin 325 mg, butalbital 50 mg, caffeine 40 mg (Fiorinal)

Disp.: 40 Tablets

Sig: Take 1 to 2 tablets q.4h. p.r.n. for pain.

Rx Aspirin 325 mg, butalbital 50 mg, caffeine 40 mg, codeine 30 mg (Fiorinal with codeine 30 mg)

Disp.: 30 Tablets

Sig: Take 1 to 2 tablets q.4h. p.r.n. for pain.

Rx Acetaminophen 650 mg, with codeine 30 mg (Margesic No. 3)

Disp.: 30 Tablets

Sig: Take 1 to 2 tablets q.4h. p.r.n. for pain.

Rx Hydrocodone bitartrate 5 mg, with acetaminophen 500 mg (Lortab 5, Anexsia 5/500, Vicodin, Zydone)

Disp.: 30 Tablets

Sig: Take 1 tablet q.4h. p.r.n. for pain.

Rx Dihydrocodeine bitartrate 16 mg, aspirin 356.4 mg, caffeine 30 mg (Synalgos-DC Capsules)

Disp.: 40 Tablets

Sig: Take 1 to 2 tablets q.4h. p.r.n. for pain.

ANALGESICS
For Relief of Moderate to Severe Pain

Rx Hydrocodone bitartrate 7.5 mg, with acetaminophen 500 mg (Lortab 7.5/500)

Disp.: 30 Tablets

Sig: Take 1 tablet q.6h. p.r.n. for pain.

Rx Hydrocodone bitartrate 7.5 mg, with acetaminophen 650 mg (Lorcet Plus)

Disp.: 30 Tablets

Sig: Take 1 tablet q.6h. p.r.n. for pain.

Rx Hydrocodone bitartrate 10 mg, with acetaminophen 650 mg (Lorcet 10/650)

Disp.: 30 Tablets

Sig: Take 1 tablet q.6h. p.r.n. for pain.

Rx   Oxycodone HCl 5 mg, with acetaminophen 325 mg (Percocet, Roxicet)

Disp.: 25 Tablets

Sig: Take 1 tablet q.6h. p.r.n. for pain.

Rx   Oxycodone HCl 5 mg, with acetaminophen 500 mg (Tylox)

Disp.: 25 Tablets

Sig: Take 1 tablet q.6h. p.r.n. for pain.

Rx   Oxycodone HCl 4.5 mg, oxycodone terephthalate 0.38 mg, aspirin 325 mg (Percodan)

Disp.: 25 Tablets

Sig: Take 1 tablet q.4h. p.r.n. for pain.

Rx   Meperidine HCl 50 mg, with promethazine HCl 25 mg (Mepergan Fortis Capsules)

Disp.: 25 Tablets

Sig: Take 1 tablet q.4 to 6h. p.r.n. for pain.

ANTIBIOTIC THERAPY
To Eliminate Pathogenic Bacterial Organisms That Cause Oral Infection

Rx   Phenoxymethyl penicillin (Penicillin V) 500 mg

Disp.: 40 Tablets

Sig: Take 2 tablets immediately and then 1 tablet q.6h. 1 hour a.c.

Rx   Penicillin V potassium liquid (Penicillin VK) 125 mg/5 mL

Disp.: 200 mL

Sig: Children should take 1 teaspoonful q.6h.

Rx   Amoxicillin (Amoxil) 500 mg

Disp.: 40 Tablets

Sig: Take one 500-mg tablet t.i.d.

Rx   Dicloxacillin sodium (Dynapen) 500 mg

Disp.: 40 Tablets

Sig: Take one 500-mg tablet q.8h.

Note: For penicillinase-resistant infection.

Rx   Trimethoprim 80 mg, with sulfamethoxazole 400 mg (Bactrim)

Disp.: 40 Tablets

Sig: Take 1 tablet q.12h.

Note: For infections with *Escherichia coli, Haemophilus influenzae,* and *Klebsiella* and *Enterobacter* species.

Rx   Metronidazole (Flagyl) 500 mg

Disp.: 40 Tablets

Sig: Take 2 tablets immediately, then 1 tablet q.6h. until gone.

Note: For febrile patients with acute necrotizing ulcerative gingivitis involving anaerobic bacteria.

Rx   Erythromycin ethylsuccinate (EES) 400 mg

Disp.: 56 Tablets

Sig: Take one 400-mg tablet q.6h. Continue for 7 days.

Rx   Tetracycline HCl (Achromycin) V 250 mg (Lederle)

Disp.: 56 Tablets

Sig: Take 1 tablet q.i.d. Continue for 7 days.

Rx   Cephalexin (Keflex) 250 mg

Disp.: 56 Tablets

Sig: Take 2 tablets q.6h. Continue for 7 days.

ANTIBIOTIC THERAPY—BACTERIAL ENDOCARDITIS PROPHYLAXIS

To Prevent Infective Endocarditis in High-Risk Patients (i.e., Prosthetic Cardiac Valves, Previous Bacterial Endocarditis, Complex Cyanotic Congenital Heart Disease, Surgically Constructed Systemic Pulmonary Shunts or Conduits) and Moderate-Risk Patients (i.e., Rheumatic, Congenital, or Other Acquired Valvular Heart Disease, Hypertrophic Cardiomyopathy, and Mitral Valve Prolapse with Regurgitation and/or Thickened Leaflets) Who are Undergoing Invasive Dental Procedures

Adult—Bacterial Endocarditis Prophylaxis

Rx	Amoxicillin 500 mg
Disp.:	4 Tablets (2 g)
Sig:	Take 4 tablets (2 g) p.o. 1 hour before dental procedure.

Note: Standard regimen for preventing bacterial endocarditis in adults and children >66 lbs (30 kg).

Adult Unable to Take Oral Medications

Rx	Ampicillin
Disp.:	2-g vial, dissolve in sterile saline
Sig:	Administer 2.0 g IM or IV within 30 minutes of procedure.

Adult Allergic to Penicillin—Bacterial Endocarditis Prophylaxis

Rx   Clindamycin 300 mg

Disp.: 2 Tablets

Sig: Take 2 tablets p.o., 1 hour before dental treatment.

OR

Rx   Cephalexin (Keflex) or cefadroxil (Duricef) 500 mg**

Disp.: 4 Tablets

Sig: Take 2 g p.o. 1 hour before dental treatment.

OR

Rx   Azithromycin (Zithromax) or clarithromycin (Biaxin) 500 mg

Disp.: 1 Tablet

Sig: Take 1 tablet p.o. 1 hour before dental treatment.

Adult Allergic to Penicillin and Unable to Take Oral Medications

Rx   Clindamycin (phosphate) 600 mg

Disp.: 600-mg vial

Sig: Administer 600 mg IM or IV within 30 minutes of procedure.

OR

Rx   Cefazolin**

Disp.: 1-g vial

Sig: Administer 1 g IM or IV within 30 minutes of procedure.

Child

Rx   Amoxicillin 250 mg/5 mL elixir

Disp.: 10 mL

Sig: Take 50 mg/kg p.o. 1 hour before dental treatment.

Note: Standard regimen for preventing infective endocarditis in children <66 lbs (30 kg). The following weight ranges may also be used for the initial pediatric dose of amoxicillin: <15 kg, 750 mg; 15–30 kg, 1,000 mg; and >30 kg, 2,000 mg.

**Avoid in patients who have a history of recent, severe or immediate type allergy (angioedema, anaphylaxis) to penicillin.

Child Unable to Take Oral Medications—Bacterial Endocarditis Prophylaxis

Rx   Ampicillin

Disp.: 2-g vial, dissolve in sterile saline

Sig: Administer 50 mg/kg IM or IV within 30 minutes of procedure.

Child Allergic to Penicillin

Rx   Clindamycin 75 mg

Disp.: By weight

Sig: Take 20 mg/kg 1 hour before dental treatment.

OR

Rx   Cephalexin or cefadroxil** 125 mg/5 mL

Disp.: By weight

Sig: Take 50 mg/kg p.o. 1 hour before dental treatment.

OR

Rx   Azithromycin or clarithromycin 125 mg

Disp.: By weight

Sig: Take 15 mg/kg p.o. 1 hour before dental treatment.

Child Allergic to Penicillin and Unable to Take Oral Medications

Rx   Clindamycin

Disp.: 600-mg vial

Sig: Administer 25 mg/kg IM or IV within 30 minutes of procedure.

OR

Rx   Cefazolin**

Disp.: 500-mg vial

Sig: Administer 25 mg/kg IM or IV within 30 minutes of procedure.

**Avoid in patients who have a history of recent, severe or immediate type allergy (angioedema, anaphylaxis) to penicillin.

ANTIMICROBIAL TOPICAL AGENTS AND RINSES

To Reduce Pathogenic Microbial Flora Often Associated with Inflammatory Oral Disease

Rx   Chlorhexidine gluconate 0.12% (Peridex, PerioGard) oral rinse

Disp.: 480-mL

Sig: Swish 1 teaspoonful for 1 minute, then expectorate. Perform twice daily (morning and evening) after brushing teeth. Avoid eating or drinking for 30 minutes.

Rx   Tetracycline HCl (Tetracyn) 250 mg

Disp.: 40 Capsules

Sig: Dissolve 1 capsule in 1 teaspoon of warm water, then swish the solution for 3 to 5 minutes and swallow. Repeat q.i.d.

Rx   Tetracycline HCl (Achromycin V) 125 mg/5 mL

Disp.: 60-mL (also available in 16 fluid oz.)

Sig: Rinse with 2 teaspoonfuls for 3 minutes and swallow. Repeat q.i.d.

Rx   Tetracycline HCl 12.7 mg, in ethylene/vinyl acetate copolymer (Actisite)

Disp.: Box of 100 fibers

Sig: Place in gingival sulcus with cyanoacrylate for 10 days, then remove.

Rx   Chlorhexidine gluconate 2.5 mg (PerioChip)

Disp.: Box of 10

Sig: (For in office use only) Place in gingival sulcus in affected areas (5 mm or greater).

Rx   Metronidazole 250 mg

Disp.: 28

Sig: Take 1 tab q.i.d.

Note: Not recommended for children.

ANTIFUNGAL THERAPY

To Eliminate Pathogenic Fungal Organisms and Reestablish Normal Oral Flora

Rx   Nystatin vaginal tablets (Nilstat) 100,000 IU

Disp.: 90 Tablets

Sig: Dissolve 1-2 tablets as a lozenge in mouth 5 times d. for 14 consecutive days.

Rx   Nystatin (Mycostatin Pastilles) 200,000 U

Disp.: 60 Tablets

Sig: Dissolve 1 pastille in mouth q.i.d. as a lozenge for 14 consecutive days.

Rx   Clotrimazole (Mycelex Troches) 10 mg

Disp.: 60 Tablets

Sig: Dissolve 1 tablet as a lozenge 5 times d. for 14 consecutive days.

Rx Ketoconazole* (Nizoral) 200 mg (Janssen Pharm)

Disp.: 14 Tablets

Sig: Take 1 tablet q.d. for 2 weeks.

Rx Fluconazole* (Diflucan) 50 or 100 mg

Disp.: 14 Tablets

Sig: Take 1 tablet q.d. for 14 consecutive days.

Rx Itraconazole* (Sporanox) 100 mg

Disp.: 14 Tablets

Sig: Take 1 tablet q.d. for 14 consecutive days.

Rx Nystatin (Mycostatin) topical powder 100,000 IU (Squibb)

Disp.: 15-g squeeze bottle

Sig: Apply liberally to tissue side of clean denture p.c. Soak the clean denture in a suspension of 1 teaspoon of powder and 8 oz. of water overnight.

Rx Nystatin (Mycostatin) ointment 100,000 IU

Disp.: 15-g (30-g) tube

Sig: Apply liberally to affected area 4–6 times d.

Rx Ketoconazole (Nizoral) cream 2%

Disp.: 15-g tube

Sig: Apply liberally to affected area after meals.

Rx Betamethasone dipropionate 0.05% and clotrimazole 1% (Lotrisone)

Disp.: 15-g (30-g) tube

Sig: Apply liberally to affected area 4 or 5 times d.

Rx Iodoquinol 10 mg, and hydrocortisone 10 mg ointment (Vytone)

Disp.: 15-g (30-g) tube

Sig: Apply liberally to affected area 4 or 5 times d.

Rx Nystatin 100,000 U and triamcinolone acetonide 0.1% (Tri-Statin II, Mycolog II)

Disp.: 15-g (30-g, 60-g) tube

Sig: Apply liberally to affected area t.i.d. to q.i.d.

Note: These drugs are most effective when dentures are removed and treated, if applicable, and when intake of fermentable carbohydrates is reduced.

*Use with caution in patients with diminished or impaired liver function.

Treatment of Oral Herpetic Infections

Rx Acyclovir ointment (Zovirax) 5%

Disp.: 15 g

Sig: Apply to oral lesions with a cotton-tip applicator 6 times daily.

Rx Acyclovir (Zovirax) 200 mg, 400 mg, 800 mg

Disp.: 50 Capsules

Sig: Take 800 mg b.i.d. for at least 4 days.

Rx Valacyclovir (Valtrex) 500 mg

Disp.: 50 Capsules

Sig: Take 2 capsules b.i.d. for at least 4 days.

Rx Famciclovir (Famvir) 500 mg

Disp.: 50 Capsules

Sig: Take 1 capsule t.i.d. for at least 4 days.

Rx L-Lysine (Enisyl) 500 mg

Disp.: 100 Tablets

Sig: Take 4 tablets q.4h. until symptoms subside.

Note: Treatment should begin during the early stage of the recurrence. Most effective if foods containing high content of arginine are avoided.

Rx Penciclovir (Denavir 1%) ointment

Disp.: 15 g

Sig: Apply to lesions with a cotton-tip applicator at least 5 times daily.

Prevention of Dentally Associated Oral Herpetic Infections

Rx Docosanol (Abreva) 10% cream [OTC]

Disp.: 2 g

Sig: Apply to lesions with a cotton-tip applicator at least 5 times daily.

Rx Valacyclovir (Valtrex) 500 mg

Disp.: 30 Capsules

Sig: Take 4 capsules b.i.d. on day of dental treatment.

ANTIVIRAL THERAPY
To Treat Oral Human Papillomavirus Infections

Rx   Podofilox (Condylox) 0.5% gel

Disp.: 3.5 g

Sig: Apply to oral lesions with a cotton-tip applicator b.i.d. for 3 days, then withdraw for the next 4 days. Repeat cycle weekly for up to four times.

Rx   Cidofovir (Vistide) 1% gel

Disp.: 5 g

Sig: Apply to oral lesions with a cotton-tip applicator on a daily basis for 2 weeks.

ANTIANXIETY AGENTS
To Manage and Provide Short-Term Relief of the Symptoms of Anxiety

Rx   Alprazolam (Xanax) 0.25 mg

Disp.: 20 Tablets

Sig: Take 1 tablet b.i.d.

Rx   Chlordiazepoxide (Librium) 10 mg

Disp.: 20 Tablets

Sig: Take 1 tablet b.i.d.

Rx   Diazepam (Valium) 5 mg

Disp.: 20 Tablets

Sig: Take 1 tablet b.i.d. or t.i.d. and 1 tablet 1 hour before dental appointments.

Rx   Oxazepam (Serax) 10 mg

Disp.: 20 Tablets

Sig: Take 1 tablet q.d.

Rx   Buspirone (BuSpar) 5 mg

Disp.: 20 Tablets

Sig: Take 1 tablet b.i.d.

Rx   Lorazepan (Ativan) 0.5 mg

Disp.: 20 Tablets

Sig: Take 1 tablet q.d.

ANTIHISTAMINES
To Relieve Symptoms of Anxiety and Anxiety-Related Skin Eruptions

Rx	Hydroxyzine (Atarax) 25 mg
Disp.:	50 Tablets
Sig:	Take 2 tablets q.i.d. p.r.n.

Rx	Hydroxyzine (Atarax) syrup 10 mg/5 mL
Disp.:	50 mL
Sig:	Take 2 teaspoonfuls 1 hour before dental appointment

Rx	Diphenhydramine HCl (Benadryl) 25 mg
Disp.:	25 Tablets
Sig:	Take 1 tablet q.i.d.

ANTIHISTAMINES
To Reduce the Effects of Histamine-Mediated Hypersensitivity and Temporarily Relieve Symptoms Associated with Minor Oral Irritations

Rx	Diphenhydramine HCl (Benadryl) 25 mg
Disp.:	40 Tablets
Sig:	Take 1 tablet q.6h. p.r.n.

Rx	Brompheniramine maleate HCl (Dimetane) 4 mg
Disp.:	40 Tablets
Sig:	Take 1 or 2 tablets q.6h. p.r.n.

Rx	Phenylpropanolamine HCl 25 mg, and brompheniramine maleate HCl 4 mg (Dimetapp)
Disp.:	40 Tablets
Sig:	Take 1 tablet q.4h. p.r.n.

Rx	Loratadine (Claritin) 10 mg
Disp.:	25 Tablets
Sig:	Take 1 tablet q.d.

Rx	Cetirizine (Reactine) 5 mg
Disp.:	25 Tablets
Sig:	Take 1 or 2 tablets q.i.d.

Rx	Fexofenadine (Allegra) 60 mg
Disp.:	36 Tablets
Sig:	Take 1 tablet b.i.d.

TOPICAL ORAL ANESTHETICS

To Relieve Symptoms Associated with Minor Irritations of the Mouth

Rx Diphenhydramine HCl
(Benadryl) elixir
12.5 mg/5 mL
OTC

Disp.: 4 fluid oz.

Sig: Rinse with 1 tablespoonful
a.c. and p.r.n. for pain.

Rx Benadryl elixir
12.5 mg/5 mL and
Kaopectate (Upjohn)
50% mixture by volume
OTC

Disp.: 4 fluid oz. of each; mix
equal parts

Sig: Rinse with 1 tablespoonful
for 2 minutes a.c. and
p.r.n. for pain.

Rx Lidocaine HCl (Xylocaine)
2% viscous solution
(Astra)

Disp.: 4 fluid oz.

Sig: Rinse with 1 teaspoonful
a.c. and p.r.n. for pain.
Expectorate after rinsing.

Rx Orabase with Benzocaine
OTC

Disp.: 5 g (15 g)

Sig: Apply to affected area
a.c. and p.r.n. for pain.

Rx Dyclonine 0.5% or 1%

Disp.: 30 mL

Sig: Apply to affected area
a.c. and p.r.n. for pain.

CORTICOSTEROIDS

Adjunctive Treatment for and Temporary Relief of Symptoms Associated with Oral Inflammatory and Ulcerative Lesions

Low Potency

Rx Hydrocortisone acetate
ointment (Orabase HCA)
0.05%
OTC

Disp.: 5-g tube

Sig: Apply to oral lesions p.c.
and h.s.

Medium Potency

Rx Triamcinolone acetonide (Kenalog in Orabase) ointment 0.1%

Disp.: 5-g tube

Sig: Apply to ulcerated area p.c. and h.s.

Rx Betamethasone valerate (Valisone) ointment 0.1%

Disp.: 15-g (45-g) tube

Sig: Apply to mouth sores p.c. and h.s.

Rx Betamethasone (Celestone) syrup 0.1%

Disp.: 50 mL

Sig: Rinse with 1 teaspoonful q.i.d, p.c. and h.s.

Rx Triamcinolone (Kenalog-40)

Disp.: 5-mL injectable vials

Sig: Mix 1 mL of steroid with 0.5 mL of anesthetic. Inject 0.25 mL at four locations around border of ulcer. Total 1 mL injected.

High Potency*

Rx Augmented betamethasone dipropionate (Diprolene) 0.05% ointment

Disp.: 15-g (45-g) tube

Sig: Apply to mouth sores p.c. and h.s.

Rx Fluocinonide (Lidex) 0.05% gel

Disp.: 15-g (30-g) tube

Sig: Apply to mouth sores p.c. and h.s.

Rx Dexamethasone elixir (Decadron) 0.5%

Disp.: 100-mL bottle

Sig: Rinse with 1 teaspoonful q.i.d. for 2 minutes, then expectorate.

*High-potency steroids should be avoided in patients with gastrointestinal ulcers, diabetes, hematologic malignancy, and hepatitis and in women who are pregnant or nursing. Imuran can be prescribed with prednisone to reduce the prednisone dose.

Very High Potency*

Rx   Dexamethasone
(Decadron) 0.75% elixir

Disp.: 100-mL bottle

Sig: Rinse with 1 teaspoonful
q.i.d. for 2 minutes, then
swallow.

Rx   Clobetasol (Temovate)
0.05% ointment

Disp.: 15 g

Sig: Apply to affected area
q.i.d.

Note: More than 2 weeks of therapy may affect normal cortisol production.

Rx   Halobetasol propionate
(Ultravate) 0.05%
ointment

Disp.: 15 g

Sig: Apply to affected area
q.i.d.

Note: More than 2 weeks of therapy may affect normal cortisol production.

Rx   Halcinonide (Halog) 0.1%
ointment

Disp.: 15 g

Sig: Apply to affected area
q.i.d.

Rx   Methylprednisolone
(Medrol 4 mg Dosepak
21s)

Disp.: 1 Dosepak (21 tablets)

Sig: Take graduated daily
doses according to the
manufacturer's directions
listed on the Dosepak.

Rx   Prednisone 10 mg

Disp.: 36 Tablets

Sig: Take 4 tablets in a.m. for
4 days.

---

*Very high-potency steroids should be avoided in patients with gastrointestinal ulcers, diabetes, hematologic malignancy, and hepatitis and in women who are pregnant or nursing. Imuran can be prescribed with prednisone to reduce the prednisone dose.

Rx   Azathioprine[a] (Imuran)
50 mg

Disp.: 30 Tablets

Sig: Take one 50-mg dose q.d.
(Patients who have not
improved in 12 weeks may
be refractory to this drug).

Caution: Chronic immunosuppression with azathioprine increases the risk for neoplasia. Doctors prescribing this drug should be familiar with this risk and the potential serious mutagenic and hematologic consequences to both men and women.

[a]Often used in combination with systemic steroids.

FLUORIDE THERAPY

To Prevent Dental Caries in Susceptible Patients

Rx Stannous fluoride 0.4%

Disp.: 4.3 fluid oz.

Sig: Apply 5–10 drops in a carrier and place carrier on teeth daily for 5 minutes.

Rx Oral fluoride (Luride) 0.125 mg per drop

Disp.: 60-mL bottle with dropper

Sig: Birth–2 years of age: apply 2 drops q.i.d.*; 2–3 years: 4 drops q.i.d.; 3–12 years: 8 drops q.i.d.*

Rx 1.1% neutral sodium fluoride (Prevident)

Disp.: 2 oz

Sig: Apply 5 drops in a custom made tray and place tray over teeth daily for 5 minutes.

*In the mouth of the child.

NUTRIENT DEFICIENCY THERAPY

To Replace Deficient Nutrients Necessary for Homeostasis

Rx Ferrous sulfate 250 mg

Disp.: 100 Tablets

Sig: Take 1 tablet q.d. for 1 month, then reassess patient's hemoglobin level.

Rx Folic acid 0.4 mg

Disp.: 30 Tablets

Sig: Take 1 tablet q.d. for 1 month, then reassess patient's folic acid level.

Caution: Medical supervision is advised.

Rx Cyanocobalamin (vitamin B_{12})

Disp: 1,000 μg/mL; 10-mL vial

Sig: Inject 0.1–1 mL IM in deltoid; reassess patient's symptoms and blood profile monthly.

Rx Water-soluble bioflavonoids 200 mg, with ascorbic acid 200 mg (Peridin-C 400 mg)

Disp.: 100 Tablets

Sig: Take 1 tablet t.i.d.

SALIVA SUBSTITUTE
To Relieve Dry Mouth

Rx   Carboxymethyl cellulose 0.5% aqueous solution [OTC]

Disp.: 8 fluid oz.

Sig: Use as a rinse p.r.n.

Rx   Carboxymethyl cellulose artificial salivas Moi-Stir[a], Orex, Sage Moist Plus, Salivart[b], Xero-Lube, MouthKote, Salix

Disp.: [a]120 mL with pump spray; [b]75 mL with pump spray

Sig: Use as a rinse p.r.n.

Rx   Hydroxyethylcellulose, xylitol, citric acid (Optimoist spray)

Disp.: 9 mL

Sig: Spray in mouth p.r.n. for dry mouth

Rx   Glucose oxidase and lactoperoxidase (Biotene)

Disp.: 120 mL

Sig: Rinse in mouth for 1 minute p.r.n. for oral dryness.

Rx   Pilocarpine (Salagen) 5 mg

Disp.: 100 Tablets

Sig: Take 1 tablet t.i.d. or q.i.d.

Rx   Bethanechol (Urecholine) 25 mg

Disp.: 100 Tablets

Sig: Take 1 or 2 tablets up to t.i.d. p.r.n. for oral dryness.

Rx   Cevimeline HCl (Evoxac) 15 mg

Disp.: 100 Tablets

Sig: Take 1 to 3 tablets up to t.i.d. p.r.n. for oral dryness.

SEDATIVE/HYPNOTICS

To Produce a Sleeplike State for the Effective Management of an Oral Disease or Condition

Rx   Triazolam (Halcion) 0.25 mg

Disp.: 30 Tablets

Sig: Take 1 tablet h.s.

Note: Not to exceed nightly use for more than 2 weeks.

Rx   Flurazepam (Dalmane) 15 mg

Disp.: 30 Tablets

Sig: Take 1 tablet h.s.

Rx   Temazepam (Restoril) 15 mg

Disp.: 30 Tablets

Sig: Take 1 tablet h.s.

Rx   Chloral hydrate (Noctec) 500 mg/5 mL

Disp.: 1 pint

Sig: Take 1 teaspoonful before bedtime or 30 minutes before surgery.

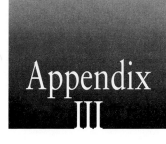

Appendix III

Guide to Diagnosis and Management of Common Oral Lesions

WHITE LESIONS

Disease	Age	Sex	Race/Ethnicity	Cause	Clinical Characteristics	Treatment
Fordyce's granules	Any	M-F	Any	Ectopic sebaceous glands	Whitish-yellow granules clustered in plaques located on buccal mucosa (bilaterally), labial mucosa, retromolar pad, lip, attached gingiva, tongue, and frenum. Lesions are nontender and rough to palpation and do not rub off. Onset after puberty; persists for life.	None required.
Linea alba buccalis	Any	M-F	Any	A type of frictional keratosis caused by persistent rubbing of buccal mucosa with interdigitating maxillary and mandibular teeth	White wavy line of varying length located on buccal mucosa, bilaterally. Lesions are nontender and smooth to palpation and do not rub off. Variable onset; persists with oral habits.	Eliminate bruxism and clenching.
Leukoedema	Any	M-F	Melano-derms	Unknown	Grayish-white patch of variable size located on buccal mucosa (bilaterally), labial mucosa, and soft palate. Lesions are nontender and smooth to palpation and disappear when the mucosa is stretched. Leukoedema becomes more evident with increasing age.	None required.
Morsicatio buccarum	Any	M-F	Any	Chronic irritation caused by cheek biting	Asymmetric white plaque located on buccal mucosa and labial mucosa, often bilaterally. Lesions are nontender and rough to palpation and peel slightly when rubbed. Variable onset; persists with cheek-biting or lip-biting habit.	Eliminate cheek-biting or lip-chewing habit.
White sponge nevus	Any	M-F	Any	Autosomal dominant condition (mutation in keratin 4 or 13 genes) that results in defect in epithelial maturation and exfoliation	Solitary or confluent raised white plaques that may appear on buccal mucosa, labial mucosa, alveolar ridge, floor of the mouth, or soft palate. Lesions are nontender and rough to palpation and do not rub off. Onset at birth; persists for life.	None required.

WHITE LESIONS *continued*

Disease	Age	Sex	Race/ Ethnicity	Cause	Clinical Characteristics	Treatment
Traumatic white lesions	Any	M–F	Any	Acute chemical or physical trauma resulting in epithelial sloughing	White surface slough (eschar) usually located on the less-keratinized alveolar mucosa. Palate common for food burns. Lesions are tender to palpation and rub off, leaving a raw or bleeding surface. Onset within hours of trauma; regression in 1–2 weeks.	Eliminate irritant; topical anesthetics and analgesics.
Leukoplakia	45–65	2:1 (M:F)	Any	Frequently related to tobacco or alcohol use	White patch that varies in size, homogeneity, and texture. High-risk locations include floor of the mouth, ventral tongue, lateral tongue, and uvulo-palatal complex. Lesions do not rub off and usually are nontender. Onset occurs after prolonged contact with an inducing agent; persists as long as the inducing agent is present.	Biopsy and histologic examination. Close follow-up mandatory.
Cigarette keratosis	Elderly	M	Any	Heat and smoke from frequent smoking non-filtered cigarettes	White pebbly circular patches located on upper and lower lips (kissing lesions). Keratoses are firm and nontender and do not rub off. Onset in conjunction with a prolonged cigarette smoking habit; persists with habit.	Use filtered cigarettes, or stop smoking. Biopsy if lesion changes in color, or becomes ulcerated or indurated.
Nicotine stomatitis	40–70	M	Any	Epithelial reaction to tobacco smoke or heat	White cobblestoned papules located on hard palate, excluding the anterior third. Papules have red centers, are nontender, and do not rub off. Onset varies according to degree of smoking; lesions are long-standing.	Stop pipe or cigar smoking, or reverse smoking habit.
Snuff dipper's patch	Teenagers and adult	M	Any	Chronic irritation of smokeless tobacco products	Corrugated whitish-yellow patch located on mucobuccal fold, most prominent unilaterally. Patch is rough and nontender and does not rub off. Long-standing habit precedes lesion; patch persists with continuation of habit.	Discontinue tobacco use. Biopsy if color changes or if lesion becomes ulcerated or indurated.

WHITE LESIONS *continued*

Disease	Age	Sex	Race/ Ethnicity	Cause	Clinical Characteristics	Treatment
Verrucous carcinoma	Over 60	M	Any	Neoplastic changes induced by long-term use of tobacco, smokeless tobacco, and human papillomavirus infection	Papulonodular whitish-red mass located on buccal mucosa, alveolar ridge, gingiva. Lesion is firm, nontender, and rough to palpation and does not rub off. Long-standing tobacco habit precedes onset; human papillomavirus present in 30%; lesion enlarges unless treated.	Biopsy to confirm diagnosis, then surgical excision. AVOID RADIATION THERAPY.
Squamous cell carcinoma (see "Red and Red-White Lesions")						

RED LESIONS

Disease	Age	Sex	Race/Ethnicity	Cause	Clinical Characteristics	Treatment
Purpura	Any	M-F	Any	Rupture of blood vessel caused by trauma or vascular abnormality	Red spot or patch consisting of extravasated blood that develops soon after trauma. Lesions do not blanch on diascopy and size varies (petechiae < ecchymosis < hematoma). Petechiae are common on soft palate; other purpura typically occur on buccal or labial mucosa, depending on site at which blood pools. Lesions fade away.	Eliminate underlying cause.
Varicosity	Over 55	F	Any	Dilated veins caused by loss of elasticity	Reddish-purple papule or nodule located on ventral tongue, lip, or labial mucosa. Lesions are asymptomatic and blanch on diascopy. Varicosities increase in size and number with increasing age and are persistent.	None necessary. Surgery for esthetics.
Thrombus	Over 30	M-F	Any	Blood clot caused by stagnating blood or clotting abnormality	Red to blue-purple nodule located on labial mucosa, lip, or tongue. Lesions are firm and may be tender to palpation. Onset after traumatic bleeding; lesion is negative on diascopy and persists until treatment. Thrombi sometime spontaneously regress.	Surgical removal and histologic examination, if persistent or symptomatic.
Hemangioma	Child-adolescent	F	Any	Congenital abnormality resulting in a network of blood vessels in bone or soft tissue	Red to purple, soft, smooth-surfaced, or multinodular exophytic mass located on dorsal tongue, buccal mucosa, or gingiva. Lesions are positive on diascopy. Develops early in life, persists until treated. Hemangiomas sometimes spontaneously regress.	No treatment is necessary if present since youth, no functional disability, and no changes in size, shape, or color. Otherwise, surgery or histologic examination.

RED LESIONS *continued*

Disease	Age	Sex	Race/ Ethnicity	Cause	Clinical Characteristics	Treatment
Hereditary hemorrhagic telangiectasia	Post- pub- erty	M-F	Any	Autosomal dominant condition associated with multiple dilated end capillaries that results from a defect in a transmembrane protein (endoglin)—a component of the receptor complex for transforming growth factor beta (TGF-β)	Multifocal red macules located on palms, fingers, nail beds, face, neck, conjunctiva, nasal septum, lips, tongue, hard palate, and gingiva. Lesions are present at birth, become more visible at puberty, and increase in number with age. Telangiectasias lack central pulsation and blanch on diascopy; if they rupture, severe bleeding may result.	Avoid trauma and intubation. Monitor for hemorrhage or anemia.
Sturge-Weber syndrome	Birth	M-F	Any	Nonhereditary congenital disorder that results in multiple venous angiomas at various anatomic sites	Syndrome associated with seizures, mental deficits, gyriform brain calcifications, and a red to purple flat or slightly raised facial hemangioma. Vascular lesion often affects lips, labial or buccal mucosa, and gingiva along branches of trigeminal nerve, stops at midline. Abnormal oral enlargements may be concurrent.	None required. Elective surgery for esthetics.
Kaposi's sarcoma	20–45*M and over 60	M	Jewish, Mediterra- nean, or *HIV- infected	Associated with human herpesvirus type 8, a virus capable of promoting angiogenesis	Asymptomatic red macule of mucocutaneous structures that enlarges and becomes raised then darkens in color. Advanced lesions are red- blue-violet nodules that ul- cerate and cause pain. The hard palate, gingiva, and buccal mucosa are the most common oral locations.	Palliative, consist- ing of radiation therapy, laser surgery, chemotherapy, sclerosing agents, or a combination thereof.
Erythroplakia	Over 50	M>F	Any	Increased vascularity associated with carcinogen- induced epithelial changes and inflammation	Red patch of variable size located on any oral mucosal site. High-risk areas include floor of the mouth, soft palate–retromolar trigone, and lateral border of tongue. Erythroplakias do not rub off and are usually asymptomatic. Lesions develop after prolonged contact with carcinogens or human papillomavirus; duration varies. Regression is rare.	Biopsy and histologic examination. Close follow-up.

RED AND RED-WHITE LESIONS

Disease	Age	Sex	Race/ Ethnicity	Cause	Clinical Characteristics	Treatment
Erythroleuko-plakia and speckled erythroplakia	Over 50	M>F	Any	Increased vascularity associated with carcinogen-induced and *Candida*-induced epithelial changes and inflammation	Red patch with multiple foci of white. Nontender, do not rub off, often superficially infected with *Candida* organisms. Common locations include lateral tongue, buccal mucosa, soft palate, and floor of the mouth. Onset after prolonged exposure to carcinogens or human papillomavirus. Regression unlikely even if inducing agent is removed.	Biopsy and histologic examination. Examine for candidiasis. Close follow-up.
Squamous cell carcinoma	Over 50	2:1 M:F	Any	Prolonged exposure to carcinogens (tobacco, alcohol, or human papillomavirus) and decreased immune surveillance	Red or red and white lesion or ulcer commonly located on lateral tongue, ventral tongue, oropharynx, floor of the mouth, gingiva, buccal mucosa, or lip. Carcinoma often asymptomatic until it becomes large, indurated, or ulcerated. Onset after prolonged exposure to carcinogens. Persistence results in metastasis, usually apparent as painless, firm, matted, fixed lymph nodes.	Biopsy and histologic examination. Complete surgical removal, radiation therapy, chemotherapy, or photodynamic therapy. Close follow-up.
Lichen planus	Over 40	F	Any	T-cell infiltration and cytokine-induced changes in epithelium; exact inducer unknown	Purple, polygonal, pruritic papules on flexor surfaces of skin; fingernails sometimes affected. Intraoral lesions are often symptomatic and consist of white linear papules, reddish patches, and ulcerated regions of mucosa. Affected surfaces are often bilateral. Most common locations: buccal mucosa, tongue, lips, palate, gingiva, and the floor of the mouth. Lesions develop with stress and liver disease, they persist for many years with periods of remission and exacerbation.	Rest, anxiolytic agents, topical corticosteroids. Evaluate for liver disease; close follow-up for occasional malignant transformation in the erosive type.

RED AND RED-WHITE LESIONS *continued*

Disease	Age	Sex	Race/ Ethnicity	Cause	Clinical Characteristics	Treatment
Electrogalvanic white lesion	Over 30	F	Any	Metal antigen of a dental restoration that induces a hyperimmune T-cell response	Reddish-white patches that resemble lichen planus located on buccal mucosa adjacent to metallic restorations. Lesions do not rub off and are usually tender or cause a burning sensation. Onset after weeks to years of exposure to metallic restoration; duration varies depending on the persistence of the allergen.	Replace metallic restoration or clasp that is causing the hypersensitive response.
Lupus erythematosus	Over 35	F	Any	Autoantibodies (antinuclear) that attack normal cells leading to perivascular inflammation	Reddish butterfly rash on bridge of nose. Maculopapular eruption with hyperkeratotic periphery and atrophic center. Affected areas may involve the lower lip, buccal mucosa, tongue, and palate. Intraoral lesions invariably have red and white radiating lines emanating from the lesion. Lesions do not rub off but are tender to palpation. Lesions often develop after short-term sun exposure. Lesions persist and require drug treatment.	Topical and systemic steroids; antimalarial agents in conjunction with adequate medical treatment.
Lichenoid and lupuslike drug eruption	Adult	M-F	Any	Drug molecules act as allergens or haptens that stimulate immune reaction	Red-white patches that resemble lichen planus and lupus. The lesions are often atrophic or ulcerated centrally. Buccal mucosa, bilaterally, is the most common site. Onset varies and may be weeks or years after an allergenic medication is begun. Regression occurs when the offending drug is eliminated.	Withdraw offending drug and substitute medication.

RED AND RED-WHITE LESIONS *continued*

Disease	Age	Sex	Race/ Ethnicity	Cause	Clinical Characteristics	Treatment
Candidiasis	Newborns, adults	M-F	Any	Opportunistic infection with *Candida* species (most commonly *C. albicans*)	Variable appearance; white curds, red patches, white patches with red margins. Any oral soft tissue site is susceptible, but the attached gingiva is rarely affected. Onset often coincides with neutropenia, or immune suppression. Lesions persist until adequate antifungal therapy is provided.	Antifungal therapy. Eliminate sucrose from diet. Medical control of diabetes, endocrinopathy, and immunosuppression.

PIGMENTED LESIONS

Disease	Age	Sex	Race/Ethnicity	Cause	Clinical Characteristics	Treatment
Melanoplakia	Any	M-F	Melano-derms	Melanin deposition in the basal layer of the mucosa and lamina propria	Generalized constant dark patch located on attached gingiva and buccal mucosa. Pigmentation varies from light brown to dark brown and is often diffuse, curvilinear, and asymptomatic and does not rub off. Melanoplakia is present at birth and persists for life.	None required.
Tattoo	Teen-agers adults	M-F	Any	Implantation of dye or metal in mucosa	Amalgam tattoo is the most common type of intraoral tattoo. Appears as a blue-black macule on gingiva, edentulous ridge, vestibule, palate, or buccal mucosa. Radiographs may demonstrate radiopaque foci. Lesions are asymptomatic, do not blanch, and persist for life.	None required.
Ephelis	Any	M-F	Light-skinned persons	Deposition of melanin triggered by exposure to sunlight	Light to dark brown macule that appears on facial skin, extremities, or lip after sun exposure. Ephelides are initially small but may enlarge and coalesce. Lesions are nontender and do not blanch or rub off.	None required.
Smoker's melanosis	Older adult	M-F	Any	Accumulation of melanocytes and deposition of melanin in association with tobacco smoking	Diffuse brown patch with diameter of several centimeters, usually on posterior buccal mucosa and soft palate. History of heavy tobacco smoking precedes development of the lesion. Features may decrease with discontinuation of the habit. Melanosis is asymptomatic and nonpalpable.	Diminish or stop smoking.
Oral melanotic macule	24–45	Slight male predi-lection	Any	Focal deposition of melanin along the basal layer, usually after trauma	Asymptomatic brown to black macule usually located on lower lip near midline; also occurs on palate, buccal mucosa, and gingiva. Onset is postinflammatory, and the lesion persists until treatment.	Biopsy and histologic examination to rule out other similar-appearing pigmented lesions.

PIGMENTED LESIONS *continued*

Disease	Age	Sex	Race/Ethnicity	Cause	Clinical Characteristics	Treatment
Nevus	Any	F	Any	Accumulation of nevus cells in a distinct location, probably controlled by genetic factors	Nevi vary greatly in appearance. They may be pink, blue, brown, or black but do not blanch on diascopy. They usually appear as a bluish or brownish smooth-surfaced papule located on the palate. Other common sites include the buccal mucosa, face, neck, and trunk. Many lesions are present at birth. They increase in size and number with increased age.	Excisional biopsy and histologic examination.
Melanoma	25–60	M	White persons, especially light-skinned persons	Malignant neoplasm of melanocytes associated with chronic ultraviolet light exposure; unknown for oral melanomas	Painless, slightly raised plaque or patch that has many colors, especially foci of brown, black, gray, or red. Ill-defined margins, satellite lesions, and inflammatory borders are characteristic. They are usually located on the maxillary alveolar ridge, palate, anterior gingiva, and labial mucosa. Thirty percent arise from preexisting pigmentations. A recent change in size, shape, or color is particularly ominous.	Excisional biopsy, surgical removal, and referral for complete medical work-up to rule out metastasis.
Peutz-Jeghers syndrome	Child, young adult	M-F	Any	Autosomal dominant condition probably caused by a germline mutation in the *LKB1* gene (19p13.3)	Multiple, asymptomatic melanotic oval macules, prominently located on the skin of the palmar or plantar surfaces of the hands and feet, around the eyes, nose, mouth, lips, and perineum. In the mouth, brown discolorations occur on the buccal mucosa, labial mucosa, and gingiva. Lesions do not increase in size, but cutaneous lesions often fade with age; mucosal pigmentation persists for life. Colicky intestinal symptoms are probable.	Oral: none required. Gastrointestinal evaluation and genetic counseling.

PIGMENTED LESIONS *continued*

Disease	Age	Sex	Race/Ethnicity	Cause	Clinical Characteristics	Treatment
Addison's disease	Adult	M-F	Any	Adrenal hypofunction	Diffuse intraoral hypermelanotic patches occurring in conjunction with bronzing of the skin, especially of the knuckles, elbows, and palmar creases. Patches are nontender and nonraised and vary in shape. The buccal mucosa and gingiva are most commonly affected. Onset of the disorder is insidious and associated with adrenal gland hypofunction. Patient may report gastrointestinal symptoms and fatigue.	Systemic corticosteroids.
Heavy metal pigmentation	Adult	M-F	Any	Prolonged exposure (vapors or ingestion) to metals (arsenic, bismuth, mercury, silver, or lead)	Blue-black linear pigmentation of marginal gingiva, prominently viewed along anterior gingiva. Spotty gray macules may be apparent on buccal mucosa. Neuralgic symptoms, headache, and hypersalivation are common. Argyria: Blue-gray skin pigmentation, especially in sun-exposed areas.	Terminate exposure to heavy metal; provide medical referral. Oral lesions require no treatment, but may be permanent.

PAPULES AND NODULES

Disease	Age	Sex	Race/Ethnicity	Cause	Clinical Characteristics	Treatment
Retrocuspid papilla	Child, young adult	M-F	Any	Developmental anomaly of connective tissue	Smooth-surfaced pink papule, 1–4 mm in diameter, located on the lingual attached gingiva apical to the marginal gingiva of the mandibular cuspids. These papules appear early in life, are often found bilaterally, and regress as the patient ages. The retrocuspid papilla is firm to palpation, asymptomatic, and nonhemorrhagic.	None required.
Lymphoepithelial cyst	Child, young adult	M-F	Any	Epithelium entrapped in lymphoid tissue that undergoes cystic transformation	Well-circumscribed, soft, fluctuant yellowish swelling that ranges in size from a few millimeters to 1 cm. Common locations for this nontender cyst include the lateral neck just anterior to the sternocleidomastoid muscle, floor of the mouth, lingual frenum, and ventral tongue. Lesion develops during childhood or adolescence and persists until treatment.	Excisional biopsy and histologic examination.
Torus, exostosis, and osteoma	Adult	F	Any	Unknown hereditary factors	Torus: bony hard nodule or multinodular mass located on the palate at the midline, or mandibular lingual alveolar ridge. Exostosis: bony hard nodule, often multiple, located on buccal or labial alveolar ridge. Osteoma: bony hard nodule located adjacent to the jaws, often embedded in soft tissue. All three types are firm, asymptomatic (unless traumatized), slow growing, and long-standing. Osteomas have the greatest growth potential.	Torus and exostosis: none required unless functional problems arise. Osteomas: gastrointestinal evaluation to rule out Gardner's syndrome. If test results are positive, then gastrointestinal surgery and genetic counseling.

PAPULES AND NODULES *continued*

Disease	Age	Sex	Race/Ethnicity	Cause	Clinical Characteristics	Treatment
Fibroma	Adult	M-F	Any	Usually a chronic irritant that produces a reactive hyperplasia of connective tissue	Irritation fibroma is a smooth-surfaced, pink, firm, symmetric papule or nodule that arises at a site of chronic irritation, such as the buccal mucosa, labial mucosa, and tongue. The gingiva is the common location for the peripheral odontogenic fibroma. Both lesions have sessile bases and are nontender and nonhemorrhagic.	Excisional biopsy and histologic examination.
Lipoma	Over 30	M-F	Any	Unknown genetic mutation possibly involving dysfunction proteins that regulate chromatin structure and function	Well-circumscribed, smooth-surfaced, dome-shaped, yellowish to pink nodule commonly located on buccal mucosa, lip, tongue, floor of the mouth, soft palate, or mucobuccal fold. Lesion is slightly doughy on palpation and grows slowly.	Excisional biopsy and histologic examination.
Lipofibroma	Over 30	M-F	Any	Unknown genetic mutation	Well-circumscribed, smooth-surfaced, dome-shaped, pinkish nodule commonly located on buccal or labial mucosa. Lesion is painless, movable, and rather firm. Slow growth and persistence are characteristic.	Excisional biopsy and histologic examination.
Traumatic neuroma	Over 25	M-F	Any	Trauma to large nerve that results in abnormal healing and aberrant neural conduction	Small, slightly raised, firm, pressure-sensitive papule that is commonly located in the mandibular mucobuccal fold near the mental foramen, facial to mandibular incisors, lingual retromolar regions, and ventral tongue. Visualization of the lesion may be difficult if the neuroma is subjacent to normal-appearing mucosa. Palpation elicits an electric shock sensation. Onset occurs after trauma; lesions persist until treated.	Excisional biopsy and histologic examination; if lesion recurs, corticosteroid injections may be effective.

PAPULES AND NODULES *continued*

Disease	Age	Sex	Race/Ethnicity	Cause	Clinical Characteristics	Treatment
Neurofibroma	Childhood	M-F	Any	Gene dysregulation resulting in uncontrolled growth of peripheral nerves and neural sheaths	Firm pink nodules that are often deep-seated. These tumors are located in skin, bones, buccal mucosa, tongue, or lips. Lesions are nontender but movable. Continued enlargement can lead to deformity. Multiple lesions and skin pigmentations are associated with von Recklinghausen's disease (neurofibromatosis).	Excisional biopsy, histologic examination, and follow-up for malignant transformation in cases of neurofibromatosis.
Papilloma	20 to 40	M	Any	Epithelial growth induced by chronic human papillomavirus infection (primarily types 6 and 11)	Small, pink, pebbly, slow-growing papule located on uvula, soft palate, tongue, frenum, lips, buccal mucosa, or gingiva. The base is pedunculated and well circumscribed, whereas the surface is most often rough to palpation.	Excisional biopsy and histologic examination.
Verruca vulgaris	Child, young adult	M-F	Any	Epithelial growth induced by chronic human papillomavirus infection (primarily types 2 and 4)	Rough, whitish-pink papule located on the skin of the hands and perilabially on the lips, labial and buccal mucosa, and attached gingiva. Lesions are slow growing and have a sessile base. Verrucae may regress spontaneously or spread to adjacent mucocutaneous surfaces.	Excisional biopsy and histologic examination.
Condyloma acuminatum	20–45	M	Any	Epithelial growth induced by chronic human papillomavirus infection (primarily types 6 and 11)	Small, pink-to-dirty gray papule with rough, papillary surface that resembles a cauliflower. Base of condyloma is sessile, and the borders are raised and rounded. Lesions occur in multiples, and onset rapidly occurs after inoculation from affected sexual partner. Most common location is genitalia, labial mucosa, labial commissure, attached gingiva, and soft palate. Lesions can spread and coalesce into extensive clusters.	Excisional biopsy and histologic examination.

PAPULES AND NODULES *continued*

Disease	Age	Sex	Race/ Ethnicity	Cause	Clinical Characteristics	Treatment
Lymphan- gioma	Child, adol- escent	M-F	Any	Congenital hamartoma of lymphatic channels	Soft, compressible, pinkish-white swelling that may be superficial or deep-seated. Superficial lesions resemble papillomas; deep-seated lesions cause diffuse enlargement. Lymphangiomas may occur in neck (cystic hygroma), dorsal or lateral tongue, lip, or labial mucosa. Long-standing lesions can cause functional problems or regress spontaneously.	Surgical excision; depending on size and location, surgery may require general anesthesia.

VESICULOBULLOUS DISEASES

Disease	Age	Sex	Race/Ethnicity	Cause	Clinical Characteristics	Treatment
Primary herpetic gingivo-stomatitis	Infant, child, young adult	M-F	Any	Primary herpes simplex virus (type 1) infection of oral epithelium, infection with type 2 is less likely	Multiple vesicles that rupture, coalesce, and form ulcers of the lip, buccal and labial mucosa, gingiva, palate, and tongue. Ulcers are painful and initially are small and yellow, and have red inflammatory borders. Onset is rapid, several days after contact with person harboring the virus. Lesions persist for 12–20 days.	Fluids, antivirals antipyretics; antibiotics to prevent secondary infection, oral anesthetic rinses, analgesics.
Recurrent herpes simplex	Teen-agers and adults	M-F	Any	Recrudescence of herpes simplex virus from sensory neuron, resulting in infection of orofacial epithelium, trauma and stress associated	Multiple small vesicles that rupture and ulcerate. Lesions occur repeatedly at same site: usually the lip, hard palate, and attached gingiva. Onset is rapid and is preceded by prodromal burning or tingling. Lesions last 5–12 days and heal spontaneously.	Antivirals (acyclovir, famciclovir, valacyclovir), bioflavonoids, sunscreens (lip), lysine.
Herpangina	Child, young adult	M-F	Any	Coxsackie virus (types A1–6, A8, A10, A22, B3) infection of oropharynx	Light gray vesicles that rupture and form many discrete shallow ulcers. Lesions have erythematous border and are limited to the anterior pillars, soft palate, uvula, and tonsils. Pharyngitis, headache, fever, and lymphadenitis are often concurrent. Lesions heal spontaneously in 1–2 weeks.	Palliative; vesicles heal spontaneously.
Chickenpox	Child	M-F	Any	Primary varicella zoster virus infection	Vesicles on skin and face that, after rupturing, resemble a dewdrop. Ulcers may be seen on soft palate, buccal mucosa, and mucobuccal fold. Skin lesions crust over and heal without scar formation. Condition often accompanied by chills, fever, nasopharyngitis, and malaise. Spontaneous healing occurs in 7–10 days.	Palliative; vesicles heal spontaneously. Avoid scratching to limit scar formation.

VESICULOBULLOUS DISEASES *continued*

Disease	Age	Sex	Race/Ethnicity	Cause	Clinical Characteristics	Treatment
Herpes zoster	Over 55, over 35 in HIV-positive	M-F	Any	Recrudescence of varicella zoster virus from sensory neuron, resulting in infection of epithelium	Unilateral vesicular and pustular eruptions that develop over 1–3 days. Lesions occur along dermatomes and especially along the trigeminal nerve tract. Lesions are vesicular, ulcerative, and intensely painful and commonly affect the lip, tongue, and buccal mucosa extending up to the midline. Neuralgia may persist after healing.	Palliative; lesions heal spontaneously. Famciclovir in severe cases or immuno-suppressed patients.
Hand-foot-and-mouth disease	Child, young adult	M-F	Any	Coxsackie virus (types A5, A9, A10, B2, B5) infection	Crops of multiple small yellowish ulcers that occur on palm and sole of hand and foot. The tongue, hard palate, and buccal and labial mucosa are affected. Total number of lesions may approach 100. Healing occurs spontaneously in about 10 days.	Palliative; ulcers heal spontaneously.
Allergic reactions immediate	Any	M-F	Any	Immediate immunologic reaction involving an allergen, IgE, and the release of histamine from mast cells	Red swellings or wheals that occur periorally or on lips, buccal mucosa, gingiva, lips, and tongue. Contact with allergen usually precedes episode by a few minutes to hours. Warmth, tenseness, and itchiness are concurrent. Lesions regress if the allergen is withdrawn.	Remove allergen; antihistamines.
Allergic reactions delayed	Any	M-F	Any	Immunologic reaction after 24 to 48 hours involving an allergen, T cells, and a cytotoxic reaction	Itchy erythematous papules orvesicles that may eventually ulcerate. May occur on any cutaneous or mucocutaneous surface. The lips, gingiva, alveolar mucosa, tongue, and palate are affected. Erythema develops slowly over 24–48 hours. Fissuring and ulceration may result.	Remove allergen; corticosteroids.

VESICULOBULLOUS DISEASES *continued*

Disease	Age	Sex	Race/ Ethnicity	Cause	Clinical Characteristics	Treatment
Erythema multiforme	Young adult	M	Any	Complement-mediated and white blood cell–mediated cytopathic effects provoked by pathogens and drug allergens	Skin: target lesions. Oral: hemorrhagic crust of the lips, painful ulcerations of the tongue, buccal mucosa and palate. Attached gingiva rarely affected. Headache, low-grade fever, and previous respiratory infection often precede lesions.	Topical analgesics, antipyretic agents, fluids, corticosteroids, antibiotics to prevent secondary infection.
Stevens-Johnson syndrome	Child, young adult	Slight preference for males	Any	Complement-mediated and white blood cell–mediated cytopathic effects provoked by pathogens and drug allergens.	Skin: target lesions. Eye: conjunctivitis. Genital: balanitis. Oral: hemorrhagic crust of the lips, painful ulcerations, and weeping bullae of the tongue and buccal mucosa. Attached gingiva rarely affected. Stevens-Johnson syndrome is the fulminant form of erythema multiforme. Eating and swallowing are often impaired.	Topical analgesics, antipyretic agents, fluids, corticosteroids, antibiotics to prevent secondary infection; hospitalization.
Toxic Epidermal Necrolysis	Older adults	F	Any	Severe complement-mediated and white blood cell–mediated cytopathic effects provoked by drugs	Severe large coalescing bullae.	IV fluids, corticosteroids, hospitalization.
Pemphigus vulgaris	40–60	2:1 (F:M)	Light skinned persons, Jewish and Mediterranean persons	Autoimmune antibodies directed against desmoglein 3 (a component of the desmosome)	Multiple skin and mucosal bullae that rupture, hemorrhage, and crust. Lesions tend to recur in the same area, have circular or serpiginous borders, and tend to spread to adjacent areas. Nikolsky's sign positive. Collapsed bullae are white and necrotic and produce fetid oris. Dehydration can occur if lesions are extensive.	Medical (and ophthalmologic) referral, systemic steroids, oral topical steroids, steroid-sparing and immuno-suppressive agents.

VESICULOBULLOUS DISEASES *continued*

Disease	Age	Sex	Race/Ethnicity	Cause	Clinical Characteristics	Treatment
Benign mucous membrane pemphigoid	Over 50	2:1 (F:M)	Any	Autoimmune antibodies directed against basement membrane antigens (laminin 5 and BP 180)	Bullous type produces blisters and ulcers on skin folds and inguinal and abdominal areas. Cicatricial type produces bullae and ulcers affecting the mucosa of the eyes, mouth, and genitals, which can lead to scarring. Bullae are often hemorrhagic and persist for days, then desquamate. Oral lesions that occur on the gingiva, palate, and buccal mucosa are painful and limit oral hygiene.	Topical steroids, occlusive topical steroids, dapsone, or tetracycline and niacinamide. Medical referral and systemic steroids if severe; rule out corneal involvement and internal malignancy.

ULCERATIVE LESIONS

Disease	Age	Sex	Race/ Ethnicity	Cause	Clinical Characteristics	Treatment
Traumatic ulcer	Any	M-F	Any	Traumatic insult to epithelium and underlying layers	Symptomatic, yellow-gray ulcer of variable size and shape, depending on inducing agent. Ulcers are often depressed and usually oval in shape, with erythematous border. Commonly located on labial and buccal mucosa, tongue at the borders, and hard palate. Ulcer lasts 1–2 weeks.	Palliative; remove traumatic influence.
Recurrent aphthous stomatitis	Young adult	F	Any	Instigating factor often unknown; related to defect in T-cell response; stress and trauma may play a role	Small yellowish oval ulcer(s) with red border, located on movable nonkeratinized mucosa. Common sites include labial mucosa, buccal mucosa, floor of the mouth, tongue, and occasionally soft palate. Ulcers are tender and may be associated with a tender lymph node. Lesions develop rapidly and disappear in 10–14 days without scar formation.	Spontaneous healing in 10–14 days. If acute symptoms or recurrent and symptomatic, topical anesthetics, coagulating agents, or topical steroids may be used.
Pseudo-aphthous	25–50	F	Any	Unknown immune defect associated with folic acid, iron, or vitamin B_{12} deficiencies, inflammatory bowel disease, Crohn's disease, gluten intolerance	Depressed yellowish round or oval ulcer located on movable nonkeratinized mucosa. Common sites include labial mucosa, buccal mucosa, floor of the mouth, tongue, and occasionally soft palate. Tongue may demonstrate atrophied papillae. Ulcers are tender, develop during deficiency state, and disappear with replacement therapy within 20 days.	Evaluate for deficiency state. If patient is deficient, then nutritional supplements (e.g., iron, vitamin B_{12}, folate) are recommended. Gluten abstinence may be required.

ULCERATIVE LESIONS *continued*

Disease	Age	Sex	Race/ Ethnicity	Cause	Clinical Characteristics	Treatment
Major aphthous stomatitis	Young adult	F	Any	Instigating factor often unknown; related to defect in T-cell response	Asymmetric unilateral large ulcer with necrotic and depressed center. Ulcers have a red inflammatory border and are extremely painful. Located on soft palate, tonsillar fauces, labial mucosa, buccal mucosa, and tongue; may extend onto attached gingiva. Rapid onset. Underlying tissue is often destroyed. Lesions heal in 15–30 days with scar formation. Recurrences are common.	Spontaneous healing, sometimes with scar formation. Topical anesthetics, topical steroids, stress management; identify allergens.
Herpetiform ulceration	Late 20s	M	Any	Variant form of recurrent aphthous stomatitis; cause unknown	Multiple pinhead-sized yellowish ulcers located on movable nonkeratinized mucosa. Common sites include anterior tip of tongue, labial mucosa, and floor of the mouth. No vesicle formation. Ulcers are painful and may be associated with several tender lymph nodes. Lesions develop rapidly and disappear in 10–14 days without scar formation.	Tetracycline rinses.
Behçet's syndrome	20–30	3:1 (M:F)	Asian, Mediterranean, Anglo	Delayed hypersensitivity reaction and vasculitis triggered by the presentation of human leukocyte antigens (HLA-B51) or environmental antigens, such as viruses, bacteria, chemicals, and heavy metals	Eye: conjunctivitis, iritis; Genital: ulcers; Oral: painful aphthous-like ulcers on labial and buccal mucosa; Skin: maculopapular rash and nodular eruptions. Oral ulcers are often an initial sign of the disease onset. Arthritis and gastrointestinal symptoms may be concurrent. Recurrences, exacerbations, and remissions are likely.	Topical and systemic steroids.

ULCERATIVE LESIONS *continued*

Disease	Age	Sex	Race/Ethnicity	Cause	Clinical Characteristics	Treatment
Granulo-matous ulcer (Tuberculosis, Histoplasmosis)	Older adult	M-F	Any	Infection by *Mycobacterium tuberculosis* or *Histoplasmosis capsulatum*	Asymptomatic, cobblestoned ulcer that usually occurs on dorsum of tongue, or labial commissure. Cervical lymphadenopathy and primary respiratory symptoms often are concurrent. Onset of oral disease follows lung infection lasting several weeks to months. Oral ulcer may persist for months to years if underlying disease not treated.	Biopsy, histologic examination. Tuberculosis: drug combination of isoniazid, rifampin, rifapentine, ethambutol, streptomycin, and pyrazinamide. Histoplasmosis: amphotericin B.
Squamous cell carcinoma	Over 50	2:1 (M:F)	Any	Mutagenesis of genes that regulate cell growth and apoptosis caused by carcinogens (tobacco, alcohol, and human papillomavirus)	Nonpainful yellowish ulcer with raised red indurated borders commonly located on posterior third of the lateral border of tongue, ventral tongue, lips, and floor of the mouth. Associated features may include numbness, leukoplakia, erythroplakia, induration, fixation, fungation, and lymphadenopathy. Carcinoma has a slow onset and is often noticed after a recent increase in size.	Surgery, radiation therapy, or chemotherapy. Smoking and alcohol cessation.
Chemo-therapeutic ulcer	15–30 and older adult	M-F	Any	Inhibition of rapidly reproducing cells by chemotherapeutic drugs	Irregular ulcerations of the lips, labial and buccal mucosa, tongue, and palate. Red inflammatory border is often lacking. Hemorrhage is likely when ulcers are deeply situated. Lesions are extremely painful and usually limit mastication and swallowing. Develops during second week of chemotherapy. Secondary infection with oral microorganisms is likely.	Antimicrobial rinses to prevent secondary infection. Topical anesthetics, palliative elixirs, and intravenous fluids.

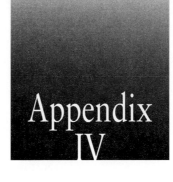

Appendix
IV

Self-Assessment Quiz

1. **(Fig. 75.1)** A 66-year-old man presents to the dental clinic with pain associated with these lesions on his tongue. He states that the lesions cropped up overnight, and the discomfort he is experiencing is limiting his ability to swallow. Although the patient has had a history of intraoral ulcerations, he says that he has never before had one in this location. The most likely diagnosis for this condition is:
   A. recurrent herpes simplex
   B. aphthous stomatitis
   C. traumatic ulceration
   D. herpangina
   E. pemphigoid

2. **(Fig. 75.2)** This ulcer appeared 8 days ago in a 31-year-old homosexual man after a vacation in the Caribbean. He claims that the lesion began as a vesicle but enlarged over the last several days; it is now quite painful. The regional lymph nodes on that side are tender to palpation. This lesion is most likely a:
   A. traumatic ulcer
   B. recurrent aphthous
   C. recurrent herpetic ulcer
   D. syphilitic ulcer
   E. granulomatous ulcer

3. **(Fig. 75.3)** Two months after you treated the patient shown in Figure 64.2, he returns for an oral surgical appointment. Examination reveals scattered white plaques on the lateral border of the tongue and persistent anterior and posterior cervical lymphadenopathy. A low-grade fever is present. This patient demonstrates clinical features most consistent with:
   A. lichen planus
   B. lupus erythematosus
   C. infectious mononucleosis
   D. syphilis
   E. HIV infection

4. **(Fig. 75.3)** The condition affecting this patient's tongue is most likely:
   A. coated tongue
   B. hairy tongue
   C. hairy leukoplakia
   D. leukoplakia
   E. erythroleukoplakia

5. **(Fig. 75.4)** A healthy 9-year-old boy appears at the dental clinic with this soft tissue mass. It has been present for 3 weeks and has progressively increased in size. The patient claims that moderate bleeding occurs every time he brushes his teeth, so he has avoided brushing that area for several days. All the adjacent teeth are asymptomatic and test vital. Periapical radiographs of the area reveal no abnormalities. The most likely diagnosis for the lesion is:

A. irritation fibroma
B. peripheral odontogenic fibroma
C. peripheral giant cell granuloma
D. peripheral fibroma with ossification
E. pyogenic granuloma

6. **(Fig. 75.5)** This 28-year-old woman presents to the dental clinic with the chief symptom of a "burning sensation in my mouth and throat." She does not report dryness. Review of her medical history reveals a recent upper respiratory infection that was treated with a 14-day course of amoxicillin. Intraorally one finds multiple red patches on buccal mucosa, soft palate, and posterior pharyngeal wall that are tender to palpation. This condition is most likely:
   A. lichen planus
   B. pemphigoid
   C. pemphigus
   D. acute atrophic candidiasis
   E. chronic atrophic candidiasis

7. **(Fig. 75.6)** These bilateral linear white plaques were discovered in a 50-year-old woman during a routine dental examination. The patient claims she has been under a lot of stress lately because of family problems. The plaques are asymptomatic and do not rub off. The most likely diagnosis is:
   A. lupus erythematosus
   B. lichen planus
   C. candidiasis
   D. frictional keratosis
   E. none of the above

8. **(Fig. 75.7)** This asymptomatic, speckled-red and white ulcerated patch of the tongue was found in a middle-aged man who admitted to heavy alcohol and tobacco use. The patient was aware of the lesion's presence but was uncertain of the duration. The lesion was firm to palpation. The most likely diagnosis of this lesion is:
   A. an accessory salivary gland tumor
   B. traumatic erythema
   C. candidiasis
   D. squamous cell carcinoma
   E. lichen planus

9. **(Fig. 75.8)** This 53-year-old woman came to the dental clinic because of burning, painful gingiva. An incisional biopsy was performed, and during the initial incision the gingiva began to slough. The biopsy report indicated that the epithelium was separating from the lamina propria below the basal cell layer. The most likely diagnosis is:
   A. pemphigus
   B. pemphigoid
   C. lichen planus
   D. lupus erythematosus
   E. erythema multiforme

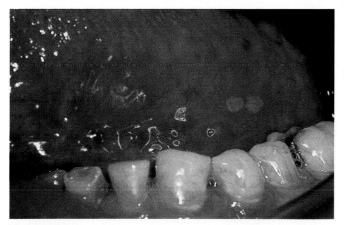

Figure 75.1.

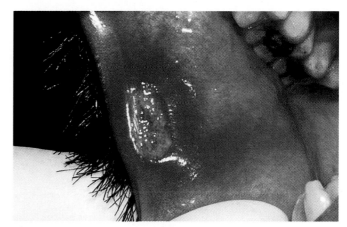

Figure 75.2.

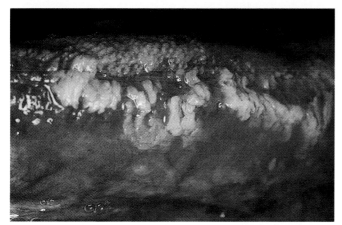

Figure 75.3.

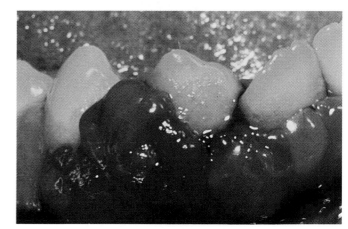

Figure 75.4.

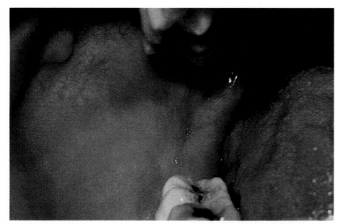

Figure 75.5.

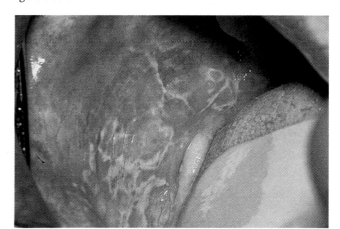

Figure 75.6.

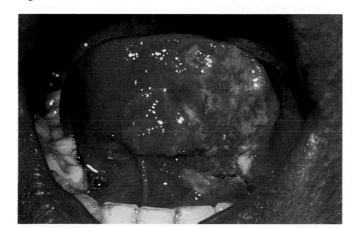

Figure 75.7.

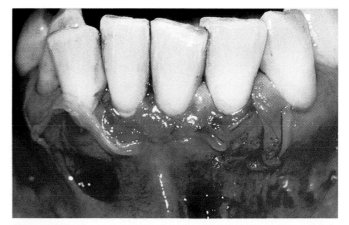

Figure 75.8.

ANSWERS TO SELF-ASSESSMENT

1. B
2. C
3. E
4. C
5. E
6. D
7. B
8. D
9. B

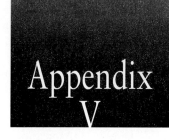

Appendix V

Glossary

Abdomen: The part of the body lying between the thorax (chest) and pelvis.

Acantholysis: Loss of coherence between epidermal or epithelial cells.

Acute: Having severe symptoms and a short course.

Adrenal gland: A small endocrine gland located near the kidney that secretes 1) endogenous glucocorticosteroids, which control digestive metabolism; 2) mineralocorticoids, which control sodium and potassium balance; 3) sex hormones; and 4) catecholamines (epinephrine and norepinephrine), which alter blood pressure and heart function.

Adrenalectomy: Surgical removal of the adrenal gland.

Afunctional: Not functioning or working.

Agenesis: Complete absence of a structure or part of a structure caused by failure of tissue development.

AIDS: Acronym for acquired immune deficiency syndrome, reserved for patients infected with HIV (human immunodeficiency virus). It also refers to the terminal stage of the disease.

Allergen: A substance that induces hypersensitivity or an allergic reaction.

Amalgam: An alloy used to restore teeth, composed mainly of silver and mercury.

Amelogenesis: The formation of the enamel portion of the tooth.

Amputation: Strictly, this term refers to the removal of a limb such as an arm or of an appendage such as a finger. With reference to a neuroma, however, amputation means a tumor of nerve tissue that results from severing of a nerve.

Analgesic: A drug or substance used to relieve pain.

Analogous: Having similar properties.

Anaplastic: Pertaining to adult cells that have changed irreversibly toward more primitive cell types. Such changes are often malignant.

Anergy: A total loss of reactivity to specific antigens.

Angioma: A tumor made up of blood or lymph vessels.

Anodontia: Congenital condition in which all the teeth fail to develop.

Anomaly: Deviation from normal.

Anorexia: A lack or loss of appetite for food.

Anterior: Located toward the front (opposite of posterior).

Antibiotic: A chemical compound that inhibits the growth or replication of certain forms of life, especially pathogenic organisms such as bacteria or fungi. Antibiotics are classified as either biostatic or biocidal.

Antibiotic sensitivity: Testing a suspected organism to see whether it is sensitive to destruction by one or more specific antibiotics.

Antibody: A protein produced in the body in response to stimulation by an antigen. Antibodies react specifically to antigens in an attempt to neutralize these foreign substances.

Antigen: A substance, usually a protein, that is recognized as foreign by the body's immune system and stimulates formation of a specific antibody to the antigen.

Antipyretic: A drug or substance used to relieve fever.

Aplasia: Absence of an organ or organ part resulting from failure of development of the embryonic tissue of origin.

Arthralgia: Pain in one or more joints.

Aspiration: The withdrawal of fluid, usually into a syringe.

Asymptomatic: A lack of symptoms in the patient.

Atherosclerosis: A condition of degeneration and hardening of the walls of arteries caused by fat deposition.

Atopy: Hypersensitivity or allergy caused by hereditary influences.

Atrophic: A normally developed tissue that has decreased in size.

Atypical: Pertaining to a deviation from the normal or typical state.

Autoinoculation: To inoculate with a pathogen such as a virus from one's own body. An example would be to spread herpesvirus from one's own mouth or lips to one's finger.

Autosomal dominant: The appearance in offspring of one of two mutually antagonistic features in association with one of the 22 pairs of chromosomes in humans that are not concerned with sexual determination.

Bacterial plaque: A collection of bacteria, growing in a deposit of material on the surface of a tooth, that can cause disease.

Bilateral: On both sides of the body, or mouth.

Biopsy: Excision of living tissue for the purpose of examination by a pathologist.

Bosselated: Covered with bosses or bumps.

Bruxism: A habit related to stress or a sleep disorder, characterized by grinding one's teeth.

Bulimia: An eating disorder characterized by frequent periods of excessive food consumption followed by the purging of the ingested food by vomiting or the use of laxatives.

Bulla: A circumscribed, fluid-containing, elevated lesion of the skin that is more than 1 cm in diameter.

Cadherin: A family of adhesion proteins that makes up the desmosome and other structures.

Carcinogen: An agent that induces cancer.

Carcinoma: A malignant growth made up of epithelial cells that are capable of infiltration and metastasis. Carcinoma is a specific form of cancer.

Cellulitis: A spreading, diffuse, edematous, and sometimes suppurative (pus-producing) inflammation in cellular tissues.

Cervical lymphadenopathy: Abnormally large lymph nodes in the neck, often caused by lymphocyte replication in response to an allergen or infectious organism.

Chemotaxis: Taxis or movement of cells in response to chemical stimulation.

Chemotherapy: Treatment by chemical substances that have a specific effect on the microorganisms causing the disease. This term is usually reserved for the treatment of cancer with the use of drugs that inhibit rapidly reproducing cells. Side effects are possible.

Choristoma: Normal tissue in an abnormal location.

Chronic: Persisting for a long time; when applied to a disease, chronic means that there has been little change or extremely slow progression for a long period.

Cicatricial: Pertaining to a scar.

Cicatrix: A scar. The fibrous tissue that is formed after a wound heals.

Cirrhosis: A chronic disease of the liver characterized by degenerative changes in the liver cells, the deposition of connective tissue, and other changes. The result is that the liver cells stop functioning and the flow of blood through the liver decreases. There are many causes of cirrhosis, including infection, toxic substances, and long-term alcohol abuse.

Clavicle: The collar bone, connecting the shoulder bone (scapula) to the chest bone (sternum).

Coagulation: The process of clotting, usually of blood. Clotting is the natural means by which bleeding ceases when a vessel has been severed.

Collagen: A protein present in the connective tissue of the body.

Coloboma: A developmental defect that may affect various parts of the eye, characterized by a missing part of the structure affected. For example, a coloboma of the lower eyelid means a missing part of the lower eyelid.

Commissure: The junction of the upper and lower lips at the corner of the mouth.

Complement: A series of enzymatic proteins in normal serum that, in the presence of a specific sensitizer, can destroy bacteria and other cells. C1 through C9 are the nine components of complement that combine with the antigen–antibody complex to produce lysis.

Concretion: A hardened mass such as calculus.

Concurrent: One or more conditions, events, or findings occurring at the same time.

Congenital: Present at or existing from the time of birth.

Constitutional symptoms: Symptoms affecting the whole body, such as fever, malaise, anorexia, nausea, and lethargy.

Cornified: A process whereby a tissue, usually epithelium, becomes rough and thickened in its outer coating.

Culture: The propagation of an organism in a medium conducive to growth.

Cyst: A pathologic epithelium-lined cavity, usually containing fluid or semisolid material.

Cytologic: Pertaining to the scientific study of cells.

Cytopathic: Pertaining to or characterized by pathologic changes in cells.

Debilitation: The process of becoming weakened.

Deciduous tooth: The primary dentition, or baby teeth. The normal number is 20.

Deglutition: The process of taking a substance through the mouth and throat into the esophagus. Deglutition is a stage of swallowing.

Dehydration: The removal of water from a substance. Prolonged fever and diarrhea cause dehydration.

Dental lamina: The embryonic tissue of origin of the teeth.

Desmosome: An intercellular bridge between epithelial cells. The bridge is made of proteins and tonofilaments.

Developmental: Pertaining to growth to full size or maturity.

Diascopy: The examination of tissue under pressure through a transparent medium. For example, suspected vascular lesions are examined by pressing a glass slide over an abnormality to see whether the reddish tissue turns white. Because blood flows through vascular lesions, pressure causes them to turn white and thus helps to confirm the diagnosis.

Distal: Furthest from a point of reference. In dentistry, distal describes the surface furthest from the midline of the patient.

Dorsal: Directed toward or situated on the back surface (opposite of ventral).

Dysphagia: Difficulty swallowing.

Dysphonia: Difficulty speaking.

Dysplasia: An abnormality of development and maturation characterized by the loss of normal cellular architecture.

Dysplastic: Pertaining to an abnormality of development. This term is often used to describe the appearance of abnormal, premalignant cells under the microscope. The cells begin to lose their normal maturation pattern and have abnormally shaped, hyperchromatic nuclei.

Dyspnea: Labored or difficult breathing.

Ecchymoses: Large reddish-blue areas caused by the escape of blood into the tissues, commonly referred to as a bruise. Ecchymoses do not blanch on diascopy.

Ecosystem: The interaction of living organisms and nonliving elements in a defined area.

Ectodermal: Pertaining to the outermost of the three primitive germ layers of an embryo. The middle layer is the mesoderm, and the innermost layer is the endoderm. Ectodermal structures include the skin, hair, nails, oral mucous membrane, and the enamel of the teeth.

Ectopic: Located in an abnormal place. The ectopic tissue or structure may or may not be normal.

Edema: Abnormal amounts of fluid in the intercellular spaces, resulting in visible swelling.

Emanate: To give off or flow away from.

Embryonic: Pertaining to the earliest stage of development of an organism.

Encephalitis: Inflammation of the brain.

Endocrinopathy: A disease or abnormal state of an endocrine gland.

Endodermal: Pertaining to the innermost of the three primitive germ layers of an embryo. Endodermal structures include the epithelium of the pharynx, respiratory tract (except the nose), and the digestive tract.

Epistaxis: Bleeding from the nose.

Epithelium: The cellular makeup of skin and mucous membranes.

Epitope: The antigenic target of antibodies (IgG, IgM, IgA).

Epulis: A nodular or tumorous enlargement of the gingiva.

Erosion: The wearing away of teeth through the action of chemical substances, or a denudation of epithelium above the basal cell layer.

Eruption: An emergence from beneath a surface. For teeth, eruption means their growth into the oral cavity; it may also refer to the development of skin lesions.

Erythematous: Characterized by a redness of the tissue because of engorgement of the capillaries in the region. Erythematous lesions blanch on diascopy.

Erythroplastic: Characterized by a reddish appearance. This term implies abnormal tissue proliferation in the reddish area.

Eschar: A slough of epithelium often caused by disease, trauma, or chemical burn.

Esthetic: Pertaining to the appearance of oral or dental structures or the pleasing effect of dental restorations or procedures.

Everted: Folded or turned outward.

Exacerbation: An increase in severity.

Exanthematic: Characterized by the development of an eruption or rash.

Excisional biopsy: To completely remove a mass of tissue for the purpose of scientific analysis.

Exophytic: An outwardly growing lesion.

Extensor surface: Because the arms and legs can be extended or tensed by the appropriate extensor or tensor muscles, the anterior surface is referred to as the extensor surface and the posterior surface is referred to as the tensor surface.

Extirpate: To completely remove or eradicate.

Extremity: A limb of the body, such as an arm or leg.

Exudate: Material that has escaped from blood vessels into tissue or onto the surface of a tissue, usually because of inflammation.

Factitial: Self-induced, as in factitial injury.

Fascial plane: Spaces between adjacent bundles of fascia that cover muscles. Infection often spreads along these planes.

Fenestration: A perforation or opening in a tissue.

Fetor oris: An unpleasant or abnormal odor emanating from the oral cavity.

Field cancerization: Malignant growths occurring in multiple sites of the oral cavity. The oral tissues have often been exposed to a carcinogen for a long time.

Fissure: A narrow slit or cleft.

Fluctuant: Strictly, this term describes a palpated, wavelike motion that is felt in a fluid-containing lesion. In this text, the term is frequently used to describe a soft, readily yielding mass on palpation.

Fontanelle: One of several soft spots on the skull of infants and children in which the bones of the skull have not yet completely united. In these areas, the brain is covered only by a membrane beneath the skin.

Frenum: A fold of mucous membrane that limits the movement of an organ or organ part. For example, the lingual frenum limits tongue movement, and the labial frenula limit lip movements.

Frontal bone: The skull bone that forms the forehead. The frontal bone contains an air space called the frontal sinus.

Furcal: Pertaining to or associated with the part of a multirooted tooth where the roots join the crown.

Ganglion: A collection of cell bodies of neurons outside of the central nervous system. A ganglion is essentially a terminal through which many peripheral circuits connect with the central nervous system.

Gastroenterologist: A medical specialist whose field is disorders of the stomach and intestines.

Gastrointestinal: Pertaining to the stomach and intestine.

Genetic counseling: A form of patient counseling in which the transmission of inherited traits is discussed.

Genodermatosis: A hereditary skin disease.

Gingivectomy: Surgical removal of gingival tissue.

Glaucoma: A disease of the eye characterized by increased intraocular pressure. This condition is often asymptomatic and, if not recognized or treated, leads to blindness.

Glossal: Pertaining to or associated with the tongue.

Glucose: A form of sugar that is the most important carbohydrate in the body's metabolism.

Glucosuria: The presence of an abnormal quantity of glucose in the urine. A sign of diabetes mellitus.

Granulomatous: Pertaining to a well-defined area that has developed as a reaction to the presence of living organisms or a foreign body. The tissue consists primarily of histiocytes.

Gravid: Pregnant.

Halitosis: An unpleasant odor of the breath or expired air.

Hamartoma: A tumorlike nodule consisting of a mixture of normal tissue usually present in an organ but existing in an unusual arrangement or an unusual site.

Hapten: An incomplete allergen. When combined with another substance to form a molecule, a hapten may stimulate a hypersensitivity or allergic reaction.

Hematoma: A large ecchymosis or bruise caused by the escape of blood into the tissues. Hematomas are blue on the skin and red on the mucous membranes. As hematomas resolve they may turn brown, green, or yellow.

Hematopoietic: Pertaining to the production of blood or of its constituent elements. Hematopoiesis is the main function of the bone marrow.

Hematuria: The presence of blood in the urine.

Hemidesmosome: An intercellular bridge between epithelial cells and the basement membrane.

Hemihypertrophy: The presence of hypertrophy on one side only of a tissue or organ. In facial hemihypertrophy, for example, one half of the face is visibly larger than the other.

Hemoglobin: The iron-containing pigment of the erythrocytes. Its function is to carry oxygen to the tissues. One of the causes of anemia is a deficiency of iron, causing patients to look pale and feel tired.

Hemolysis: Generally speaking, this term refers to the disintegration of elements in the blood. A common form of hemolysis occurs during anemia and involves lysis or the dissolution of erythrocytes.

Hemorrhage: Bleeding; the escape of blood from a severed blood vessel.

Hemostasis: The stoppage of blood flow. This can occur naturally by clotting or artificially by the application of pressure or the placement of sutures.

Hereditary: Transmitted or transmissible from parent to offspring; determined genetically.

Hiatal hernia: Protrusion of any structure through the hiatus of the diaphragm. Affected patients are prone to indigestion.

Histiocyte: A large phagocytic cell from the reticuloendothelial system. The reticuloendothelial system is a network made up of all of the phagocytic cells in the body, which include macrophages, Kupffer cells in the liver, and the microglia of the brain.

Histology: The microscopic study of the structure and form of the various tissues making up a living organism.

Hyperdontia: A condition or circumstance characterized by one or more extra, or supernumerary teeth.

Hyperemia: The presence of excess blood in a tissue area.

Hyperglycemia: The presence of excessive sugar or glucose in the bloodstream.

Hypermenorrhea: Excessive uterine bleeding of unusually long duration at regular intervals.

Hyperorthokeratosis: Keratin is the outermost layer of epithelium as seen under the microscope and is seen in two forms: orthokeratin and parakeratin. Orthokeratin has no visible nuclei within the outer layer, whereas nuclei are present in parakeratin. Hyperorthokeratosis is the presence of excess orthokeratin.

Hyperplasia: An increase in the size of a tissue or organ caused by an increase in the number of constituent cells.

Hypersensitivity: Generally, this term means an abnormal sensitivity to a stimulus of any kind. The term, however, is often used with specific reference to some form of allergic response.

Hypertension: High blood pressure.

Hypertrophy: An increase in the size of a tissue or organ caused by an increase in the size of constituent cells.

Hypocalcification: Less than normal amount of calcification.

Hypodontia: The congenital absence of one or several teeth as a result of agenesis.

Hypoplasia: Incomplete development of a tissue or organ; a tissue reduced in size because of a decreased number of constituent cells.

Hypopyon: Pus in the anterior chamber of the eye.

Hypotension: Low blood pressure.

Ileum: The distal or terminal portion of the small intestine, ending at the cecum, which is a blind pouch forming the proximal or first part of the large intestine.

Ilium: The lateral or flaring part of the pelvic bone, otherwise known as the hip.

Immunofluorescence: A laboratory assay used by pathologists and researchers that applies known antibodies (IgG, IgM, IgA) to tissue to identify the presence and location of specific antigens or proteins.

Incisional biopsy: The removal of a portion of suspected abnormal tissue for microscopic study.

Incisive papilla: A slightly elevated papule of normal tissue on the palate in the midline immediately posterior to the central incisors. Immediately beneath this structure lies the incisive canal.

Induration: Characterized by being hard; an abnormally hard portion of a tissue with respect to the surrounding similar tissue, often used to describe the feel of locally invasive malignant tissue on palpation.

Infant: A human baby from birth to 2 years of age.

Infarct: A localized area of ischemic necrosis resulting from a blockage of the arterial supply or the venous drainage of tissue. Ischemic necrosis is dead tissue resulting from an inadequate blood supply. An example is a heart attack, which is an infarct of heart muscle.

Insulin: A protein hormone secreted by the islets of Langerhans of the pancreas; insulin deficiency produces hyperglycemia, otherwise known as diabetes mellitus.

Integrins: A large group of heterodimeric transmembrane proteins that serve as receptors for extracellular matrix and cell surface proteins.

Invaginate: To fold and grow within, in the manner of a pouch.

Iris: The part of the eye that is blue, gray, green, or brown. It is a muscular tissue, and its function is to constrict and dilate the pupil. The pupil is the black appearing portion in the middle of the iris that allows light into the eye.

Iritis: Inflammation of the iris that is often caused by viral infection or rheumatoid disease. The main symptom of iritis is photophobia (aversion to light).

Ischemia: A deficiency of blood to a body part, usually caused by constriction or blockage of a blood vessel.

Kaposi's sarcoma: A malignant tumor of vascular tissue. Once rare in the Americas, it is now seen frequently in patients with AIDS. The lesions are red-purple in appearance and may be seen anywhere on the skin, especially on the face and in the oral cavity.

Keratinization: The formation of microscopic fibrils of keratin in the keratinocytes (keratin-forming cells). In the oral cavity, the term is used to describe changes in the outer layer of the epithelium.

Keratotic: A condition of the skin characterized by the presence of horny growths. On the oral mucous membrane, keratotic tissue usually looks white; the term implies a thickening of the outer layer of the oral epithelium.

Kilodalton: A unit of mass being one thousand times that of a dalton. A dalton is one sixteenth the mass of an oxygen atom.

Lamina propria: The layer of connective tissue immediately beneath the epithelium of the oral mucosa.

Laryngeal: Pertaining to the larynx, which is a part of the airway. It is located between the pharynx at the back of the oral cavity and the trachea at the beginning of the lungs. The larynx contains the vocal cords, which make audible sounds.

Lateral: Pertaining to or situated at the side.

Leptomeninges: The two more-delicate components of the meninges, the pia mater and the arachnoid.

Lesion: A site of structural or functional change in body tissues that is produced by disease or injury.

Leukoplakia: A white patch that cannot be rubbed off and that does not clinically represent any other condition.

Lipid: Fat or fatty; a naturally occurring substance made up of fatty acids.

Lobulated: Made up of lobules, which are smaller divisions of lobes. Many structures are divided into lobes and lobules, such as the brain, lung, and salivary glands. Some pathologic lesions are described as lobulated when the lesion is divided into smaller parts.

Lymphadenitis: Inflammation of lymph nodes generally resulting in enlargement and tenderness.

Lymphadenopathy: Enlarged lymph nodes that may or may not be tender. The enlargement results from increased number of lymphocytes presenting in the node.

Lymphoblastic: Pertaining to a cell of the lymphocytic series; the term implies proliferation. Lymphoblastic is one of the forms of leukemic cancer of the leukocytes characterized by the presence of malignant lymphoblasts or immature lymphocytes.

Lymphocyte: A variety of leukocyte that is important to the immune response and that arises in the lymph nodes. Lymphocytes can be large or small; they are round and nongranular and are classified as either T or B lymphocytes.

Macrocheilia: Abnormally large lips.

Macrodontia: Teeth that are considerably larger than normal.

Macule: A spot or stain on the skin or mucous membrane that is neither raised nor depressed. Some examples of macules include café au lait spots, hyperemia, erythema, petechiae, ecchymoses, purpura, oral melanotic macules, and many others illustrated in this atlas.

Malaise: A constitutional symptom that describes a feeling of uneasiness, discomfort, or indisposition.

Malignant: A neoplastic growth that is not usually encapsulated, grows rapidly, and can readily metastasize.

Mastication: Chewing.

Medial: Situated toward the midline (opposite of lateral).

Melena: Darkened or black feces that are caused by the presence of blood pigments; a sign of intestinal bleeding.

Meningitis: Inflammation of the meninges, which are the three membranes covering the brain and spinal cord (the dura mater, arachnoid, and pia mater). Meningitis produces both motor and mental signs, such as difficulty in walking and confusion.

Mesenchymal: The meshwork of embryonic connective tissue in the mesoderm that gives rise to the connective tissue of the body, blood vessels, and lymph vessels.

Mesial: Toward the front, anterior, or midline. The mesial surface of teeth is the side of the tooth closest to the midline. The five surfaces of teeth are mesial, distal, occlusal or incisal, labial or facial, and lingual or palatal.

Metastasize: To spread or travel from one part of the body to another; a term usually reserved to describe the spread of malignant tumors.

Microdontia: Teeth that are considerably smaller than normal.

Mineralized: Characterized by the deposition of mineral, often calcium and other organic salts, in a tissue. The term calcified is used when the mineral content is known to be calcium, whereas the term mineralized is more general and does not specify the exact nature of the mineral.

Monocytic leukemia: Leukemia is cancer of the leukocytes; in this condition the predominating leukocytes are monocytes.

Morphology: Descriptive of shape, form, or structure, or the science thereof.

Mucopurulent: Consisting of both mucus and pus.

Mutagenesis: The induction of genetic mutation.

Myelogenous leukemia: Leukemia is cancer of the leukocytes; in this instance the predominating leukocytes are myeloid or granular (polymorphonuclear leukocytes).

Nasopharyngitis: Inflammation of the nasopharynx (the back of the nasal complex and upper throat). Sore throat, postnasal drip, and fever are common signs.

Necrosis: The death of a cell as a result of injury or disease.

Neocapillary: New growth of capillaries, which are the smallest blood vessels and connect small arterioles to small venules.

Neoplasia: Characterized by the presence of new and uncontrolled cellular growth.

Neoplasm: A mass of newly formed tissue; a tumor.

Neurogenic: Originating in or from nerve tissue.

Neuropathy: Any abnormality of nerve tissue.

Neutrophil: A medium-sized leukocyte with a nucleus consisting of three to five lobes and a cytoplasm containing small granules; one group of leukocytes is called granulocytes, and the others are eosinophils and basophils. Neutrophils make up about 65% of the leukocytes in normal blood. Also known as polymorphonuclear leukocyte, PMN, or "poly."

Neutrophil chemotaxis: Taxis or movement of neutrophils in response to chemical substances or agents.

Nevus: A small tumor of the skin containing aggregations or theques of nevus cells; a mole. It may be flat or elevated and pigmented or nonpigmented; it may or may not contain hair.

Nodule: A circumscribed, usually solid lesion having the dimension of depth. Nodules are less than 1 cm in diameter.

Noncaseating: A tissue-degenerative process that forms a dry, shapeless mass resembling cheese.

Occipital bone: One of the bones that make up the skull; a thick bone at the back of the head.

Oligodontia: Presence of fewer than the normal number of teeth.

Oncogenic: Capable of causing tumor formation.

Opportunistic microorganism: Microorganisms that usually are not pathogenic but become so under certain circumstances, such as an environment altered by the action of antibiotics or long-term steroid therapy. Opportunistic microorganisms cause opportunistic infections.

Organism: Any viable life form, such as animals, plants, and microorganisms, including bacteria, fungi, and viruses.

Otorhinolaryngologist: An ear, nose, and throat specialist.

Palliative: Treatment to relieve symptoms; not the cause of a condition.

Pallor: Paleness of the skin or mucous membrane; an absence of a healthy color. This sign often accompanies constitutional symptoms and anemia.

Palpate: To feel with the fingers or hand.

Papule: A small mass, without the dimension of depth, that is smaller than 1 cm in diameter. When described as pedunculated, a papule is on a stalk; when described as sessile, a papule is attached at its base and does not have a stalk.

Parturition: The delivery of the fetus from the mother; to give birth.

Patch: Similar to a macule but larger; a large stain or spot, usually neither raised nor depressed, which may be textured.

Patent: The condition of being open; this term is often applied to ducts, vessels, and passages to indicate that they are not blocked.

Pathognomonic: Uniquely distinctive of a specific disease or condition; usually consists of signs or findings that, when present and recognized, enable the diagnosis to be made.

Pathologic: Pertaining to or caused by disease.

Pathosis: An abnormal state or condition.

Parietal bone: One of the bones that make up the skull; there is one parietal bone on each side of the skull, forming the skull's top and upper sides.

Pedunculated: A tissue mass originating by a stalk from its base.

Periapical: Pertaining to or located at the apex (root end) of a tooth.

Perifurcal: Pertaining to or located at the furcum of a tooth; below the cementoenamel junction where the roots fuse together.

Perilabial: Pertaining to the region around or near the lips.

Perineum: The lower surface of the trunk; when a patient is lying down with legs spread apart, the perineum is the area from the base of the spine to the anal region to the genital area and, finally, to the crest of the mons pubis.

Perioral: In the proximity of or around the oral cavity.

Periorbital: In the proximity of or around the orbit, which is the bony socket of the eye.

Peripheral: Pertaining to the outer part, such as the edge or margin.

Permanent dentition: Succedaneous (adult) teeth, which follow the primary teeth. Because there are no replacements for the permanent teeth, they must last a lifetime. There are 32 permanent teeth.

Petechiae: Little red spots, ranging in size from pinpoint to several millimeters in diameter. Petechiae consist of extravasated capillary blood.

Physiologic: Refers to normal body function (opposite of pathologic).

Pilocarpine: A drug used to stimulate salivary flow or to produce constriction of the pupil of the eye.

Plaque: An area with a flat surface and raised edges.

Platelet: One of the elements found in circulating blood. A platelet has a circular or disklike shape and is small; hence the term platelet. Platelets aid in blood coagulation and clot retraction.

Polydipsia: Excessive thirst. A sign of disease.

Polypoid: A polyplike protruding growth with a base that is equal in diameter to the surface of the mucosal lesion.

Polyuria: Excessive amounts of urine. A sign of disease.

Posterior: Directed toward or situated at the back (opposite of anterior).

Primary tooth: Deciduous (baby) tooth; there are 20 primary teeth.

Prognathism: A developmental deformity of the mandible that causes it to protrude abnormally.

Pruritus: Itching.

Pseudohyphae: Long, filamentous forms that can be seen under the microscope when *Candida albicans*, a fungal microorganism, assumes its pathogenic form.

Pulse: A patient's heartbeat, as felt through palpation of a blood vessel.

Punctate: Spotted; characterized by small points or punctures.

Purpuric: Pertaining to purpura, which are large bruises consisting of blood extravasated into the tissues. Bruises are bluish-purple in color.

Purulent: Containing pus.

Pustule: A well-circumscribed, pus-containing lesion, usually less than 1 cm in diameter.

Qualitative: Of or pertaining to quality; descriptive information about what something looks and feels like.

Quantitative: Of or pertaining to quantity; descriptive information about how much of something there is or how big something is.

Radiation: In dentistry, electromagnetic energy or x-rays transmitted through space. Radiation also means divergence from a common center; one of the properties of x-rays is that, like a beam of light, they diverge from their source.

Radiotherapy: Radiation therapy; the use of radiation from various sources to treat or cure malignant disorders.

Recrudescence: Recurrence of signs and symptoms of a disease after temporary abatement.

Refractory: Not readily responsive to treatment.

Remission: Improvement or abatement of the symptoms of a disease; the period during which symptoms abate.

Renal failure: Inability of the kidneys to function properly. A patient whose kidneys completely fail will die without renal dialysis or a kidney transplantation. One of the causes of kidney failure is prolonged hypertension (high blood pressure).

Retinopathy: A disease or abnormality of the retina of the eye. The retina cannot be seen without special instruments and is the part of the eye that receives and transmits visual information coming in from the pupil and lens onto the brain via the optic nerve.

Sarcoma: A malignant growth of cells of embryonic connective tissue origin. This condition is highly capable of infiltration and metastasis.

Sarcomatous: Pertaining to sarcoma, which is a malignant tumor of mesenchymal tissue origin.

Scar: A mark or cicatrix remaining after the healing of a wound or other morbid process.

Sclera: The strong outer tunic of the eye, or whites of the eyes. When the sclera turns blue or yellow, it is a sign of systemic abnormality.

Sepsis: A morbid state resulting from the presence of pathogenic microorganisms, usually in the bloodstream.

Septicemia: The presence of pathogenic bacteria in the blood.

Sequestration: Abnormal separation of a part from the whole, such as when a piece of bone sequestrates from the mandible because of osteomyelitis; the act of isolating a patient.

Serosal: Pertaining to the lining of internal organs such as the intestines.

Serpiginous: Characterized by a wavy or undulating margin.

Serum: The watery fluid remaining after coagulation of the blood. If clotted blood is left long enough, the clot shrinks and the fibrinogen is depleted; the remaining fluid is the serum.

Sessile: Attached to a surface on a broad base; does not have a stalk.

Sign: An objective finding or observation made by the examiner that the patient may be unaware of or does not report.

Sinus: An airspace inside the skull, such as the maxillary sinus; an abnormal channel, fistula, or tract allowing the escape of pus.

Splenic: Of or pertaining to the spleen, which is a structure in the upper left abdomen just behind and under the stomach. The spleen contains the largest collection of reticuloendothelial cells in the whole body; its functions include blood formation, blood storage, and blood filtration.

Spontaneous: Occurring unaided or without apparent cause; voluntary.

Superficial: Located on or near the surface.

Supernumerary: In excess of the regular number.

Symptom: A manifestation of disease that the patient is usually aware of and frequently reports.

Syndrome: A combination of signs and symptoms occurring commonly enough to constitute a distinct clinical entity.

Taurodont: A malformed multirooted tooth characterized by an altered crown-to-root ratio, the crown being of normal length, the roots being abnormally short, and the pulp chamber being abnormally large.

Telangiectasia: The formation of capillaries near the surface of a tissue. Telangiectasia may be a sign of hereditary disorder, alcohol abuse, or malignancy in the region.

Template bleeding time: The amount of time necessary for bleeding to stop after a skin incision of consistent length and depth.

Texture: Pertains to the characteristics of the surface of an area or lesion. Some descriptions of texture are as follows: smooth, rough, lumpy, and vegetative. The tiny bumps on the surface of a wart cause it to have a vegetative texture.

Therapeutic: Of or pertaining to therapy or treatment; beneficial. Therapy has as its goal the elimination or control of a disease or other abnormal state.

Thorax: That part of the body between the neck and abdomen, enclosed by the spine, ribs, and sternum. In the vernacular, the thorax is referred to as the chest. The main contents of the thorax are the heart and lungs.

Thrombophlebitis: The development of venous thrombi in the presence of inflammatory changes in the vessel wall.

Thrombosis: Formation of thrombi within the lumen of the heart or a blood vessel. A lumen is the space within a passage; a thrombus is a solid mass that can form within the heart or blood vessels from constituents in the circulating blood. Patients prone to the formation of thrombi should receive anticoagulant therapy.

Tooth bud: The embryonic tissue of origin of the teeth; tooth buds develop from the more primitive tissue of the dental lamina.

Torus: A bony nodule on the hard palate or on the lingual aspect of the premolars.

Tourniquet test: When pressure is applied to the blood vessels of the upper arm using a blood pressure cuff, a bleeding tendency is detected when petechiae develop in the region.

Transient: Temporary; of short duration.

Translucent: Somewhat penetrable by rays of light.

Trauma: A wound or injury; damage produced by an external force.

Trismus: Tonic contraction of the muscles of mastication; commonly referred to as lockjaw. Trismus is caused by oral infections, salivary gland infections, tetanus, trauma, and encephalitis.

Trunk: The main part of the body, to which the limbs are attached. The trunk consists of the thorax and abdomen and contains all of the internal organs. This term is also used to describe the main part of a nerve or blood vessel.

Tumor: A solid, raised mass that is larger than 1 cm in diameter and has the dimension of depth. This term also describes a mass consisting of neoplastic cells.

Ulcer: Loss of surface tissue caused by a sloughing of necrotic inflammatory tissue; the defect extends into the underlying lamina propria.

Unilateral: Affecting only one side of the body.

Uremia: A toxic condition caused by the accumulation of nitrogenous substances in the blood that are normally eliminated in the urine.

Urticaria: A vascular reaction of the skin characterized by the appearance of slightly elevated patches that are either more red or paler than the surrounding skin. Urticaria is also known as hives and may be caused by allergy, excitement, or exercise. These patches are sometimes intensely itchy.

Vasoconstriction: To decrease the diameter or caliber of a blood vessel.

Ventral: Directed toward or situated on the belly surface (opposite of dorsal).

Vermilion: That part of the lip that has a naturally pinkish red color and is exposed to the extraoral environment. The vermilion contains neither sweat glands nor accessory salivary glands.

Vermilion border: The mucocutaneous margin of the lip.

Vermilionectomy: Surgical removal of the vermilion border of the lip.

Vertigo: An unpleasant sensation characterized mainly by a feeling of dizziness or that one's surroundings are spinning or moving.

Vesicle: A well-defined lesion of the skin and mucous membranes that resembles a sac, contains fluid, and is less than 1 cm in diameter.

Visceral: Pertaining to body organs.

Viscous: Thick or sticky.

Wheal: A localized area of edema on the skin. The area is usually raised and smooth-surfaced and is often very itchy.

Xerostomia: Dry mouth.

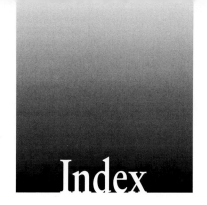

Index

Page numbers in *italics* denote figures.

Index

Index